Nurses' Aids Series

SURGICAL NURSING

NURSES' AIDS SERIES

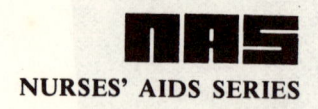

ANAESTHESIA AND RECOVERY ROOM TECHNIQUES
ANATOMY AND PHYSIOLOGY FOR NURSES
EAR, NOSE AND THROAT NURSING
GASTROENTEROLOGICAL NURSING
GERIATRIC NURSING
MATHEMATICS IN NURSING
MEDICAL NURSING
MICROBIOLOGY FOR NURSES
MULTIPLE CHOICE QUESTIONS, BOOK 1
MULTIPLE CHOICE QUESTIONS, BOOK 2
NEUROMEDICAL AND NEUROSURGICAL NURSING
OBSTETRIC AND GYNAECOLOGICAL NURSING
OPHTHALMIC NURSING
ORTHOPAEDICS FOR NURSES
PAEDIATRIC NURSING
PERSONAL AND COMMUNITY HEALTH
PHARMACOLOGY FOR NURSES
PRACTICAL NURSING
PRACTICAL PROCEDURES FOR NURSES
PSYCHIATRIC NURSING
PSYCHOLOGY FOR NURSES
SOCIOLOGY FOR NURSES
SURGICAL NURSING
THEATRE TECHNIQUE

NURSES' AIDS SERIES

Surgical Nursing

TENTH EDITION

Elizabeth J. Fish

SRN, ONC, RCNT, RNT

*Senior Tutor (Post-basic Education),
South Glamorgan School of Nursing*

Baillière Tindall · London

A BAILLIÈRE TINDALL *book published by*
Cassell Ltd,
35 Red Lion Square, London WC1R 4SG

and at Sydney, Auckland, Toronto, Johannesburg

an affiliate of
Macmillan Publishing Co. Inc.
New York

© *1979 Baillière Tindall*
a division of Cassell Ltd

All rights reserved. No part of this publication may be reproduced, stored in a retrieval system or transmitted in any form or by any means, electronic, mechanical, photocopying or otherwise, without the prior permission of Baillière Tindall, 35 Red Lion Square, London WC1R 4SG

First published 1938
Ninth edition 1974
 Reprinted 1975, 1978
Tenth edition 1979

ISBN 0 7020 0748 X
Sinhala edition (Ceylon Government)
Spanish edition (CESCA, Mexico)
Turkish edition (Turkish Government)
Portuguese edition (Publicacoes Europa-America, Mira-Sintra)
Dutch edition (Stafler, Leiden)

Published in an English Language Book Society edition

Printed in Great Britain by Spottiswoode Ballantyne Ltd., Colchester and London

---

British Library Cataloguing in Publication Data

Fish, Elizabeth Janice
 Surgical nursing.—10th ed.—
 (Nurses' aids series).
 1. Surgical nursing
 I. Title
 II. Series
 610.73'677   RD99

ISBN 0-7020-0748-X

Contents

	Preface	*vii*
1	Control of Infection in Hospitals	1
2	Wounds: Shock: Haemorrhage: Fluid Balance: Transfusion	10
3	Inflammation and Infection	44
4	Burns and Scalds	66
5	Tumours	77
6	Preparation of the Patient for Operation	92
7	Anaesthesia	101
8	Postoperative Care	115
9	Surgery of the Head and Neck	129
10	Surgery of the Oesophagus	160
11	Thoracic Surgery	170
12	Surgery of the Heart and Great Vessels	186
13	Vascular Surgery	205
14	Surgery of the Breast	217
15	Abdominal Surgery	223
16	Gastric and Duodenal Surgery	233

vi CONTENTS

17	Conditions affecting the Intestines	249
18	Conditions affecting the Gall-bladder, Liver, Pancreas and Spleen	263
19	Hernia	274
20	Surgery of the Rectum	282
21	Surgery of the Sympathetic Nervous System	291
22	Diseases of the Genitourinary System	296
23	Surgery in Bone and Joint Diseases	321
24	Fractures: Dislocations: Sprains and Strains	334
25	Plastic Surgery	365
26	X-ray Examinations	371
	Further Reading	381
	Index	383

List of Plates

between pp. 200 and 201

1. Equipment for general anaesthesia
2. Intensive care unit
3. Total patient care at a bed station
4. Goitre
5. Exophthalmos
6. Position of the hand in tetany
7. Day patient theatre
8. Cardiac catheterization (radiograph)
9. Barium meal
10. Varicose veins
11. Physiotherapy
12. Pedicle graft

Preface to the Tenth Edition

Since the publication of the last edition of this popular textbook, many changes have taken place in nursing and these are reflected in the care required by the patients.

Nurses following a general training leading to registration within countries that are members of the European Economic Community will, as a result of the European Economic Community Nursing Directive signed on 27 June 1977, follow a pattern of training that is recognized by all member countries, together with recognition of her qualifications and the associated freedom of movement and employment as a registered general nurse within these member countries. As a result the 'competent authorities' (General Nursing Council in the United Kingdom) have had to initiate certain changes in their patterns of training. One of these is that nurses must become more familiar with the 'social, cultural and economic factors, which influence the promotion of health, the incidence of disease and health care provisions in society'.

This means that training will encourage nurses to look at the patient as a whole person—a social being—and not merely as a surgical problem with its associated medical and nursing care. The nursing process is at the same time being introduced, this being a method of assessing a patient's needs and problems and then planning care from this base-line. Chapter 6 on Preparation of the Patient for Operation explains this in more detail.

The authors of previous editions have included a paragraph in their preface which I should like to repeat, since it states so clearly what they and I have striven to accomplish: 'We hope that with these changes the new edition will prove of greater value to the student nurse in promoting a sure understanding of the basic principles of surgical treatment and nursing, and particularly in the practical application of them to the patient during his stay in hospital and afterwards. The nurse plays an increasingly important part in this interesting and constantly expanding and changing field of work, and must be able to carry out her duties with intelligent

viii PREFACE

understanding so that she can adapt her technique to the varying conditions she is sure to meet.'

I would like to thank all my professional colleagues in South Glamorgan for their invaluable assistance in updating this text; without their specialist knowledge the value of this new edition would have been greatly reduced.

June 1979   E. J. FISH

1

Control of Infection in Hospitals

A nurse's duty is to see that the patient comes to no harm while in her care, which means, amongst other things, that he must be protected from infection. This presents a problem which is urgent in hospitals all over the world because of the development of pathogenic organisms that have become resistant to antibiotics by mutation. The problem is also intensified as totally new antibiotics are no longer being discovered, only structured variations of those already in use. Many patients attend hospital on account of the invasion of their bodies by pathogenic organisms. This produces a high bacterial population in hospital even when standards of hygiene are high. In consequence, many of the hospital staff, as many as 95% in certain environments, carry pathogenic bacteria and most of the staff are of an age, and enjoy a standard of health, which enables them to resist such infection. Many patients are not so fortunate and are liable to suffer damage, if not death, as a result of infection they contract after admission to hospital. This is one reason why increasing efforts are being made today to treat infants and young children in their own homes.

The main reservoirs of infection in a surgical ward are the patients' wounds and the skin and hands of all people in the environment. Skin and hands can become further contaminated from alimentary and genitourinary tracts. Micro-organisms from patients and staff pass into the ward environment via the hands and in the skin scales that are being continually shed; this is the main reason why the centre of each bed must be 2·5 m from the centre of the next bed. The organisms are also transmitted by direct contact from contaminated hands and by droplet infection.

Indiscriminate use of antibiotics, either in inadequate dosage or for trivial infections, has led to the development of strains of bacteria, especially staphylococci and Gram-negative organisms, which are resistant to these antibiotics. These resistant organisms are found very commonly in hospitals and when they are involved in cross-infection, treatment with antibiotics may be completely ineffective. Furniture and all ward utensils become contaminated and many micro-organisms accumulate in the dust on the floor. Every effort should be made to isolate an infected patient effectively, since hands, instruments, basins, furniture and floor can all readily become contaminated by organisms from a wound.

HYGIENE

In 1959 a subcommittee of the Central Health Services Council reported to the Minister of Health on the subject of *Staphylococcal Infections in Hospitals*. A number of recommendations were made, including the appointment of Infection Control Officers. In hospitals both medical and nursing staff can assist greatly by understanding the problem and in consequence maintaining the highest standards of personal and ward hygiene and by being scrupulous in their surgical technique.

Personal Hygiene

The surgical nurse will already be quite familiar with the subject of personal hygiene, but certain points require emphasis in relation to surgical nursing.

1. *The hair* should always be kept clean and neat. If hair is worn long it should be effectively controlled so that it neither 'flops' forward nor needs frequent brushing back with the hand.

2. *Nails and hands* must be well cared for. The nurse should come on duty with hands and nails thoroughly clean. Scrubbing is not advocated immediately prior to surgical procedures because this tends to damage the epidermis. Instead the hands are thoroughly washed, rinsed and dried on a clean fabric or disposable towel.

3. *Uniform.* The same uniform should not be worn indiscriminately for clean and dirty duties in the ward. Protective plastic aprons should be worn at appropriate times and aprons never worn outside the ward. Skin scales pass through cotton in less than five minutes so cotton gowns do not form an effective barrier.

4. Organisms may be disseminated from the respiratory tract by *coughing, sneezing and speaking*, etc.; most people carry micro-organisms in this area.

5. All staff, including non-professional personnel, should receive 'in-service training' which includes the prevention of *cross-infection*.

6. Laboratory tests have proved that *men* shed staphylococci much more profusely than women. The reason is not fully understood.

7. All staff on duty must be free from any form of *active infection*. If infection such as skin sepsis or a gastrointestinal infection is recognized, the member of staff must not remain on duty. This also applies if a member of staff has eczema, especially in a surgical environment.

Patients' Hygiene

The nurse is responsible for the patients' hygiene when they are unable to care for themselves. Hand-washing after toilet rounds is very important as wounds can readily become contaminated by organisms from the colon and these infections tend to become chronic. It is important to remember that auto-infection can occur as well as cross-infection, so the wounds of confused patients will require extra protection.

Ward hygiene and administration

Good ventilation is essential to minimize the bacteria content of the ward atmosphere. A nurse should always notice this when she enters a ward, a time when she will be most sensitive to any defects. Ideally surgical wards should have artificial ventilation by means of a vacuum extraction system with filtration for the periods of time when the windows cannot be left open, e.g. mid-winter. *Sunshine* has excellent bactericidal properties because of the infra-red and ultra-violet rays.

Adequate bed spacing will help to maintain good atmospheric conditions. The minimum permissible space between bed centres in a surgical ward is 2·5 m. Overcrowding by putting up extra beds, as well as having an adverse effect on ventilation, is almost always accompanied by shortage of equipment, shortage of staff and lowering of staff morale. This leads to a breakdown in surgical technique and increases the likelihood of cross-infection, which in turn delays the discharge of patients and thus a vicious circle is set up.

Cupboard space. Every effort should be made to see that there is sufficient cupboard space for storage, especially as disposable equipment is rather bulky. CSSD packs must be kept in easily cleaned racks in an area specially allocated for this purpose—a clean utility room, next door to a treatment room. A clearly defined labelling system for the various compartments is useful for new nurses.

Ward design and furnishings. As far as possible dark corners should be avoided. Surfaces should be smooth and easily cleaned, and corners rounded. Ward utensils should be kept in good repair; cracks and chips make perfect breeding grounds for bacteria. Cellular cotton blankets are now in use in hospital wards as they can be disinfected and laundered frequently; they do not cause very much blanket fluff. Mattresses should be covered with impermeable material and the surface thoroughly washed on each patient's discharge. Pillows should be made from material that is washable, such as Dacron. Foam is also an improvement over feathers as it does not produce dust, but is not washable.

Ward cleaning. Only the highest standards are acceptable and cleaning methods should be used which are designed to prevent the scattering of dust; surfaces must be cleaned using cleaning solutions and detergents as recommended by the Control of Infection Committee. New solutions must also be tested by the Infection Control Officer before they are introduced. Suction apparatus for floor cleaning and damp dusting is satisfactory. Ward cleaners must have sufficient instruction in the importance of their duties and in the use, care and maintenance of apparatus. Many hospitals employ contract cleaners who are trained to do this work in the most efficient manner. Alternatively 'in-service training' is arranged for hospital cleaners.

Bedmaking must be carried out in a manner designed to produce the minimum scattering of dust: however, it always results in an increase in the contamination of the ward air and must be timed so that the dust created settles before dressings are begun. In *Staphylococcal Infections in Hospitals* it is recommended that bedmaking should be completed 15 minutes before dressings are taken down. Some hospital authorities are now introducing duvets as they cause much less dust to enter the ward environment. This is because hospital duvets are totally washable.

Dressings should be taken down as infrequently as possible. Dressings should be done only when dust from cleaning, bed-making and toilet rounds has had time to subside and when all traffic and movement of air is at a minimum. This means that all doors and windows should be closed while dressings are in progress and the ward closed to all traffic—very difficult conditions to achieve. Clean wounds should always be dressed first and isolation technique used for infected ones. Great care should be taken in the disposal of all contaminated articles. Soiled dressings are best collected in disposable bags which are subsequently burnt. Ideally the patients should only be given treatment involving the aseptic technique in a treatment room, and not in the ward where the risk of cross-infection is much higher.

STERILIZATION

Sterilization is the destruction of all micro-organisms in or on the article to be sterilized and is a very difficult process, as the slightest degree of carelessness can result in the production of infected articles, so it is essential that all nurses consider their own technique carefully.

Preliminary Cleaning

This must be carried out before the sterilization of instruments and receivers. If this is not done carefully particles of organic matter may be left on the article; when this is exposed to heat they will coagulate and prevent the sterilization process taking place.

If the articles are known to be grossly infected they may be immersed in a chemical disinfectant before the actual cleansing process is carried out.

The article may be cleansed in a variety of ways. It can be cleansed automatically by an ultrasonic washer or be allowed to pass through an automatic spray washer which contains a detergent and has a thermostatic temperature control. Alternatively, the articles may be scrubbed, first in cold water, then in warm soapy water, using an instrument brush, especially on the serrated blades of instruments; this is a much used method when cleansing delicate instruments, even when automatic equipment is available.

6 SURGICAL NURSING

Methods of Sterilization

Moist heat

Boiling for five minutes. The articles must be immersed separately in boiling water. Small articles are best held in a wire tray so that they will not 'get lost' and breakable articles should be placed individually in containers to that they will not roll about during the boiling process. Cheatle's and Harrison's bowl-holding forceps, which are used for removing the articles from the sterilizer, must be handled very carefully to prevent them becoming contaminated. They should be sterilized frequently and stored upright with the handles protruding from the container; The container must also be sterilized frequently and always immediately afterwards if there is any suspicion that the forceps may have been infected. The forceps will either have its blades immersed in a reliable sterilizing agent or be stored dry.

Autoclaving. This method uses steam under pressure and is one of the most widely used and efficient methods in the hospital service. The articles for sterilization are pre-cleaned and then, if required, are assembled into packs. These articles are then enclosed in one of the following: a sterilization box, linen wraps, paper wraps or metal drums. They are then placed in the autoclave and the process is commenced; this consists of the creation of a pre-vacuum to withdraw the air from the chamber, then the introduction of steam under pressure for the required length of time (32 lb/in^2 at 135°C for 5 minutes) and this sterilizes the articles. This is followed by the creation of another vacuum to withdraw the steam from the chamber and by the drying process, which lasts five minutes.

Pasteurization. This method is sometimes used to sterilize cytoscopes, but it does allow organisms to survive, so other methods are much more reliable, e.g. ethylene oxide.

Dry heat

Hot dry air. An electric hot air oven is often used to sterilize glass-ware, metal-ware and syringes. A temperature of 160°C is used for a period of one hour. The oven contains a fan which circulates the heat through the whole of the interior and has a graph which continually records the temperature and the time factor. This is a precaution to ensure that sterilization is taking place.

Flaming. This method is used in the laboratories to sterilize loops, before spreading a culture for example. It is rarely used in hospital wards, but the inside of metal receivers can be rendered safe by pouring a small quantity of methylated spirit into them, placing the bottle well away from the receiver, and lighting the spirit in the receiver. This will be sterile when the flames burn out. However, this is a very dangerous method and the greatest care must be taken should it be required in an emergency.

Gas

Ethylene oxide. A 12% mixture of ethylene oxide with carbon dioxide (to reduce its explosive tendency) and water vapour is often used to sterilize equipment that would be damaged by exposure to heat. The water vapour increases the efficiency of the gas. This method is often used to sterilize the inside of rooms, e.g. operating theatres, when the gas is atomized into the atmosphere of the room. This is usually done overnight so the theatre is ready for use the next day.

Formalin and steam. This has been proved to be much more effective than formalin alone. A 40% humidity is used.

Irradiation

Infra-red. The articles to be sterilized are usually packed in black non-reflecting metal tubes which absorb and do not reflect the rays of heat. These then are placed on a conveyor belt which passes through an infra-red tunnel. The temperature used is 180°C for 20 minutes. Glass syringes and instruments are sometimes sterilized in this way, but it has one disadvantage in that the equipment occupies a lot of space.

Ultra-violet. This has powerful sterilizing properties, but is of little practical use as its power of penetration is limited. Even specks of dust will prevent the passage of the rays. So it is only used for surface sterilization, e.g. the inside of a spotlessly clean cabinet.

Ionizing radiation, Gamma radiation is used commercially and most prepacked articles are sterilized in this way, such as suture materials, rubber articles, plastic equipment and very delicate substances which may be used for transplantation surgery.

SURGICAL NURSING

Chemicals

There are a great number of chemicals which destroy microorganisms or prevent them multiplying. However, their use must be very carefully controlled as it is important to ensure that the correct chemical is used in the correct concentration for the specified period of time.

Central Sterile Supplies Departments

Central departments now provide most of the equipment previously prepared by nurses in surgical wards.

Some hospitals prepare their own packs for various specific purposes; others use commercially prepared packs. Where the services of a CSSD are not available, equipment for such special procedures as 'cut down' blood transfusions, chest aspiration or tracheostomy is almost always obtained from an operating theatre, where it is likely to have been sterilized in an autoclave apparatus, ward facilities rarely being adequate for efficient preparation of such specialized equipment. This also means that every ward does not have to keep its own 'set', thus saving duplication of expensive equipment.

To Prepare the Hands

Before assisting or doing dressings a nurse should see that her nails are filed reasonably short and to the shape of her fingertips, that they are clean and that her hands are free from any injury or infection. She must then wash her hands and forearms under running water using either good quality soap or one of the available preparations such as Hibiscrub, pHisoHex or Betadine. The fingers should then be held uppermost so that the hands and arms can be rinsed. This method prevents the contaminated water from the arms running over the hands and fingers. The hands and arms are then dried on a freshly laundered or disposable towel, using a different part of the towel for the different parts of the hands and arms.

Once the hands have been prepared they must not be allowed to come into contact with anything that is not sterile. If sterile gloves are to be worn, the hands should be dusted with sterilized powder after drying and the nurse should put on the sterile gloves without touching the outside of the glove with the hand. The nurse should hold the first glove by the turned-back cuff and slip it on, then insert the gloved fingers under the turned-back cuff of the second glove and slip it on. When turned back the cuffs of the gloves must completely envelop the sleeves of the sterile gown. A 'leak' at the wrist can be disastrous. Without gloves the hands are never sterile and must not touch wounds.

Nail and instrument brushes. Polypropylene brushes should be used as they can be autoclaved each day. Otherwise all brushes must be sterilized by some other means, the most common method being immersion in boiling water for five minutes. However, this is not reliable as spores are not destroyed.

Nail brushes should only be used for nails, not for the skin of the hands as their repeated use will damage the skin and so expose the nurse to the risk of infection and discomfort.

2

Wounds: Shock: Haemorrhage: Fluid Balance: Transfusion

WOUNDS

A wound is caused by damage to tissue, internal or external.

Open wounds

These may be:

1. Incised.
2. Lacerated and contused.
3. Punctured, which includes gun shot wounds.
4. Poisoned.
5. Due to burns or scalds.

Incised wounds. These are produced by sharp cutting instruments. An incised wound gapes if the deep fascia is also incised. In the scalp the aponeurotic fascia is nearly always split as well as the skin and the wound gapes; an incised wound of the finger seldom gapes as the fascia is usually intact. The wound may bleed freely, but the pain is seldom great. There is no bruising of the edges. Most operation wounds are in this category.

Lacerated and contused wounds. These may be produced in road accidents, by factory machinery or by a jagged fragment of shell or bomb. There is a ragged cut on the surface. This type of wound is frequently contaminated and it supplies an excellent culture medium for micro-organisms. There is more pain than in an incised wound, but bleeding may not be severe due to constriction of the blood vessels.

Punctured wounds. These may be inflicted by sharp instruments, nails, dogs' teeth, knives and bullets. Although superficially they may appear trifling, deeper structures such as blood vessels and nerves or an internal organ may have been damaged and contamination carried into deep tissues. These wounds are specially susceptible to infection from anaerobic organisms, for example those causing tetanus and gas gangrene, which start thriving when the aerobic organisms such as staphylococci and streptococci have used up the available oxygen in the deep tissues.

Poisoned wounds. These include insect stings, snake bites and dog bites where hydrophobia is present. *Insect bites* produce swelling, irritation and discomfort, but are only serious at the back of the mouth where swelling may obstruct the airway if suitable treatment is not undertaken and also when the stings are multiple, e.g. arising from disturbance of a wasps' nest. Cold may be applied as a compress round the throat, antihistamine drugs ordered and in emergency a tracheostomy may be necessary to save life. *Snake and dog bites* can be serious if the snake is venomous or the dog hydrophobic. Most snakes and dogs are not; the only venomous snake native to Great Britain is the adder or viper and *rabies* is not found in the United Kingdom because of the rigid quarantine laws. Where this is not the case special precautions must be taken.

Burns and scalds. These and compound fractures will be considered in later chapters.

Closed injuries

Closed injuries to tissues can take the form of:
1. A bruise or contusion.
2. A haematoma.
3. A sprain.

A bruise or contusion. This is a superficial injury without damage to the skin: the swelling, pain and discomfort are due to the extravasation of blood into the tissues. When there is much loose subcutaneous tissue, such as the eyelids and scrotum, bleeding is more severe and the part becomes black. Colour changes occur as the haemoglobin is oxidized.

A haematoma. This is a collection of blood in the tissues, which causes a swelling and may press on surrounding structures. In favourable circumstances the blood is gradually absorbed, if it is

SURGICAL NURSING

not evacuated surgically. The danger is that the haematoma can readily become infected by micro-organisms entering from devitalized overlying skin or reaching it via the blood stream. Once there the haematoma provides an excellent breeding ground for bacteria and an abscess may develop.

A sprain. This involves the tearing of the capsule and ligaments round a joint with consequent exudation of fluid.

Wound Healing

Noxious or harmful agents when applied to the body excite two reactions: inflammation followed by repair. The stage of inflammation may be long or short and will be considered in detail in a later chapter. It persists as long as the harmful agent is present and only when its action ceases does repair begin. Harmful agents are of two kinds, animate and inanimate. Inanimate agents are usually physical, for example heat or the friction caused by a surgeon's knife or bedclothes. Their action is usually brief and the stage of inflammation is short. Animate, harmful agents are bacteria and viruses; they remain active longer as they are able to breed, and some time elapses before the body can destroy them all, and consequently repair tends to be delayed.

Wounds heal by forming fibrous scar tissue over which epidermis grows. Wounds are said to heal by first intention or by second intention or granulation, but the process is identical and it is merely a question of the quantity of new tissue required to heal a wound.

Healing by first intention occurs in incised wounds where the skin edges are in apposition (for example, operation wounds) and only a thin line of new tissue is required to procure healing.

Healing by second intention occurs in gaping wounds where tissue has been lost by injury or disease, so that the edges cannot be approximated and a mass of new tissue is required to fill the gap.

Repair proceeds by stages. In the first few days the wound is filled by a variable amount of blood (which quickly clots) and tissue fluid. At about the fourth day fibroblasts grow out into this exudate forming a type of 'scaffolding' to capillary buds which sprout out. These fibroblasts cannot multiply if the plasma protein level is low, hence the importance of adequate protein intake for efficient wound healing. This almost jelly-like tissue or precollagen now contained in the wound turns into fibrillar collagen in the presence of vitamin

C and it is this which gives strength to the scar, maximum tensile strength being achieved towards the end of the second week. Gradually the fibrous tissue contracts, 'strangling' the capillaries which continue to atrophy for about a year; the scar changes over the months from pink to white and becomes, in the case of incised wounds, less noticeable. In the case of incised wounds the amount of epithelial tissue needed to bridge the gap between the cut edges of skin is minimal, but with wounds of the ulcer type much more is needed and it will grow out from healthy epithelium as soon as granulation tissue has filled in the defect. If granulation tissue grows too exuberantly and rises above the level of the surrounding epithelium, this epithelialization does not take place normally and the over-granulations have to be burnt down by being gently touched with a caustic stick, e.g. of silver nitrate.

All wounds heal much more rapidly where there is a good blood supply.

Treatment of Wounds

Little can be done to hasten healing in a simple wound, but complications which might delay healing can be treated.

Gaping. A wound usually gapes open when the deep fascia has been cut. When a wound is clean, skin edges should be approximated as soon as possible in order to minimize scar tissue and prevent infection. To obtain rapid healing it is important that the skin edges should not turn in, otherwise the cut epithelium of one edge does not come in contact with the cut epithelium of the other. In surgical sewing care is taken to pass the cutting needle through the skin at right angles, which ensures that the cut edges are brought into good apposition.

Excessive tissue loss. This can lead to severe contractures owing to shrinkage of scar tissue. It is therefore important to splint the area in extension and to apply a skin graft as soon as possible. A large area of scar tissue is undesirable also because it is more readily damaged than normal skin, the dermis is never renewed and the scar tissue contains no sweat glands, sebaceous glands, hair follicles or tactile sense organs.

Contamination. Contamination of the wound must be treated with the minimum delay in order to prevent infection.

14 SURGICAL NURSING

The wound must be cleansed. Bleeding in moderation should not be discouraged in order to wash out any micro-organisms and foreign material that have gained entrance and the surrounding skin should be washed with a lotion such as Savlon 1/100 or aqueous Hibitane 1/1000, and shaved if necessary.

Whenever tissue is damaged *wound toilet* is essential. A clean cut destroys little tissue, whereas a crush injury may devitalize much tissue. Wound toilet is required for the latter but not the former wound. It means that after thorough washing of the wound, all foreign bodies, dead and dying tissues are removed and the wound is again thoroughly irrigated with a solution such as sterile normal saline. This removes from the wound micro-organisms and the material they like to feed on in order to multiply. The presence of dead or devitalized tissue predisposes to the development of gas gangrene.

After-care of Wounds

Local

All patients must be reassured that the wound will heal, no matter how serious it appears initially, and must be given advice concerning the avoidance of secondary infection or injury such as may occur if the wound is allowed to become contaminated by dirty fingers.

Dressings. A dressing is usually applied to protect a wound from contamination, to give pressure and support and to keep the wound edges in good apposition. Traditionally it consists of such materials as sterile gauze, cotton wool and a bandage or adhesive plaster. The wound should always be kept as dry as possible as bacteria thrive in warmth and moisture and the skin under a dressing can readily become moist and soggy. This is the reason why some surgeons like all dressings removed at an early date after surgery. Exposure to the atmosphere stimulates the skin and they consider the danger of air-borne bacteria less than the danger of their multiplication under warm moist dressings. Recently sterile transparent plastic dressings, which can be sprayed on, have been introduced. The wound can be seen through them and they are left undisturbed until the stitches are due to come out, when a special solution is applied to aid in the removal of the dressing. When such a dressing is used the part can safely be immersed when the patient has a bath.

Drainage. This may be required to enable the escape of blood, tissue fluid or pus or to ensure that a wound heals from the depths of the wound upwards, otherwise fluid may collect in the wound and cause it to break down. Rubber or plastic drainage tubes or a strip of corrugated or glove rubber may be used. They are usually anchored with a skin stitch and a stout safety pin is inserted crosswise to prevent them from slipping into the wound once the stitch is removed. Gentle suction may be applied to the tube when there is likely to be much oozing of blood, lymph or serum, e.g. to the wound drain after a radical mastectomy when lymph drainage from the arm is impaired. A wound should only be plugged lightly if ribbon gauze is used as a wick instead of a drainage tube, so that the secretions are not dammed back, and the surrounding skin should be protected.

The sterile gauze and cotton-wool over the drain while dry acts as a germ filter; once it is soaked with blood and serum infection can, and does, pass through it and the dressing should be changed or at least repacked. For this reason when there is a drain in a wound the dressing requires frequent attention, possibly several times daily.

General

A nurse must also pay attention to a patient's general health if she wishes to see wounds healing rapidly.

Diet. This is important as healing cannot occur unless there are sufficient repair substances in the body. The patient therefore requires a high-protein diet, a generous supply of vitamin C, which promotes the formation of scar tissue, and sufficient fluids to assist the excretion of waste products.

Many diseases impair nutrition and consequently affect the rate of healing, e.g. cancer.

A good blood supply to the injured part. This brings essential nutrients and carries away waste substances. Areas with a rich blood supply are always quickest to heal and this is one reason why stitches are commonly removed much earlier from wounds of the face and neck than from, say, the limbs or the abdomen.

Rest. This, both general and local, helps to promote rapid healing. Areas that are not easily immobilized, such as the knuckles, heal slowly. When a wound traverses the surface of a

16 SURGICAL NURSING

large joint, some *gentle* movement may be necessary to prevent permanent stiffening of the joint or deformity; this is unlikely to do harm and by improving the blood circulation may encourage healing. It is movement which produces a shearing force at the wound edges that is harmful.

The conditions which most frequently complicate a severe wound are shock, haemorrhage and infection. These complications also frequently follow surgery and they will be considered in turn below.

Wound Drainage

Drains of different types are inserted into the area of operation by the surgeon. These are used to allow blood and excess fluid to drain away from the wound and so reduce the risk of infection and promote healing.

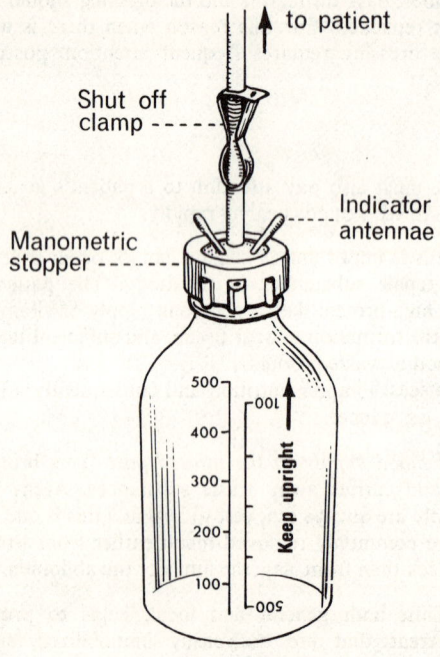

Fig. 1. A Redivac drain.

The Redivac drain is often used in the care of patients who have had partial thyroidectomies or surgery to the hip joint. The bottle has a vacuum of 600 mmHg within it, so waste fluid is gently drawn from the tissues into the bottle. When an efficient vacuum is present the indicator antennae are positioned as in Fig. 1, but when the vacuum drops to 40–50 mmHg the antenna adduct instead of abduct and this shows that the bottle requires changing. The instructions are clearly stated on the bottle and must be carefully followed.

SHOCK

Shock is a clinical state that is characterized by a fall in blood pressure. The patient is pale and cold, the skin feels clammy and the pulse is weak and rapid.

The blood volume of an average adult is about 6 litres. If all the blood vessels were open at the same time there would be insufficient blood to fill them all and the circulation would cease. The body manages with this relatively small volume of blood by controlling the muscles in the walls of the arterioles; by this means it can narrow or widen the lumen of the small arteries and so allow less or more blood to the part; unnecessary supplies are cut down. The control is very exact and normally the total volume of blood exactly equals the cubic capacity of the vessels that are open. At times the equation becomes unbalanced and the volume of blood is not enough to fill the vessels that must remain open if the blood is to circulate. This is the condition called shock, a state of circulatory failure when blood is insufficient to fill the main blood vessels.

Compensation. When shock occurs compensation is immediate. Vessels supplying parts that can survive temporarily with little blood are shut. Vessels supplying essential organs, like brain, heart and kidneys, continue to receive their blood supply, while blood supply to muscle, skin, stomach and intestines is severely rationed. As a result the patient feels prostrated, his body temperature falls and he complains of cold. The skin is grey, cold and moist and there is delay in the stomach emptying. If this reaction is satisfactory shock will be compensated; the main blood vessels will be filled and blood pressure and pulse will remain normal. These are therefore the signs and symptoms of compensated shock.

SURGICAL NURSING

Uncompensated shock. Compensation may fail, or the normal reflexes may be unable to produce compensation, or secondary shock may develop and again there is insufficient blood to fill the blood vessels. Less blood returns to the heart and, therefore, the cardiac output is reduced, blood pressure falls and the pulse rate increases. These are the most important signs of uncompensated shock.

The most important causes of shock are the inhibition of the vasoconstrictors by such stimuli as severe pain or fright, loss of blood, plasma or electrolytes and altered permeability of the capillaries.

Types of Shock

The two *main* types of shock are cardiogenic and hypovolaemic, but other kinds may also occur.

Cardiogenic shock

This type is recognized when a patient is in a shocked state following severe pain or an emotionally traumatic experience, e.g. a myocardial infarction or pulmonary embolism. This is caused by stimulation of the vagus nerve (sometimes called vasovagal or neurogenic) which acts on the sino-atrial node and slows down the heart beat, so causing a drop in the patient's normal blood pressure.

Hypovolaemic (oligaemic) shock

Hypovalaemic shock is due to a reduction in the volume of circulating blood such as occurs following a severe haemorrhage, burns or dehydration. In this type of shock the low volume of blood reduces the stroke volume of the heart and results in a drop in the blood pressure.

Anaphylactic shock

A sudden widespread increase in capillary permeability (causing hypovolaemia) and severe bronchospasm occur in this type of shock. This may arise following the introduction of a foreign protein such as antitetanus serum into the person's body

Bacteraemic (endotoxic) shock

In this type the endothelium forming the walls of the blood vessels is damaged by the bacterial toxins. This causes them to dilate, resulting in hypotension. Irreversible shock will result if the normal blood flow is not restored. This occurs because poor blood flow damages the endothelium in the capillaries and this allows plasma proteins to escape into the tissues causing a total disruption of the tissue cell environment and resulting in death.

Clinical Assessment of Shock

The patient's condition will be very carefully monitored by:

1. Central venous pressure. This is normally between +5 and +15 mmHg and falls in shock.
2. Left arterial pressure by means of an arterial pressure line. Normally the pressure is 5 mmHg.
3. Blood pressure.
4. Electrocardiogram.
5. Urinary output.
6. Blood pH, electrolytes and blood gases.
7. The haematocrit, especially if the patient has been burnt.

Signs and symptoms of shock have all been mentioned but may usefully be listed as:

1. A low blood pressure continuing to fall.
2. A pulse becoming weak, imperceptible, irregular and increasing in rate.
3. Respirations shallow and almost imperceptible.
4. Face pale or grey with lips and ear lobes cyanosed.
5. Skin cold and clammy.
6. Temperature subnormal.
7. Muscles relaxed and atonic.
8. Patient unconscious or quite apathetic.

Factors which aggravate surgical shock are loss of fluid from whatever cause, fear, pain, starvation and exposure.

A nurse looking after patients before and after operations must remember these factors. Fluid intake should be high, an unconscious or injured patient should never be overheated so that fluid is lost through perspiration and patients should not be excessively purged before operation nor kept without fluids for more than five hours. A nurse allays fears and anxiety by making time to listen to the patient, by giving suitable explanations and by the calm and efficient performance of all her duties. This is very important because, as previously mentioned, fear is one of the causes of shock. Fear associated with the accident, for instance, cannot be rectified at this time, but further fear-inducing situations can be avoided or at least compensated for. The doctor will order analgesic drugs, but it is often left to the nurse to determine the best time to give them. Pain undermines morale as well as aggravating shock and should be relieved by nursing measures in addition to drugs—this on grounds of humanity as well as in relation to preventing and treating shock. Long periods of starvation before surgery should be avoided, especially for children, and the patient carefully observed during meals to ensure that his diet is sufficient and enjoyed. At no time before, during or after surgery should a patient be unnecessarily exposed and chilled, unless hypothermia is being used, when the chilling is carefully controlled.

Curative Treatment of Shock

1. The patient is nursed flat with *blocks to the foot of the bed* or couch, so that the blood circulates to the vital centres of the medulla, that is particularly to the vasomotor, cardiac and respiratory centres. 'Flat' is meant to describe a horizontal position on the bed; the patient need not necessarily lie flat on his back but may lie on his side if he is more comfortable, the important point being to keep his head low.

2. *Reassurance* is given.

3. The patient *rests* undisturbed, with the *minimum of handling* or questioning. If the patient must be moved this must be done very gently.

4. *Pain* is relieved by making the patient as comfortable as possible and giving morphine, 15–30 mg, if this is ordered. It should be given intramuscularly on account of the depressed circulation in the subcutaneous tissue or may be given intravenously by the doctor.

5. *Warmth* in moderation may be applied in primary shock. In secondary shock there may be danger of drawing the blood away from the deep vital structures like the heart and kidneys to the surface tissues, which can better withstand a diminished blood

WOULDS 21

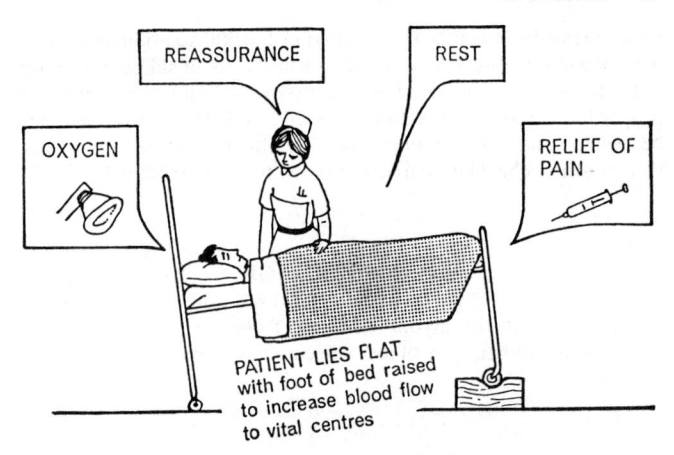

Fig. 2. The treatment of shock.

supply. If warmth is applied in excess it causes perspiration, further fluid and electrolyte loss, and consequently aggravates shock.

6. Fluids are administered as prescribed. A patient loses 600–1000 ml of fluid a day from skin and lungs, besides the quantity of urine passed. If this fluid cannot be taken by mouth, the patient will rapidly become dehydrated and shock is aggravated. Blood should be given if it has been lost and plasma or serum in the treatment of burns. When these fluids are not immediately available dextran is a good substitute. It is a carbohydrate solution with molecules about the size of plasma proteins; it therefore remains in the blood vessels and helps to restore blood pressure. This is a form of carbohydrate which is never available for oxidation as is glucose. It tends to cause rouleaux formation of the red blood cells and therefore makes grouping and cross-matching difficult later. If these procedures are likely to be required later, it is advisable to take a specimen of blood for laboratory use before the dextran is infused. Plasmosan has the advantage over dextran in that it does not cause this rouleaux formation.

7. The nurse may give *oxygen* to a cyanosed patient, in a 80–95% concentration, through a polythene mask. A satisfactory concentration is achieved by allowing the oxygen to flow at 8 litres per minute, providing there are no contraindications.

8. *Stimulants* are given only on the surgeon's instructions. *Noradrenaline* may be run into the intravenous infusion to raise the

blood pressure. It is usually prepared in 1 : 1000 solution and a 4 ml ampoule containing 4 mg is given in a litre flask of saline. This gives a 1 : 250 000 solution for slow intravenous infusion. Levophed is a proprietary preparation which is widely used. *Hydrocortisone* may be used in place of noradrenaline. The effects of these drugs must be repeatedly checked by frequent blood pressure readings.

HAEMORRHAGE

Haemorrhage is the escape of blood from the blood vessels. It results from damage to blood vessels caused by either injury or disease.

Types of Haemorrhage

Haemorrhage may be classified as:

1. Arterial
2. Venous
3. Capillary

   } According to the vessel from which it comes

4. Primary
5. Reactionary
6. Secondary

   } According to the time at which it occurs

7. External or obvious
8. Internal or concealed

   } According to whether the bleeding can or cannot be seen

Arterial haemorrhage is characterized by:

1. The bright red colour of the blood.
2. The blood 'spurts' out under considerable pressure.
3. The blood spurts from the proximal side of the wound only, except where there is free anastomosis, as in the radial and ulnar arteries, where the blood will flow from both sides.

Venous haemorrhage is characterized by:

1. The dark purplish colour of the blood.
2. The blood welling up in an even, gentle stream from the wound.

3. The blood coming from the distal side of the wound, except where the veins are varicose, when blood flows from both sides.

Capillary haemorrhage is the oozing of blood from a raw surface.

Primary haemorrhage is haemorrhage occurring at the time of injury and continuing until it is stopped by natural or artificial means.

Reactionary haemorrhage is bleeding which begins a few hours after injury or operation, generally within 12–24 hours. It is due to the fact that shock and haemorrhage or drugs given at the time of injury or operation reduced the blood pressure so much that small vessels that were cut did not bleed at the time; bleeding begins when the blood pressure rises as the shock passes off. The rise may cause dislodging of clots or ligatures. Another possible cause is slipping of a ligature as the result of clumsy lifting or violent vomiting. Because of this danger anything likely to lead to sudden rise in blood pressure, such as excitement and stimulants, must be avoided for 24 hours after operation. The patient should be kept quiet and visitors excluded or reduced to the minimum, as the surgeon orders. Stimulants must only be given when ordered to raise a dangerously low blood pressure.

Secondary haemorrhage occurs about ten days from the time of injury or operation and is always due to sepsis. Infection of the wound affects the blood clots in several vessels, causing them to break down instead of becoming organized so as to seal them permanently. It is most frequently met with in the mouth, where complete asepsis is impracticable, and following amputations.

External haemorrhage is bleeding from a wound or orifice, in which case the blood is visible.

Internal haemorrhage is bleeding into an internal cavity such as the peritoneum, the bowel, the pleura or the tissues of a limb in cases of fractures. In these cases the blood cannot be seen and diagnosis depends on the general signs and symptoms of haemorrhage, which are present in all cases. These signs and symptoms are of the utmost importance, as early diagnosis and treatment should result in the saving of life, which may otherwise be lost. It is therefore the duty of every nurse to know them with absolute accuracy.

SURGICAL NURSING

Signs and Symptoms of Internal Haemorrhage

1. Rise in pulse rate, and pulse becoming small and rapid, termed the 'running' or 'haemorrhagic' pulse.
2. Sudden or gradual fall in blood pressure.
3. Pallor, spreading to the lips and mucous membranes.
4. Subnormal temperature.
5. Restlessness. } These are the symptoms of
6. Rapid sighing respirations. } 'air hunger'.
7. Skin which is cold and clammy to the touch and the patient may complain of feeling cold.
8. Faintness or actual fainting.
9. Thirst.
10. Dilated pupils.
11. A 'sinking' feeling and possible dimness of vision.

Pain will be present if the bleeding is in the peritoneal cavity, as in ruptured ectopic gestation, ruptured spleen or liver. Haemorrhage occurring into the tissues when there is no break in the skin, i.e. subcutaneous bleeding, results in bruising or haematoma. The colour change in a bruise occurs as the red blood cells break down: blue/black = reduced haemoglobin, green = biliverdin, yellow = bilirubin.

Arrest of Haemorrhage

Arrest of haemorrhage may be natural or artificial.

Natural arrest

Natural arrest results from both local and general changes. The local processes may be divided into temporary and permanent.

Temporary local arrest is due to:

1. The clotting of blood in the mouth of the severed vessel, which takes place in the following manner: the damaged tissue and platelets produce thromboplastin. In the presence of calcium salts and prothrombin, which is always present in the blood, this produces thrombin. The thrombin, in the presence of fibrinogen (also always present in the blood), then produces fibrin. This traps the cells in the blood and forms a clot.
2. The contraction of the vessel wall.

3. The retraction of the vessel in its sheath because of its elasticity, which results in the blood stagnating and clotting around the mouth of the cut vessel.

Permanent arrest is due to the conversion of the blood clot into fibrous tissue occluding the mouth of the vessel.

The general effect, which is of great assistance to this local process, is a fall in blood pressure, which makes the blood more liable to clot in the mouth of the cut vessel and lessens the risk of the clot being dislodged. The fall in blood pressure may result in fainting, which still further reduces the pressure; this is beneficial where the surgeon is depending upon the natural processes of arrest and should not be treated by stimulation, provided the blood pressure is sufficient to maintain life.

Aids to natural arrest. All these natural processes can be assisted by various treatments.

The process of *clotting* can be hastened by:

1. The application of heat, 48–71°C. Care must be taken not to burn the patient but temperatures much lower than this may dilate vessels and so increase the bleeding. Hence this is a dangerous 'aid'.
2. The application of drugs, e.g. tannic acid or thrombin.
3. The giving of calcium salts or vitamin K, where these are deficient, or, less often, coagulen or snake venom (Russell's viper).
4. Contact with a rough surface, particularly cellulose alginate wool, cellulose or gauze. Cellulose alginate is prepared from seaweed and is supplied ready sterilized for use. It is particularly used for application to the cut surface of the liver or on the brain. It is absorbed without producing local irritation. It can also be used for bleeding sockets after tooth extraction and in prostatectomy.

The *contraction of the vessel wall* may be, temporarily, increased by:

1. The application of cold.
2. The application of adrenaline—not very satisfactory, as the effects pass off quickly.
3. The application of pressure.

The *reduction of the blood pressure* can be assisted by:

1. Absolute rest.
2. Avoidance of excitement.
3. Reassuring the patient and allaying fears.
4. Avoiding all stimulants.

Artificial arrest

This may be either temporary or permanent.

Temporary arrest may be secured by:

1. Direct pressure on the bleeding point with the thumb covered with a sterile gauze or clean rag, or the application of a sterile pad and firm bandage to exert sufficient pressure to stop the bleeding.
2. Digital pressure on the main artery supplying the part at a pressure point.
3. Application of a tourniquet to a limb, if the above fails.

Permanent artifical arrest is obtained either by ligature of the bleeding vessel or twisting of the vessel, if small, or by the application of alginate wool or gauze, or by cauterization.

Treatment of External Haemorrhage

The treatment of haemorrhage may be considered under the following headings:

1. First aid.
2. Operative treatment.
3. Clinical treatment.
4. General management.

First-aid treatment consists of any of the following:

1. Digital pressure on the bleeding point; this will stop all haemorrhage, however furious, provided no foreign body is present; it is the most efficient method where practicable, but cannot be applied by the same person for more than a short period.
2. Application of a sterile pad over the bleeding point, secured by a firm bandage. This is a better method than the application of a tourniquet and will often be sufficient. It does not deprive the tissues of any part of their blood supply.
3. Digital pressure on the main artery supplying the part at the pressure points. For the hand the ulnar and radial arteries may be compressed with the two thumbs just above the wrist. The brachial artery can be pressed against the humerus by grasping the arm from behind, so that the fingers lie over the artery between the biceps and triceps muscles in the middle of the arm, and giving an outward twist to the arm, or by placing a roll of material in front of

the elbow and flexing the joint fully; the subclavian artery can be pressed against the first rib by placing the thumb above the clavicle at the root of the neck with the fingers over the back of the spine and pressing downwards and backwards; the carotid can be compressed against the transverse processes of the vertebrae just above the sternomastoid muscle, but is of little value owing to the free anastomosis in the neck and head; the femoral can be compressed against the innominate bone in the centre of the groin, using two thumbs, one over the other, with the hip very slightly flexed.

4. Application of a tourniquet. Theoretically this is available as a last resort; in practice it is almost never needed since a really firm pad *tightly* bandaged over the wound will stop even severe arterial bleeding, the possible exception being if, say, a fragment of glass is embedded in the wound. Especially if applied to the arm a tourniquet can damage nerves, its use can lead to gangrene and subsequent need for amputation of the limb and if applied not quite tightly enough it can increase the bleeding by impeding the venous return without obstructing the arterial inflow of blood.

As well as the alternatives mentioned above, the first aid treatment should *always* begin by raising the bleeding part well above the level of the heart, the exception being when the bleeding occurs from a wound on head, neck or shoulder, when the patient should lie *flat*.

Operative treatment consists of opening up the part and securing the bleeding vessel with artery forceps or ligature. In a few cases it may be necessary to leave the artery forceps on for 48 hours, incorporating them in the dressings. A ruptured organ may need to be removed, e.g. the spleen. A ruptured liver may be sewn up or a damaged part removed and the surface covered quickly with alginate gauze, with successful results in skilled hands.

Operative treatment is sometimes needed to control prolonged slight bleeding rather than to control a single torrential haemorrhage; in such instances cauterization may be carried out.

Clinical treatment includes:

1. Applications of cold, e.g. after simple nasal operations or dental extraction in patients with bleeding diseases, ice packs or poultices.

2. Applications of heat (not merely warmth, which will only make the bleeding more copious), e.g. hot bladder wash-out or hot

irrigation for an oozing wound at temperatures from 48 to 71°C. These hasten the enzyme action essential for clotting.

3. Application of the cautery; this must be dull red to sear the tissues; when glowing brightly it cuts like a knife and causes bleeding.

4. Application of styptics, i.e. drugs which, applied to the wound, assist in arresting haemorrhage, e.g. tannic acid, adrenaline, thrombin or snake venom.

5. Administration of haemostatics, e.g. morphine 8–15 mg, vitamin K and calcium salts such as calcium lactate or calcium gluconate.

General management includes:

1. Providing absolute rest to reduce the blood pressure and lessen the demand for oxygen.

2. Nursing the patient flat with the foot of the bed elevated to send blood the vital centres.

3. Keeping the patient quiet, avoiding all excitement, reassuring the patient. This will lower the blood pressure and reduce blood loss while hastening clotting.

4. Protecting the patient from chill, but without applying warmth to such a degree as to induce sweating. Lowering of the temperature lessens the oxygen needs of the tissues and is a natural protective reaction; if, therefore, it is not excessive, it should be allowed to continue, especially in the limbs.

5. Giving non-stimulating fluids by mouth to relieve thirst.

Arterial haemorrhage is the most difficult to control and may require any of these treatments.

Venous haemorrhage is slightly more readily stopped but can nevertheless be very severe; elevation of the part, with direct pressure by pad and bandage at the bleeding point, together with a firm bandage on the distal side of the wound, will control it.

Capillary haemorrhage can be controlled by digital pressure on the bleeding point.

Treatment of Internal Haemorrhage

Local treatment of internal haemorrhage, other than by operative means, is impossible, but the above general measures are helpful pending operation or as part of conservative treatment. When there is haemorrhage into the peritoneal cavity from ruptured spleen, kidney or ectopic gestation, operation for the removal of the ruptured organ is generally necessary to save life, since, although bleeding may stop naturally when the blood pressure becomes very low, the subsequent rise as the general condition improves may dislodge the clots, with grave risk of a fatal result. In preparation for operation the patient should be treated for shock, nursed lying flat with blocks at the foot of the bed to send blood to the brain and kept quiet and reassured. Stimulants should be avoided, as by increasing the blood pressure they increase the loss of blood. Morphine will be ordered and the operation will probably be undertaken as soon as possible.

A blood transfusion is likely to be started just before and continued during and after the operation.

In caring for the patient after operation there are three main considerations:

1. Protect the patient from chill.
2. Keep the patient flat with the legs elevated until the blood pressure has risen.
3. Replace lost fluid by
    a. Fluids by mouth (if allowed).
    b. Transfusion of blood or plasma.
    c. Intravenous infusion of saline or dextran.

Medical or conservative treatment of internal haemorrhage

This consists of the measures described under General Management (p. 28). In addition the doctor is likely to order morphine in a dosage of up to 15 mg intramuscularly or it may be given intravenously. He may have some difficulty in weighing up the pros and cons of giving a blood transfusion since the loss of blood from circulation is often such as to make one highly desirable; on the other hand its administration may so raise the blood pressure, back towards normal, as to increase the bleeding. A frequent compromise is to give a transfusion but at a slower rate than usual. In most instances the patient is given nothing to eat and if fluids are allowed by mouth they are usually given in small amounts at a time.

Special Types of Haemorrhage

A number of special types of haemorrhage may be seen in the surgical ward.

Epistaxis

Spontaneous epistaxis (Greek: *epi* = upon; *stazein* = to drip) is common in cases of high blood pressure, where it may afford relief provided it does not continue excessively; it is also common in patients where there is undue fragility of the capillaries near the tip of the nose. It is also an expected complication of a blow on the face!

Treatment. The patient should be seated, with his head held slightly forward. The whole of his face should be liberally sponged with the coldest water available, and the nostril on the bleeding side pressed firmly against the septum. Bleeding generally occurs from the front of the septum called Little's area, where the blood vessels are very numerous. If this fails, plugging with ribbon gauze will probably be necessary. It must be sterile and should be spread with sterile soft paraffin wax or other oily material, so that it does not stick and cause bleeding to restart when it is removed. Iodoform is often employed to lessen the risk of sepsis, as infection may spread from the nasal cavity the meninges, producing meningitis. Adrenaline is not recommended, as the temporary constriction of the vessels is liable to be followed by dilatation. Russell's viper venom, strength 1 : 10 000, may be applied. The plugging is only left in for 12–24 hours because of the danger of sepsis and preparation for plugging should be made in case of a recurrence, which is particularly likely if the plug had not been impregnated with a greasy material. Recurrent bleeding may be treated by cauterization.

Haemoptysis

Haemoptysis (Greek: *haima* = blood; *ptuein* = to spit) is the coughing-up of blood from the lungs. The blood is bright red, frothy, mixed with sputum and alkaline in reaction. It must be carefully distinguished from haematemesis. It may be seen in the late stages of bronchial carcinoma or pulmonary tuberculosis. Large haemoptyses are relatively rare; coughing up of small amounts which do little more than stain sputum or a handkerchief is much more likely. These small haemoptyses often occur fairly early in the disease and may be valuable in drawing attention to a serious condition; the patient usually needs no immediate attention beyond reassurance.

Treatment of severe haemoptysis. The nurse should:

1. Place the patient either sitting up to cough out the blood or with the head right down below body level so that the blood runs out, or asphyxiation will result.
2. Reassure the patient, as he suffers from the terrifying sensation of choking, in addition to the sense of weakness from sudden loss of blood.
3. Give frequent mouth-washes and fluids of a non-stimulating type to drink.
4. Keep the patient warm, quiet and at absolute rest.
5. Withhold all stimulants.
6. Prepare to give blood transfusion in severe cases.

When the attack subsides the patient may be placed in a semi-recumbent position with two or three pillows to enable him to expectorate with moderate ease, while also improving the blood supply to the brain, if the loss has been serious.

Haematemesis

Haematemesis (Greek: *haima* = blood; *emeein* = to vomit) is the vomiting of blood. The blood may be bright in colour, but is more often brown and granular, as a result of the action of digestive juices on it and is called 'coffee-ground' vomit. It is acid in reaction and probably mixed with food. The common cause is gastric ulcer, but it may be due to gastric polyps, malignant growth, cirrhosis of the liver or oesophageal varices.

Treatment may be either medical or surgical, with the use of blood transfusion, as for internal haemorrhage. Nowadays patients are usually allowed at least milky drinks quite early in the course of treatment since it is considered better not to leave the acid gastric juice undiluted and unbuffered.

Melaena

Melaena (Greek: *melas* = black) is a black, tarry stool due to changed blood. It is due to bleeding high up in the alimentary canal, usually from duodenal ulcer. A single melaena can result from swallowing a large amount of blood, e.g. after a severe epistaxis. In this case no treatment is needed. It must be carefully distinguished from the black stool due to the taking of iron, bismuth or charcoal by mouth.

Treatment is that for internal haemorrhage, though immediate operative treatment is rare.

Haematuria

Haematuria (Greek: *haima* = blood; *ouron* = urine) is blood in the urine and is a common symptom of kidney and bladder diseases, including inflammations, trauma, growths, tuberculosis and stone. The amount is often slight and disappears with treatment of the disease. Bleeding is most likely to be severe after operations on the kidney and bladder and in cases of growth, when it is continuous and results in progressive anaemia unless the growth is removable. Slight haematuria, with all symptoms of internal haemorrhage in accident cases, may indicate ruptured kidney, necessitating immediate operation to remove the damaged kidney if the bleeding is sufficient to endanger life.

Treatment. If the bleeding is less severe, rest in bed and the giving of morphine will, in the majority of cases, be followed by cure, with absorption of the blood clot. Watch must be kept in case infection follows.

FLUID BALANCE

Man left the sea quite recently in geological time. He has adapted himself to a gaseous external environment, but the cells of the body still require to be bathed in saline fluid to survive.

The total water of the body amounts to 70% of its complete weight. An average adult 'contains' about 45 litres of water. Of this, intracellular fluid, that is fluid within the cells, accounts for about two-thirds of the total (30 litres). The remainder is outside the cells, being partly the plasma and partly the interstitial fluid which 'bathes' all the tissue cells (15 litres: 12 of these forming tissue fluid and 3 litres forming plasma). The body water and its several divisions remain remarkably constant in a healthy adult and depend upon an exact balance of water intake and output. During growth and during periods of convalescence from illness, when new tissue is being formed and the body weight is increasing, the output of water is less than the intake because a large volume of water is laid down with the protein of the newly formed tissue.

In a temperate climate the average adult takes in about 2500 ml of water a day. Part of this is taken in fluid form and part as the water of metabolism derived from the digestion of the food he eats. He loses about 500 ml by insensible perspiration from the skin, 350 ml in saturated expired air from his lungs (these figures vary

about 70% of total body weight is WATER = 45 Litres

$\frac{2}{3}$ intracellular = 30 Litres

$\frac{1}{3}$ interstitial fluid and plasma = 15 Litres

2500 ml. fluid per day
350 ml. is expired
500 ml. perspired
1500 ml. excreted in urine
150 ml. excreted in faeces

INTRACELLULAR FLUID   EXTRACELLULAR FLUID

—potassium—

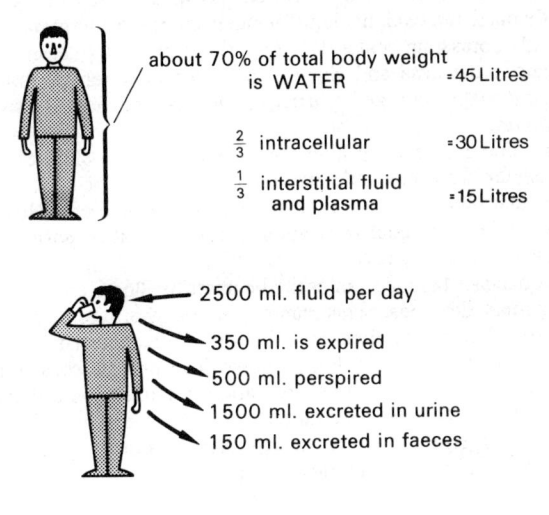

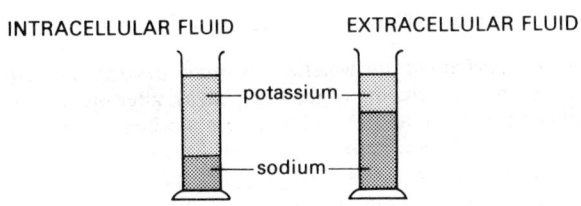

—sodium—

FIG. 3. The distribution of body fluids and the electrolyte balance.

considerably and sometimes the combined loss from the skin and lungs is estimated as low as 600 ml), 1500 ml in urine and 150 ml in faeces.

In maintaining a correct balance between fluid taken in and fluid eliminated from the body, more than water itself has to be considered. At one time it was thought that mineral salts were of major importance; in recent years an increasing importance has been attached to maintaining the electrolyte balance.

SURGICAL NURSING

An electrolyte is a substance which when dissolved in water dissociates into electrically charged particles called ions, some carrying a positive and some a negative charge. Sodium chloride is one of the best examples; a molecule of sodium chloride in solution dissociates into sodium particles, each having a positive charge, and chloride particles, each having a negative charge. Sodium bicarbonate and potassium chloride are other important electrolytes. Substances like urea and glucose, dissolved in water, do not split into electrically charged particles and so are not classed as electrolytes.

Intra- and extracellular fluids are very different in character, e.g. extracellular fluid has little potassium and a lot of sodium and intracellular fluid a lot of potassium and little sodium. However the two fluids are equal in relation to the amount of positive and negative charges they carry.

This delicate balance can easily be upset by illness and a state of *dehydration* develops. This simply means that the tissues are deprived of sufficient fluid and the state is manifested by a dry mouth and thirst as everybody knows. The oral mucosa is most sensitive to the body's state of hydration; a nurse should therefore always observe her patient's mouth carefully. A dry wrinkled skin, sunken eyes and a low or absent urinary output give further evidence of marked dehydration.

Causes of Dehydration

Simple deprivation of water. This may develop in certain illnesses such as carcinoma of the oesophagus, after operations on the alimentary tract and in unconsciousnss when the patient is unable to take sufficient water by the normal route.

Excessive loss of water. This occurs in severe vomiting, diarrhoea, excessive discharge from wounds and fevers, where much water is lost from lungs and skin.

Salt loss. Water can be held in the body only as an isotonic solution, that is its osmotic pressure due to dissolved salts must be the same as plasma. Thus, if much salt is lost from the body, for example in gastric aspiration, water must also be lost in order to keep the fluids isotonic. (An isotonic solution contains 9 mg *of salt in each litre of water*—a 0·9% solution.)

Water and salt loss. This is what most frequently occurs, and it is particularly the salt loss which upsets the electrolyte balance.

Fluid Balance Charts

The accurate maintenance of fluid balance charts is an important and an exacting part of a nurse's duties. On the intake side the nurse must measure everything taken by mouth, intragastric tube, rectally, subcutaneously or intravenously. On the output side she charts the measure for urine, faeces, vomit, gastric aspiration and drainage tube. Occasionally dressings must be weighed to measure fluid lost. A surgeon tries to keep the patient's fluid balance as near normal as possible; he therefore seldom orders more than 3 litres of fluid for the patient per day. A good fluid intake is important in order to permit necessary repair after surgery and elimination of waste substances. A dry mouth and low urinary output are often the first indication of dehydration, but a low urinary output is normal during the first 24 hours after surgery.

Intravenous Infusions

Intravenous therapy is used when it is impossible to introduce fluids and electrolytes required by the body by other routes, but it should never be forgotten that fluids are safest given by mouth. The natural safeguard is that if a person is not thirsty, he will not drink. If he drinks to excess the extra liquids and electrolytes are excreted by the kidney. In intravenous therapy the body has to accept the fluid injected and immediately after surgery the action of the kidney is depressed. It is therefore easy to produce a condition of overhydration.

The *isotonic solutions* most frequently used are 5% dextrose and normal saline which is a 0·9% solution of sodium chloride. In determining the quantity and the nature of fluids used, consideration has to be given to both water balance and electrolyte balance. The latter is estimated in the laboratory after samples of the patient's blood have been taken. The fluid intake in uncomplicated cases will be kept near the normal level of 2–3 litres in 24 hours. If, however, vast quantities of fluids are being lost by gastric aspiration, through drainage tubes or from a large raw surface as in severe burns, much greater quantities may be required in 24 hours. In this case it will be necessary to make good abnormal loss of electrolytes. Normally not more than 500 ml normal saline is required in 24 hours unless there is abnormal loss from the alimentary tract. In addition some patients undergoing surgical operations may require additional potassium in the intravenous fluid to replace potassium lost from tissue damage. This is safer if given by mouth and is not given intravenously if renal function is impaired, as a high concentration in the blood may cause cardiac arrest. Not more than 6 g potassium chloride is given in 24 hours. If needed it is always added to one of the other infusion fluids and given as a weak solution. Intravenous therapy may be used to correct the condition of acidosis, when the blood is less alkaline than normal, or alkalosis, when the blood is more alkaline than normal. In acidosis the patient has deep sighing respirations as in diabetic coma and the fluids ordered will be normal saline, sodium lactate or saline lactate. In alkalosis the patient has a severe headache, is very irritable, and suffers from nausea, vomiting and anorexia. Sodium or potassium chloride with lactate may be ordered. These saline infusions are not very valuable in conditions of shock unless they are given with plasma, as, owing to the increased permeability of the capillaries, the infused fluid rapidly leaves them and the blood pressure is consequently not improved.

Complications of intravenous therapy

Thrombophlebitis is by no means uncommon, but as only superficial veins are affected there is little danger of embolus formation. The condition can be very painful, but may be somewhat relieved by kaolin poultices, glycerine and ichthyol. In this case the thrombosis is initiated by inflammation caused by the intravenous therapy.

Local oedema may be very painful and necessitate the removal of the infusion to another site. Appliction of a kaolin poultice may hasten absorption of the fluid.

Air embolus. An entry of air into the vein may be fatal. It has been suggested that as little as 10 ml can be fatal in severely ill patients if it enters the heart, but this would require about 100 ml to be introduced into the circulation.

Over-hydration may result from the introduction of excess fluids or salt. A 'bubbly' cough, rising pulse and respiratory rate with dyspnoea are signs of excessive fluid intake, or the patient may start to become oedematous. There is a grave risk of this complication in infants and young children. If these signs are noticed the infusion must be slowed down and the doctor called immediately. He will probably stop the infusion and may start to treat the patient by postural drainage to free the lungs of excess fluid.

Acute heart failure may occur if the circulation is suddenly overloaded, especially in patients whose hearts are already damaged. These last two complications are especially liable to affect elderly patients.

Infection, due to faulty sterilization or technique, may occur.

TRANSFUSION

When human blood, or a derivative of human blood, is transferred into the vascular system of another individual the procedure is spoken of as a transfusion. It may be of whole blood, plasma, serum, packed cells or platelets. Blood transfusion is invaluable in the treatment of severe haemorrhage, certain forms of anaemia and as supportive treatment before, during and after surgery. First of all the blood must be *compatible*, that is blood which will mix with the patient's blood without causing agglutination of the corpuscles. Agglutination is the clumping together of red blood corpuscles which have become sticky. They may thus block the lumen of small blood vessels in vital organs; the cells are then haemolysed, the haemoglobin is released and has to be excreted by the kidneys and may fatally damage the delicate uriniferous tubules, so urine production fails.

Grouping of Blood

Red blood cells may contain agglutinogens or antigens. (N.B. The suffix -ogen means 'the forerunner of something else'—in this case the forerunner of agglutination.) These are referred to by the capital letters A and B. Blood serum may contain agglutinins, referred to by the small letters a and b. If cells containing agglutinogen A are mixed with serum containing agglutinin a, then the cells will clump together, i.e. there will be agglutination.

Blood group	Red cells	Serum
A	Agglutinogen A	Agglutinin b
B	Agglutinogen B	Agglutinin a
AB	Agglutinogen A and B	No agglutinins
O	No agglutinogens	Agglutinins a and b

38 SURGICAL NURSING

In considering compatibility the important factors are the donor's cells and the recipient's serum; since it is so quickly and markedly diluted the donor's serum is not of such great importance.

Theoretically a Group AB recipient can *receive* blood from a donor of any group since his serum contains no agglutinins and therefore no clumping of the donor's cells could be produced. Theoretically also a Group O donor can *give* blood to a recipient of any group since his cells contain no agglutinogens and could not therefore be caused to clump by either agglutinin. A recipient of Group A must always be given blood from a Group A donor. A recipient of Group B must always be given blood from a Group B donor. Since in Great Britain the National Blood Transfusion Service can supply blood from any of these groups at extremely short notice, in practice Group AB recipients are always given blood from Group AB donors and Group O donors give blood, always and only to Group O recipients. Where less developed services exist this may not always be possible.

There are other blood factors (apart from the rhesus factor) in addition which are comparatively rarely found, but because of the risk of their presence the blood about to be transfused is always *cross-matched*, i.e. a drop is mixed with a little of the recipient's serum to ensure that when the transfusion is given there will be no agglutination.

The rhesus factor is a complex substance (consisting of at least six parts) found in the red cells of the rhesus monkey and in 85% of the white population, being absent from the blood of the remaining 15%. The six parts of the complex are described as C, D, E, c, d, e, the most powerful one being D. If blood containing this factor is donated to a recipient not possessing it, he or she will be stimulated to produce antibodies. In certain instances, if a pregnant woman's blood should contain these antibodies there is grave risk of damage to the unborn baby's red cells. Consequently no rhesus-negative girl, or woman prior to the menopause, would be given rhesus-positive blood (i.e. containing the rhesus factor) but instead would be transfused with blood of the appropriate ABO grouping, rhesus-negative (i.e. not containing the rhesus factor). In practice, no patients, including boys and post-menopausal women, are given rhesus-positive blood if they themselves are rhesus-negative, since complications could arise in relation to future transfusions if they were ever needed. Although it would not matter if rhesus-positive patients were transfused with rhesus-negative blood, this is not generally done since it would cause too great a drain on the relatively small supply of rhesus-negative blood, which might then be unavailable for those people who desperately need it and for whom rhesus-positive blood is harmful.

Blood Donors

The United Kingdom is fortunate in the blood banks maintained at the various Department of Health transfusion depots, which are kept supplied with blood from volunteer donors. The donors are recruited by local advertising campaigns and nurses can help by being well informed about transfusion services in their district. Frequently relatives are very ready to give blood, especially after a member of their family has benefited from a transfusion. A donor must be adult and healthy and submit to a complete blood test before being accepted as a donor. Diseases like syphilis, malaria and infective hepatitis permanently exclude a person from the donor panel.

The National Blood Transfusion Service maintains lists of would-be donors and organizes 'taking sessions' in a wide variety of places, e.g. works canteens, village halls and hospitals themselves in most towns and villages up and down the country. Disposable giving sets are in universal use for all patients receiving blood transfusions and also disposable taking sets for use on the rare occasions when a donor is required to go to hospital to give blood for immediate use for a specific patient; this need almost never arises on a surgical ward.

Storage of Blood

Blood is stored in special refrigerators maintained at a temperature of 4°C until required. Blood should not be fetched long before it is needed and it should not be heated before use; standing for an hour at room temperature is quite adequate. Ordinary refrigerators are quite unsuitable for blood storage as their temperatures vary and frozen cells disintegrate on thawing.

On storage the cells settle and the supernatant plasma should be a uniform colour; if it is a deep orange or red, haemolysis has occurred and the blood should not be used. Normally blood can be used for three weeks after it has been taken. After that the plasma can be taken off, freeze dried, and stored for long periods. Blood

40 SURGICAL NURSING

should be checked carefully before it is transfused: two people must read and check the label on the bottle and the patient's notes as to full name and address, the patient's age, the number of the bottle to be given, the blood group, and whether it has been signed as having been cross-matched and found compatible.

The blood must be used within 24 hours of breaking the seal, and after use the remnants in the bottle must be conserved for 24 hours in case a reaction occurs and investigation proves necessary.

Giving Blood

The giving set is a *plastic, disposable, single-use type*, made to Department of Health specifications based on recommendations of a Medical Research Council subcommittee. It is made almost entirely of polyvinyl chloride, but the piercing needle assembly, filter and adapters are made of nylon. A short piece of rubber tubing is included in the length of plastic tubing near the adapter to which the needle is attached in order that drugs may be injected through this tubing if necessary. The set is put up in a cardboard box with instructions for use printed on the outside and the warning that the exterior of the set is not sterile except where protected by a sheath. If the container of the set has been damaged and there is doubt about sterility it should be discarded.

Transfusion Dangers

There are many dangers associated with blood transfusions; briefly these are:

1. *Infection*, caused either by the donor blood carrying an infection, e.g. malaria, or by the blood or equipment being contaminated.

2. *Allergic reactions* of an urticarial type. These are controlled by antihistamines.

3. *Pyrexial reaction*, which is seen in 5–10% of cases.

4. The circulation can be overloaded, so producing *heart failure*, most commonly encountered when the patient has a chronic anaemia. To prevent this packed cells should be given.

5. The patient may develop a *citrated plasma toxicity*, due to the high levels of potassium present in old blood and especially in plasma.

6. An *incompatible blood transfusion* may be given, usually owing to a clerical error.

7. *Cold blood* may cause death due to ventricular fibrillation.

Signs and symptoms of transfusion reaction

A transfusion reaction is most likely to develop within minutes of the transfusion having been started. Common features are:

1. *Fever*, ranging from a transient slight rise of temperature, 37–38°C, to a severe rigor, 40·5–41°C.
2. *Headache*.
3. *Backache*, tending to occur later.
4. *Complete or partial reduction of urine volume*. This together with pain in the loins is the most important observation for it may indicate severe renal damage; it also tends to develop later.
5. *Vomiting*.
6. *Urticaria and other rashes*.
7. *Jaundice*. This may occur in days if there has been any haemolysis or in months if it is due to a virus contained in the serum of the donated blood.

All evidence of an early transfusion reaction except reduction and suppression of urine may be masked in patients who receive unsuitable blood during an operation or while anaesthetized. Any postoperative reduction in urine volumes in these patients may therefore be of vital significance and must be reported to the doctor.

Treatment of transfusion reaction

If there is a rapid rise in temperature, particularly in the early stage of transfusion, with backache and with or without rigor, the transfusion should be stopped immediately, but not taken down, and the doctor called. Rigor and headaches should receive symptomatic treatment. If there is a less striking rise in temperature, with or without other evidence of a reaction, the drip should be slowed to 10 drops a minute and the doctor called. He may order an antihistamine drug, such as chlorpheniramine (Piriton) made up in 10 mg in 1 ml ampoules.

Further action is the responsibility of the doctor, but when a transfusion reaction is suspected, certain evidence is essential to determine the cause so that the appropriate treatment may be given:

1. Venous samples of the patient's blood in plain and heparin tubes should be sent to the laboratory for blood urea estimation, evidence of haemolysis and Coombs's test, etc.
2. All urine passed should be measured and specimens sent to the laboratory for examination for free haemoglobin, albumin, etc.
3. All bottles of blood used and partly used should be sent to the laboratory labelled and unwashed for checking.

When anuria has developed a satisfactory treatment has recently been evolved and has much reduced the high mortality previously associated with these disasters. The patient is given a protein-free, mineral-free diet containing an adequate number of calories and having a water content of approximately 600 ml a day (corresponding to the amount being lost by lungs, skin and faeces). 600 ml of 50% glucose solution are given daily by intragastric drip during the phase of anuria and two days after diuresis begins. Additional potassium may be added to make good what the patient has lost in the urine. Thereafter the patient is allowed as much fluid by mouth as is passed in the urine, and later a low-protein, high-carbohydrate diet is substituted for the intragastric drip. Provided this conservative regimen, which is aimed at resting the kidney during the initial period of damage, is instituted early and over-hydration is avoided, the recovery rate, even in severe cases, exceeds 90%. Gone are the days of administering alkalis and trying to flush the kidneys by 'pushing fluids'.

Transfusion of Blood Derivatives

Plasma may be obtained from a bottle of blood that has been in store for more than three weeks, in which case it is dried and must be reconstituted before use. Alternatively when the blood is in a plastic blood pack it may be centrifuged so that the plasma spins off, and this is given to the patient in its liquid state. The cells from the blood may be given to a patient or to the donor (especially if he repeatedly gives blood). The liquid plasma may again be treated and after freezing cryoprecipitate can be removed. Albumen and fibrinogen may also be obtained. Liquid plasma may be stored as fresh frozen plasma.

Dextran may be used as a plasma substitute in emergencies until supplies are available. The large molecules of this carbohydrate solution keep it in the blood vessels and therefore it helps to restore blood pressure. A sample of the patient's blood should be taken for grouping and cross-matching before the Dextran is given, as Dextran causes rouleaux formation and makes these tests difficult subsequently.

Packed cells from which the fluid portion of the blood has been removed are valuable when the doctor wishes to raise the patient's haemoglobin level without increasing the blood volume so much, for example in conditions of severe anaemia following toxaemia.

Platelets are extremely fragile, but they can with special precautions be transfused in the treatment of certain haemorrhagic conditions.

Autotransfusion is sometimes carried out if blood loss is expected during surgery and the patient will not give permission for blood from a donor to be transfused.

Cryoprecipitate is used in the treatment of patients suffering from haemophilia and is given intravenously.

Albumen is given in the treatment of oedematous patients when salts may not be administered.

Fibrinogen is used when the defibrination syndrome occurs, e.g. following lung, prostatic and uterine surgery, due to fibrinolysin digesting the fibrinogen.

3

Inflammation and Infection

INFLAMMATION

Inflammation is the reaction of the tissues to an irritant. The irritant may be inanimate, for example physical agents such as heat, cold, radiation, friction or a foreign body, or chemical agents such as strong acids or alkalis, for example hydrochloric acid or caustic soda. Inanimate agents, especially things like the surgeon's knife, exert their irritant action only very briefly; the inflammatory action is therefore transient and trivial and inflammation is rapidly followed by the process of repair.

The irritant more frequently is animate, that is bacteria or viruses which can breed and survive long periods of time in the tissues and therefore produce a prolonged inflammatory reaction. Repair cannot be complete until the irritant has been removed.

The *local signs and symptoms of inflammation* were described by Celsus, a Roman physician who lived in the first century A.D., as '*rubor, calor, tumor et dolor*', that is *redness, heat, swelling* and *pain*. The signs are what the doctor or nurse can observe when they examine the patient; the symptoms are what the patient complains about. Since the time of Celsus, *loss of function* has been added to the list. These signs and symptoms can all be attributed to the altered blood supply to the inflamed area. First the volume of blood to the part is increased, the arterioles dilate and the capillaries consequently swell up, which accounts for the redness and heat. The venules and veins cannot carry the blood away as quickly as it is arriving, the circulation is therefore slowed down and fluid leaves the capillaries and distends the tisssue spaces. This accounts for the swelling or inflammatory oedema which increases the tension in the tissues so that pressure and tension are exerted on the sensory nerve endings, thus causing pain. The pain of acute inflammation is usually throbbing in character; each beat of the heart sends a fresh jet of blood to the part, increasing the tension and thus accentuating the pain. To minimize the pain the patient keeps the inflamed part as still as possible, while inflammatory oedema and reflex muscle spasm also inhibit movement, hence the loss of function. With the fluid leucocytes emigrate from the blood vessels to fight any infection that may be present, and finally macrophages appear which are large cells that eat up the debris.

Aseptic inflammation may cause a *local* reaction, as after a small incised wound, or a *general* reaction. The general reaction is characterized by a rise in temperature, pulse and respiration; the skin feels dry and hot, or sweating occurs, the mouth is dry, urine scanty and the patient frequently suffers from headache, general malaise and constipation. For example, after stripping out varicose veins, although the wounds remain aseptic, there is considerable tissue damage and a generalized inflammatory reaction while the débris from the damaged tissue is being absorbed. This occurs also after thrombosis of femoral veins or coronary artery.

A very common cause of inflammation is *infection*. Infection occurs when pathogenic, that is disease-producing, microorganisms gain access to the tissues and start multiplying in them. The inflammatory reaction persists until the polymorphonuclear leucocytes have destroyed the invading organisms, when repair can begin.

Resolution

Resolution is the most frequent result of bacterial invasion. The white cells do their work so efficiently that we are unaware of their activities. They engulf the bacteria, macrophages clear away the débris and repair takes the place of inflammation of which we have been unaware. When white cells are deficient in numbers, as in radiation sickness and after taking certain drugs such as sulphonamides or carbimazole, their beneficent activities will be sadly missed and the patient may be overwhelmed by a quite trivial infection.

LOCAL INFECTIONS

A local infective reaction may occur if the invading organisms are more numerous and virulent and the patient's resistance, both local and general, is weaker.

46 SURGICAL NURSING

Frequently there is *suppuration*, i.e. *pus* is formed; it is composed of dead leucocytes, dead bacteria, dead tissue cells and tissue fluid which have formed a foul liquid of a creamy consistency. Pus varies in appearance according to the organisms producing it. A nurse must always observe carefully the nature of pus on a dressing; these observations may be particularly helpful when immediate laboratory facilities are not available. The staphylococcus produces a creamy yellow pus and the streptococcus a more watery pus. *Pseudomonas pyocyanea*, which frequently gets into cross-infected wounds, gives a characteristic blue pus.

Cellulitis is inflammation of connective tissue and is usually subcutaneous. However, it does arise in deeper tissues, such as the perinephric or pelvic areas. The haemolytic streptococci are the usual causative organisms: they are able to spread through the cells as they produce substances called streptokinase and hyaluronidase which 'dissolve' the barriers. When cellulitis occurs the tissues are hot, deep red and swollen and death of tissue may occur. The lymphatic vessels and glands are often involved.

Examples of local infective reactions

An acute abscess (Fig. 4) is a collection of pus in a cavity lined with granulation tissue. It may be caused by a pyogenic (pus-forming) organism, but it can be sterile, as occurs from the mechanical irritation caused by an injection. It can occur anywhere in the body. The usual signs of local inflammation will be present and, after pus has formed, *fluctuation* may be felt if the abscess is palpable and the investigation not too painful. An abscess may be complicated by *sinus* formation. This is a track lined with granulation tissue leading from a focus of infection.

A fistula may also form in association with an abscess. This is an abnormal track, lined with granulation tissue, running between two epithelial surfaces, for example a vesicovaginal fistula between bladder and vagina or an anal fistula between anal canal and skin surface.

A whitlow is a septic infection of the finger-tip often associated with the nail.

A boil (Fig. 4) is usually due to the staphylococcal infection of the deep part of a hair follicle. Friction predisposes to its development. A boil affects only one hair follicle, although it is frequently followed by others in the neighbourhood. It starts with a

INFLAMMATION AND INFECTION

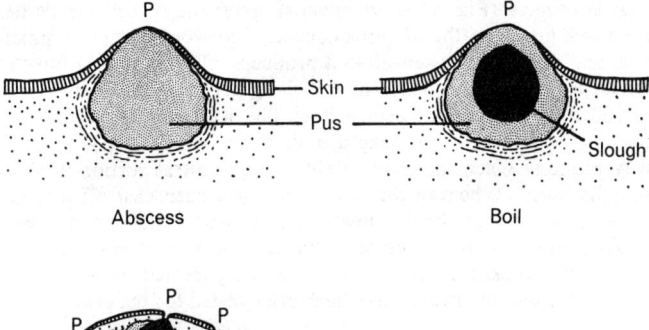

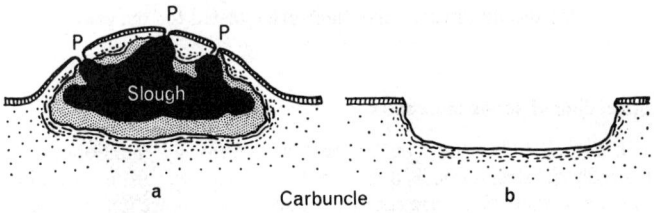

Fig. 4. *Above*, An abscess and a boil. Both are pointing and pus is about to burst through the skin. *Below*, A carbuncle pointing on to the skin in several places (*a*) and after separation of the slough (*b*), showing extensive tissue destruction.

red, hot, tender lump in the skin; pain and tenderness are intense, until a bead of pus erupts and relieves the tension. A day or two later a slough or core of necrotic material is extruded. After this healing is rapid. Those who have suffered from a series of boils will confirm that no treatment greatly affects the evolution of a boil. Nevertheless an attempt should be made to prevent its spread by cleansing the surrounding skin with an antiseptic such as cetrimide 1%. Ultra-violet light may also be used, if available, as it hastens the body's healing processes. Boils are better not dressed except when discharging, as dressings are usually painful and create a warm moist skin on which staphylococci thrive. The doctor may decide that it is advisable to incise the boil and to administer an antibiotic, e.g. oxytetracycline 150 mg four times a day. The worst treatment is to squeeze a boil to hasten the separation of the slough. This breaks down the delicate fibrous tissue walling off the infection and may convert a local infection into a general one.

A *furuncle* is, strictly speaking, the same thing as a boil, but the term is usually reserved for those tiny, but extremely painful, 'boils' which develop in the external auditory meatus and in the nose.

48 SURGICAL NURSING

A carbuncle (Fig. 4) is an infective gangrene of cellular tissue usually caused by the staphylococcus. The word means a small coal and describes the sensation it produces. Clinically, a carbuncle looks like a multiple boil, but the slough is large and cannot be extruded through a small central hole. The necrotic mass presses on the skin from below, depleting it of its blood supply; the skin gives way in many places and ultimately a large central portion of skin sloughs away. When all the dead tissue has been cast off a large ulcer is left which heals slowly, unless early excision or skin grafting hastens the process. Diabetes makes a person very susceptible to skin infections. Patients being treated for boils and carbuncles should always have their urine tested for the presence of sugar.

Spreading of septic infections

Cellulitis. This may be caused (as previously mentioned) by haemolytic streptococci but can be caused by an insect bite. Constitutional effects are rarely produced and intense itching rather than pain is the patient's main complaint. This gives rise to scratching and then secondary infection by bacteria can easily occur.

Lymphangitis occurs when the body defences have not been entirely successful in localizing an infection: it may spread up the lymphatic channels and the condition manifests itself as angry red lines on the skin overlying the lymphatic vessels. These can often be seen on the arm when infection is spreading from a septic finger.

Lymphadenitis occurs when the lymph nodes also are affected. At first the nodes exercise their normal function as filters, but eventually they are overwhelmed and become fresh foci of infection. Next the glands become easily palpable and the usual signs of inflammation are present. Most people have suffered at some time from cervical adenitis following a sore throat.

A SPREADING INFECTION READILY BECOMES GENERALIZED

Septicaemia is an acute infection of the blood stream when bacteria are not merely circulating but are actively multiplying in the blood stream. The arrival of bacteria in the blood stream frequently causes rigor and this may be repeated if the condition persists. The patient has a high, swinging temperature and a full, bounding, rapid pulse at first which, later, may become weak and irregular. The patient may be flushed and anxious at first, but may rapidly become delirious and comatose. The skin is hot and dry, the tongue furred and anorexia and constipation are present. Urine is scanty and concentrated. Headaches and vomiting are common. The condition is confirmed by a blood culture. In the old days the condition was almost invariably fatal. Nowadays it will sometimes respond to energetic treatment, but unfortunately when it occurs, the original cause of infection is usually an organism resistant to antibiotics.

Pyaemia means pus in the blood stream. It is a condition in which secondary abscesses form in various parts of the body. It is specially liable to follow the breaking up of a septic thrombus. Small septic emboli are carried to other parts of the body. The primary abscess is usually painful, but the secondary ones are often painless, although they manifest the other signs and symptoms of local inflammation. Rigors and a swinging temperature are common. There may be much septic absorption. The abscess cavities must be drained. General treatment is likely to have to be prolonged. Fortunately this condition is rare today. When it does occur, these pyaemic abscesses usually develop in the liver or lungs.

Bacteraemia is a term sometimes used to denote the transient presence of bacteria in the blood stream; they are not multiplying there as in septicaemia and their presence is much more difficult to demonstrate by means of blood culture.

Principles of Treatment of Acute Inflammation

Prevention

The nurse has an important part to play in the prevention of infection of patients in her care. She does this by careful attention to the state of their general health which raises their general immunity; she also does it by her care of the hygiene of the ward and its equipment, by her practice of aseptic technique and by her care in relation to her own standards of personal hygiene.

When a wound is likely to have been contaminated by certain organisms, it is sometimes possible to give an inoculation to prevent the development of those organisms. A common example of this has been in the use of antitetanus serum, e.g. for patients who have been involved in road accidents. However, nowadays, a large number of civilians as well as members of the armed forces

50 SURGICAL NURSING

are actively immunized with an antitetanus toxoid. Unfortunately there are, as yet, no specific vaccines for most of the organisms causing sepsis. Some surgeons use antibiotics prophylactically; others condemn this practice.

An infection of any grade of severity is the result of a battle between the defences of the body and the attacking micro-organisms. If prevention fails, the rational line of treatment therefore lies in (*a*) *strengthening the defences* and (*b*) *weakening the attack*.

Strengthening the defences

Rest assists the body to fight infection. Rest should be both local, to the affected area, and general. Even a common cold, nasopharyngitis, will clear more quickly if the sufferer goes to bed. This counsel is seldom followed and so the cold is spread. Rest also slows down the flow of lymph from the infected areas, and the slower the lymph flows, the more efficiently the nodes act as filters.

To achieve *local rest*, splints, slings and sandbags may be required.

A nurse can do much to promote *general rest*. Patients must have sufficient sleep if recovery is to be rapid. Analgesics and hypnotics should be given as required, but natural sleep is always most beneficial and a nurse should do all in her power to promote this by eliminating all external stimuli like noise, light and unpleasant smells and by seeing that the patient is comfortable physically and relaxed mentally. Infectious conditions have a depressing effect on morale and the patient will require much encouragement and sympathy.

Gravity should be used to assist venous drainage from an inflamed area. This is difficult to achieve if the patient is not in bed. An arm can be supported on a pillow or a sling can be arranged by passing a roller towel over a blood transfusion pole. For a leg infection the foot of the bed should be raised on blocks. This nearly always gives relief and reduces throbbing pain.

Diet. A high fluid intake will help the body during the febrile stage, and during the period of repair building materials in the form of fluid, protein, salts and vitamins, especially vitamin C, will be required in generous quantities.

Heat has traditionally been used to aid the normal defences of the body; it is undoubtedly soothing and helps to relax muscle spasm and relieve pain and tension, but poultices and fomentations are seldom used today as they create warm moist conditions in which bacteria can thrive. Electric pads do not have these disadvantages and often are comforting. Infra-red and ultra-violet rays may be ordered by the surgeon and may hasten repair.

Analgesics should be given as required, but it is sometimes necessary to withhold them until a diagnosis has been made. In any case their prescription is a doctor's responsibility.

Antitoxic sera. In certain forms of infection, for example tetanus and gas gangrene, antitoxic sera can be introduced ready-made into the circulation to raise the body defences.

Weakening the attack

Antibiotics are the best method of weakening the attack of the micro-organisms. These should never be used in trivial infections when the defences of the body are likely to prove adequate on their own and ideally they are only used after sensitivity tests have been carried out. Many inflammatory conditions are far less serious today because we are able to use these drugs. Usually antibiotics are given systemically, but some surgeons use them locally also, introducing them into wounds in the form of powders.

Adequate surgery, where appropriate, will also weaken the attack of the micro-organisms and minimize the harmful effects of inflammation. In certain conditions, like acute appendicitis, the whole inflamed area can be excised. In most inflammatory conditions the damage to cells is local. Some of this damage is due to the direct action of micro-organisms on the tissues in which they are present, but most of the tissue destruction is due to inflammatory oedema cutting off the blood supply. The tension in the tissue spaces rises so high that the blood can no longer flow freely through the area; the danger of ischaemia and subsequent death of tissue is particularly serious in areas surrounded by rigid walls, such as bone and tendon sheaths. Tension can be relieved by incision, but incision greatly increases the risk of spreading infection, especially in conditions like cellulitis. All surgeons agree that when pus has formed it should be evacuated. Antibiotics will sterilize pus, but healing will not occur until it has been removed. The presence of pus is indicated by leucocytosis, i.e. an increase in the leucocyte count, locally tender oedema, and fluctuation—a sign it may only be possible to elicit after the patient has been anaesthetized.

52 SURGICAL NURSING

The *incision of an abscess* must always be sufficient to permit free drainage. The surgeon explores the cavity for the presence of sinuses or fistulas and a nurse must always provide a silver probe and sinus forceps for this purpose. The abscess cavity will usually be drained by a piece of corrugated rubber or a piece of rubber glove inserted into the most dependent part of the abscess, which is determined by the position in which the patient is to be nursed. A drain is usually attached to the skin by a stitch and a safety-pin at right angles through the drain prevents it from disappearing into the abscess cavity. The surgeon will give directions about shortening the drain. For example, in a large breast abscess the stitch may be removed after two days and the drain shortened 1 cm every two days. Each time the drain is shortened a sterile safety-pin is introduced aseptically 1 cm lower and the protruding 1 cm of drain cut off. If a drain is removed too soon the surface tissues may heal over and an abscess re-form below. A drain kept in too long delays healing. A tubular drain may also require to be rotated in order to prevent pocketing of pus. Wicks of ribbon gauze are sometimes used instead of rubber drains; they must extend into the depths of the abscess cavity, but should not be packed in tightly; such a drain is likely to be removed and renewed daily.

When *dressing a discharging wound or abscess,* the surrounding skin should be cleansed with an antiseptic, such as cetrimide 1%, then dried, and the skin may require protection with an ointment such as silicone barrier cream such as Vasogen. The dressing usually requires to be changed frequently. The nurse must see that the patient is comfortably supported in a position in which satisfactory drainage can occur.

Rehabilitation may be slow after an acute infection. When the inflammatory condition has subsided movement should be encouraged. When an internal organ has been involved, restoration of function may be slow and diet and activity will have to be modified until recovery is complete.

CHRONIC INFLAMMATION

Chronic inflammation is caused by different organisms and produces a different reaction from the body. *Mycobacterium tuberculosis*, *Mycobacterium leprae*, the spirochaete of syphilis and the actinomyces are the principal organisms causing chronic inflammation.

The reaction of the body is much less violent and there is no redness, heat or pain in the area. Lymphocytes rather than polymorphs emigrate to the infected tissue. Their method of defence is not fully understood, but the main defence appears to be the laying down of an *encircling band of fibrous tissue* which by shrinking cuts off the blood supply.

In *tuberculosis*, if the focus of an infection is small, *fibrosis* is all that occurs; later *calcium salts* are sometimes deposited in the fibrous nodules, and the body has successfully overcome the invading organism. If the attack is more virulent and the defence poorer, everything within the sphere of fibrous tissue disintegrates into a cheesy mass. The process is called *caseation*. Presently liquefaction occurs and a *cold abscess* forms. A cold abscess differs from a hot one in that there is no redness, heat, pain or tenderness. There may or may not be impairment of function. A cold abscess is a well-circumscribed, cold, painless, fluctuant lump. With the much better treatment of tuberculosis in recent years, however, cold abscesses are rarely seen. It is important for the nurse to observe any abnormal lumps as the patient may be unaware of them. The *general symptoms and signs* may also be mild. There may be slight pyrexia and general lethargy.

Principles of Treatment

The principles of treatment are the same as for acute infection.

Prevention of tuberculosis can be successfully accomplished by the use of *bacille Calmette–Guérin* vaccine which has been proved to increase greatly the body's resistance to this infection.

Strengthening the body's defences is assisted by a sanatorium regimen; that is, rest of the affected part to preserve the fibrous barrier, general rest, good food, fresh air and the promotion of mental and psychological well-being by suitable occupation and the assistance of the social services, if they are required.

The organism is weakened by the administration of *chemotherapy*, which today is effective in the treatment of almost all types of chronic infection. *Surgery* is occasionally required to excise an area of chronic inflammation, for example a tuberculous kidney.

A cold abscess requires incision and evacuation. The great danger is cross-infection as there are few leucocytes in the area to destroy any organism introduced. In the past these abscesses were frequently aspirated in order to avoid this complication and, since healing tended to be slow, to prevent the formation of a persistent sinus. As the contents of the cavity often remain cheesy rather than liquid, this is not always a satisfactory form of treatment and nowadays cold abscesses are usually incised and their contents evacuated; they are sewn up again immediately. Chemotherapy is used in conjunction with surgery.

GANGRENE

Gangrene is death of tissue in bulk, often with putrefaction.

Causes

This condition may be caused by vascular lesions, commonly thrombosis, spasm, embolism and external pressure. Other causes may be trauma, infection, extremes of temperature, chemicals and lesions of the nervous system.

Conditions which cause gangrene due to *gradual cutting off of the blood supply* are frostbite, Raynaud's disease (in which blood vessels go into spasm when exposed to only moderate degrees of cold) and, on the Continent of Europe or in other places where rye bread is eaten, ergot poisoning. Ergot poisoning is occasionally seen in Great Britain when it has been taken in a misguided attempt to terminate an unwanted pregnancy; gangrene can then be an added complication.

The second group of conditions which can produce gangrene are those in which there is a *sudden cutting off of the blood supply*. This can occur from an embolus or thrombosis. An embolus frequently sticks at a bifurcation of the vessels, thus occluding two and rendering more difficult the opening up of a collateral circulation. If the collateral circulation opens up, as it usually does in the arm, which has a rich collateral supply, the limb will be saved. If collaterals fail to open, massive death of tissue will occur and a line of demarcation appears; but the surgeon may anticipate this by amputation. A strangulated hernia causes a sudden cutting off of blood supply to a portion of the gut, and unless the condition is rapidly diagnosed and the intestine released a portion of necrotic tissue will have to be resected.

INFLAMMATION AND INFECTION

Trauma can also cause gangrene, especially those injuries which produce crush fractures. The blood vessels in the injured area go into spasm and if this is near the knee or elbow many of the collateral vessels may be involved in the spasm, which spreads a little way up and down the vessels. Bedsores and splint sores are forms of traumatic gangrene which should always be prevented. Traumatic gangrene can also be produced by chemical and physical agents such as corrosives or radiation.

Myocardial infarction resulting from coronary thrombosis is, in effect, gangrene of the heart muscle, though it is never described as that.

Gas gangrene is the most dreaded form of gangrene as it is invariably a moist or spreading gangrene. It was a fairly frequent complication of war wounds received in areas where there was manured soil and in peace can occur as the result of road accidents on country roads. *Clostridium perfringens* (or *welchii*) enters the wound. It is anaerobic and usually thrives best where mixed infection has used up the available oxygen. The organism causes thrombosis of the vessels in the damaged muscle and evolves a gas which spreads between the tissues and further impedes the blood supply. It causes shock, tachycardia, vomiting, intense pain, discoloration and foul-smelling pus. In the old days it was almost invariably fatal.

An *acute appendix* can produce another type of moist gangrene. The blood supply to the appendix is poor and acute inflammation can produce septic thrombophlebitis leading to gangrene. This is why acute appendicitis is operated on early, if a diagnosis is made before an appendix mass has formed.

Signs and Symptoms

The symptoms are first of all pain on exercise, then pain on rest, relieved by hanging down the legs. The signs are paleness of the leg in elevation, duskiness when hung down and a steep temperature gradient between these two positions. The leg pulses are feeble or absent. Finally a small patch of gangrene, black shrivelled tissue, will appear on one toe, but the underlying tissues do not have sufficient vitality to produce a line of demarcation. If such a patient is admitted to the ward, the nurse should keep the limb level with the body, protect it by a large cradle, keep it cool with air

56 SURGICAL NURSING

circulating freely round it, keep it dry and protect it from injury until she receives further instruction from the surgeon. By this means metabolism in the limb is lowered, the minimum demands are made on a failing circulation, and it is protected from injury and infection. Application of heat locally must *never* be allowed.

Once gangrene has developed fully it is characterized by:

1. Loss of pulsation in the vessels.
2. Coldness which does not respond to heating.
3. Loss of sensation, although the part is very painful during onset.
4. Loss of function.
5. Change of colour—first white, then mottled bluish and finally black.
6. Ultimately a line of demarcation occurs between dead and healthy tissue which is a narrow ulcerated area where the dead tissue has acted as an irritant to the healthy tissue.

Treatment

Conservative treatment may take the form of drugs, such as tolazoline (Priscol), and Buerger's exercises designed to open up the collateral circulation. These measures are not usually very successful. Various forms of *surgery* have been employed, of which the most satisfactory is probably arterial grafting when the arteriosclerosis is confined to a small area.

When a patient suffers from arterial insufficiency he must take *special care of his feet* and wear only soft well-fitting shoes and soft woollen socks with no holes, hard seams or knobbly darns, and he must visit a chiropodist regularly and not attempt to cut his own toe-nails or, worse still, his corns. Injury to the feet must be prevented as the blood supply is not sufficient to permit healing.

Surgical treatment. The surgeon will excise all the affected tissue and this may mean that an amputation is necessary if the spread has been extensive. Following surgery a hyperbaric oxygen chamber (if available) is used to increase the amount of oxygen in the circulating blood. Antibiotics and blood transfusion are given.

Prevention is better than cure, so if a patient's wound is suspect, i.e. there is a risk of anaerobic infection developing, excision is carried out in the first instance. Antibiotics and anti-gas-gangrene serum are also administered.

ULCERS

Causes

An ulcer is produced by the cellular death of tissue from an internal or external surface; for example, peptic ulcers which occur in the stomach or duodenum, and bedsores which occur on the surface skin. The cells die off singly or in small groups that are not visible to the naked eye until the process is advanced. They occur more readily in patients with general diseases, such as tuberculosis, diabetes and arteriosclerosis, when the tissues are poorly nourished. The fundamental cause of ulceration is lessening of the blood supply to the surface tissues.

The blood supply may be arrested by pressure from without. Bedsores and plaster sores are commonly caused in this way. *Trophic ulcers* are caused by pressure or other harmful agents acting on the skin, whose nutrition has been affected by damage to its nerve supply. These ulcers are the most difficult of all to prevent and cure, but great advances in their treatment have been made in recent years. Examples are the ulcers that readily occur on the pressure areas of the lower limbs of paraplegic patients, who are at special risk when both movement and sensation are lost. Ulcers occur on the feet of patients suffering from locomotor ataxia of tertiary syphilis, because the sensory pathways from the soles of the feet are diseased and they are insensitive to pain stimuli resulting from, say, pressure or friction from an ill-fitting shoe.

Pressure from within can also cut the blood supply to surface tissues. This occurs with rapidly growing neoplasms. They distend the skin from within and cut off the blood supply; the skin then dies and ulcerates, and 'fungation' of the neoplasms is said to occur. The gummatous ulcers of tertiary syphilis are produced similarly; as the gumma enlarges it compresses surface vessels and ulceration occurs.

Arterial insufficiency caused by degenerative changes in the arteries often advances until gangrene occurs, but the condition is usually heralded by ulceration of the surface tissues.

Poor venous return, resulting from varicose veins or a post-thrombotic syndrome, affects the nutrition of surface tissues and causes ulceration.

58 *SURGICAL NURSING*

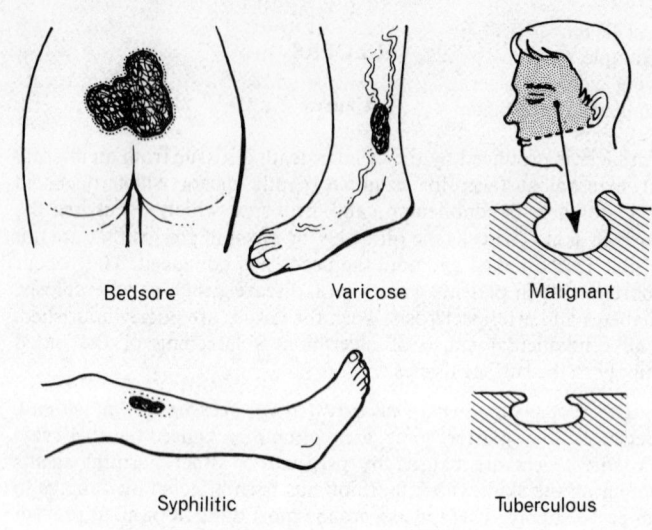

Bedsore Varicose Malignant

Syphilitic Tuberculous

Fig. 5. Some common ulcers in characteristic positions.

Physical and chemical agents like heat and cold and strong chemicals can destroy surface tissues and produce ulceration.

Acute infection, as in carbuncle, can cut off blood supply to the surface by an acute inflammatory oedema and lead to ulceration.

Chronic infection, particularly by *Mycobacterium tuberculosis*, can cause ulceration.

Neoplasms, epithelioma, carcinoma and rodent ulcers are all new growths of surface tissue. They frequently outgrow their blood supply and ulceration occurs.

Principles of Treatment of Ulcers

Prevention. Bedsores, plaster sores and trophic sores can normally be prevented. Their presence is a reflection on the medical and nursing care that the patient has received. However, it must in fairness be remembered that today physicians and surgeons are able to save, or at any rate prolong, the lives of many patients who, even a generation ago, would have died in a matter of days before they could have developed bedsores.

INFLAMMATION AND INFECTION 59

The initial cause of ulceration must be found and treated, for example tuberculosis, syphilis or varicose veins. When the underlying cause of ulceration has been treated, it is difficult to prevent an ulcer from healing.

A good blood supply to the surface tissues must be promoted. When an ulcer has become chronic it is usually surrounded by an area of induration, i.e. hard fibrous tissue which contracts and reduces the blood supply to the area. Massage and physiotherapy may be required to break this down, or curettage of the base of the ulcer may be required. Elastic bandages and exercise aid venous return from the legs and so remove waste substances and promote freer circulation in the surface tissues. For the same reason, keeping the patient who has a leg ulcer in bed, so that the part is not dependent, helps.

Infection must be eliminated or prevented, otherwise healing will be delayed. Whenever possible ulcers are dressed with bland ointments because topical antibiotics and hypochlorites tend to sensitize the skin.

Rest will usually hasten healing, but it is not always an appropriate form of treatment.

Ultra-violet light hastens the processes of repair.

Skin grafting may greatly accelerate healing, but it cannot be undertaken unless the ulcer is clean, or, alternatively, all infected tissue can be excised.

Bedsores

Patients with neurological diseases and elderly patients are the most prone to develop bedsores. They can occur in any patient lying in bed over a long period of time, but the nature of the individual's skin does seem to be an important factor: sores develop much more readily in some patients than in others. They may develop whereever a bone lies near the surface of the body: over the spines of the scapulae and thoracic vertebrae, over the sacrum and iliac crests, over the shoulder-tips and elbows, on the sides of the knees and over the malleoli and heels. A great deal of research into this subject has been carried out, e.g. by Doreen Norton. As a result, 'scales' are available for assessing each patient with reference to his individual risk of developing a pressure sore. This has now become part of the nursing process: the patient is assessed, the pattern of care required is specified, the ultimate goal being to prevent pressure sores developing.

A bedsore develops by stages. The skin first appears red and there is a burning pain; the skin may then crack and thus become exposed to infection; ulceration and then gangrene may follow.

Prevention of bedsores

Position. The patient should be turned two-hourly. To do this the patient must be lifted gently and not dragged over the bedclothes. The *position must be adjusted* so that there is no pressure on susceptible areas. Small pillows, air or sorbo rings, foam rubber wedges and pads, nursing sheepskins, ripple mattresses and ripple pads are all extremely useful in relieving pressure. Cradles should be used to take the weight of the bedclothes, the cantilever pattern being the better type.

Diet. The patient, especially if elderly, must have an *adequate dietary intake* to maintain tissue repair, particularly in relation to protein and vitamins. Milk and eggs are usually well tolerated and if necessary Casilan can be added. Complan or Carnation Instant Breakfast can be added too as they contain all essential nutrients.

Frequent *change of position* and feeding the patient properly are the two most important measures in the prevention of bedsores.

The sheets must be kept smooth, clean, dry and free from crumbs and bits of plaster.

Massage over pressure areas providing this is not done over damaged tissue is said to help to promote a good blood supply. This is most effective when done with a smooth bland powder, like starch, using the palm of the hand and kneading the superficial over the deep tissues. The skin does not require washing more than twice a day unless soiled with excreta; constant washing, especially with soap containing a strong alkali, tends to remove the natural oil from the skin and lower its resistance. Various barrier creams, such as silicone (Vasogen), are helpful in protecting the skin around discharging wounds and Drapolene will protect the skin of an incontinent patient from ammonia dermatitis. Some authorities contend that by producing a localized shearing force, massage can do more harm than good.

Bedpans. Patients must always be carefully put on and taken off bedpans and not left on for too long. Incontinence may be controlled by indwelling catheter and periodic enemas.

Treatment of bedsores

When a bedsore is present this should be treated with aseptic precautions as any other wound. The surrounding skin should be cleansed and protected from irritation by the discharge from the sore. In many hospitals massage is also carried out, but this is of doubtful value as it can cause a shearing force and result in damage to the deeper structures. The varieties of treatment for the actual sore are legion; each method has its advocates. Today skin grafting is used to hasten recovery.

Observations to Make when Dressing an Ulcer

A nurse is often the first person to see an ulcer and may be the only person dressing it regularly. She should be able to record her observations accurately, as these will assist diagnosis and treatment. First she should notice the *position of the ulcer*. Varicose ulcers frequently occur just above the medial malleolus. Gummatous ulcers are usually closer to the knee. Then she should notice the *skin surrounding the ulcer*: in varicose ulcers the skin is often pigmented; in pyogenic ulcers, inflamed; and in gummatous ulcers, normal. The *shape of the ulcer* is usually irregular in pyogenic infections and spherical in gummatous ulcers. Next she should note the *edge of the ulcer*. Malignant ulcers have a piled-up everted edge; gummatous, a straight clean-cut edge; and tuberculous ulcers, an undermined edge. Finally the *floor of the ulcer* should be observed—the nature of the granulation tissue and the presence or absence of slough and pus.

If an ulcer is healing, the edge will be flat, the walls sloping down to the crater will appear faintly blue due to the growth of fresh epithelium, and the granulation tissue on the floor, a healthy bright red colour.

If the ulcer is spreading, the surrounding skin is likely to be inflamed, the sides straight or undermined, and the floor covered with pus. When an ulcer is callous, neither healing nor spreading, the edges may be raised, the walls indefinite and the floor pale pink, indicating a poor blood supply. There is likely to be much induration, that is hard fibrous tissue, in the region.

AMPUTATION OF LEG

An amputation may be performed in the treatment of acute and chronic infections, injuries and tumours; many are due to vascular disease.

If time allows, careful psychological preparation of the patient should be undertaken, as this operation can be devastating to the patient, resulting in a completely changed life-style. Some patients, however, e.g. when severe ischaemic pain is present, welcome the removal of the limb.

Amputation may also be performed in the treatment of some cases of congenital deformities, but this is usually only when the patient requests it. The preparation for amputation is as for any other surgical operation. Present-day technique (myoplastic) is such that the cut muscles are sutured together over the distal end of cut bone, thus producing a stump with equal muscle balance, a muscular pad over the cut bone, an improved circulation and a cylindrical stump. In emergency a guillotine amputation may be performed when the limb is simply cut off. Skin traction is then applied to prevent retraction of the skin. Later, a further amputation may be performed to provide the patient with a stump more suitable for artificial limb wearing.

The amputation bed. A divided bed may be prepared to allow easy observation and access to the stump, but many surgeons state that this is not necessary and the bed should be made up in the usual way with the addition of a bed cradle to take the weight of the bed clothes off the operation site. All nurses should know how to arrest arterial haemorrhage, but the need to practise this skill is most unlikely.

Bed posture. The position of the stump is very important as flexion–abduction contractures must be prevented. Under no circumstances should a nurse place a pillow under the stump unless instructed to do so by the surgeon. It must be understood that any form of passive pressure applied to the hip flexor muscles of the amputated side will tend to make the patient resist this by flexing his hip, thus encouraging a flexion contracture. The stump should be left free in bed and repeated instructions given to the patient to keep his stump flat on the mattress; the nurse should explain why this is so important. To encourage correct bed posture fracture boards should be placed under the mattress of all amputees. This will also provide a firm base for the patient to move himself about the bed. It is helpful if the patient is nursed in the prone position for predetermined periods of time as this ensures extension of the hips and prevents a flexion deformity developing. For below-knee amputees a back splint may be used at night to prevent flexion deformities of the knee, but in some cases of very short below-knee stumps this may prove fruitless and it is far more important to maintain full hip extension.

Rehabilitation. The nurse is a vital member of the rehabilitation team. It is not suggested that the nurse should do the work of the physiotherapist, but she should understand some of the basic aims of exercise therapy, a knowledge gained only by forming a working relationship with the therapist working on the ward. The modern concept of rehabilitation for amputees is *early* rehabilitation and the patient will greatly benefit from the nurse who has some understanding of the following requirements:

1. Full active movement of the hip and knee joint of the amputated side.
2. Improvement of the muscle tone of the extensors of the hip and knee joints of the amputated side.
3. General active movements of the sound leg, arms and trunk.
4. Correct chair and bed posture.
5. Correct position of the stump during crutch walking.
6. Correct standing balance on the sound leg.
7. Correct stump bandaging.

The patient must be encouraged to become independent. In the early stages this involves much hard work and there will almost certainly be stump sores, setbacks and frustrations, but the skin gradually hardens and sympathetic interest, help and encouragement can do much to assist progress and hasten return to normal life and work.

The physiotherapist is, in the main, solely responsible for the programme of exercise and will arrange this in accordance with the views and wishes of the surgeon in charge.

Stump bandaging. Incorrect stump bandaging has been, and still is in many cases, the biggest cause of delayed rehabilitation. It is therefore necessary for the nurse to understand the particular technique of stump bandaging requested by the Limb Fitting Ser-

64 SURGICAL NURSING

vice. The stump is bandaged to condition it for limb wearing—*not to shape it*. The remedial aims are:

1. To prevent any terminal oedema.
2. To help encourage a healthy venous return.
3. To help tone up flabby tissue.

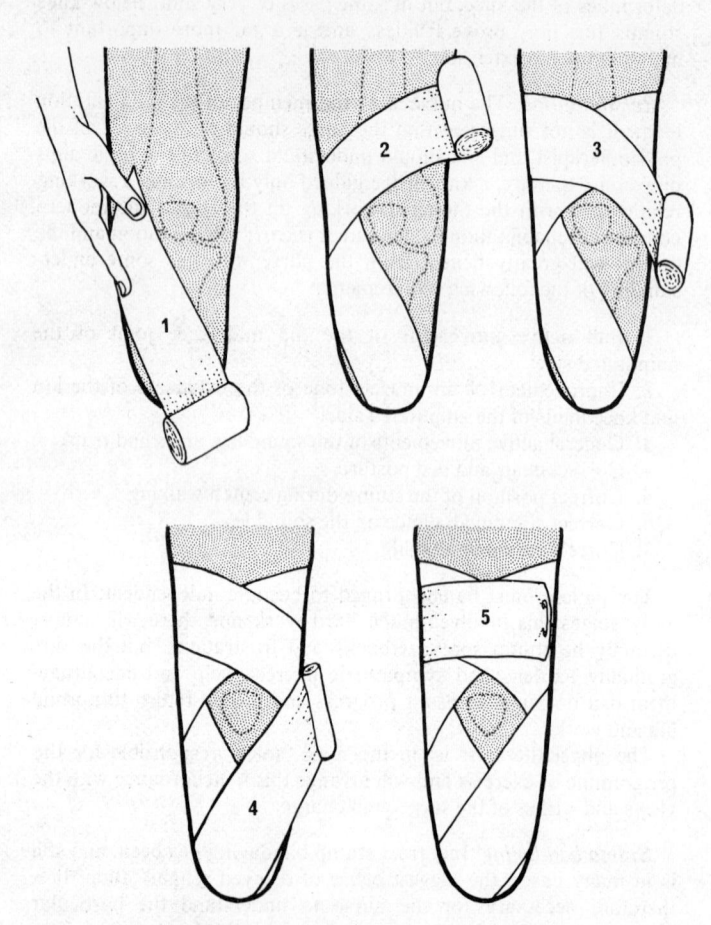

FIG. 6. Bandaging a below-knee stump. For full details see text.

4. To help prevent an adductor roll of flesh in the groin, which would cause great discomfort to the patient when wearing an artificial limb.

5. To accustom the stump to a constant covering.

Fig. 6 shows how the bandage should be applied to the below-knee stump. It is applied in figure-of-eight turns, with the fixing turns *above* the joint. The patella must not be covered as this will result in limitation of movement and the presence of fixing turns below the joint will result in a very badly formed stump, which will greatly hinder rehabilitation.

Commence just above the lateral tibial condyle, then bring the rayon and elastic bandage diagonally across the anterior aspect of the stump to the medial distal corner. Then bring it back across the stump posteriorly and swing across the beginning of the bandage. Anchor it with a circular turn above the patella. The bandage is then brought down around the medial tibial condyle and across the posterior aspect of the stump to the lateral distal corner. Figure-of-eight turns are then continued for the rest of the bandage, care being taken to cross the crest of the tibia in an angular manner. The final fixing turn is made above the patella.

The degree of pressure from the bandage that the patient can stand must be carefully observed, but it must be applied from the time of amputation.

Prostheses. The tendency today is to fit artificial limbs early. A light temporary pylon is usually supplied in the first instance to all amputees, followed by the first permanent limb when the patient is fully independent and safe—any time between the fourth and sixth week if the stump is ready. In many cases when the patient is wearing the pylon he will be weight-bearing on his ischial tuberosity. With a correct programme of rehabilitation, and a myoplastic amputation stump, many patients finally manage to wear a total-contact weight-bearing socket whereby the body weight is spread over the whole area of the stump.

4

Burns and Scalds

A burn is the destruction of tissue by dry heat, friction, electricity, radiation or corrosive fluid. A scald is the destruction of tissue by moist heat. The results, symptoms and treatment of the two conditions are similar and can be considered together. Mucous membrane is more tolerant of heat than skin and fluids which can be easily drunk would burn the skin if poured over it.

Prevention of Burns

About 14 000 people require hospital treatment every year as a result of burns and, of these, at least 600 die and many more are cared for at home. The majority occur in the home but it must be remembered that they also occur in industry and in road accidents. It has been estimated that 80% of all burns in the home could be prevented by an ordinary exercise of common sense. Those aged under three years experience mainly scalds; from three to fourteen years burns due to clothing catching fire; from 15 to 60 industrial and household burns; and 60 years and over heat injuries often due to blackouts, clothing catching fire and leaking hot-water bottles. In the United Kingdom it is a civil offence to leave a child under the age of 12 years alone in a house where any heating appliance is installed, e.g. a paraffin heater, but prosecutions are seldom undertaken.

Nurses, especially district nurses, health visitors and those working in antenatal and postnatal clinics, can do much to educate the public and so help to prevent many tragedies. Too many children's clothes are still made of inflammable material: flannelette is particularly dangerous if untreated. The statutory regulations about fire guards are not always sufficient where the old and young are concerned. Hanging tablecloths are a hazard to the toddler when a teapot is sitting on top of the table. Excellent pamphlets concerning the prevention of accidents in the home are published by the Department of Health and Social Security. A busy housewife does not always have time, or inclination, to read them, but a friendly nurse can see that she understands their contents.

Classification of Burns

A burn can be of any degree of severity from a mild erythema, such as one may acquire while sunbathing, to the charring of part of the body, as when, for example, a person during a fit falls with a limb in the fire and, being unconscious, does not move. For practical purposes burns are classified today as:

Superficial burns, involving only *partial skin loss*, which means that over the burnt area islands of epithelium are left, from which regeneration can take place.

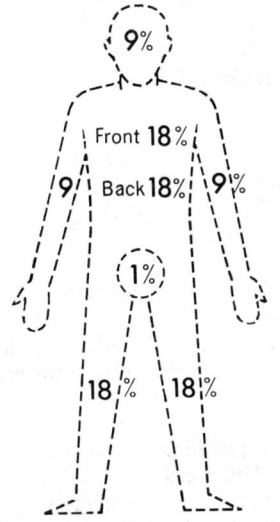

FIG. 7. Wallace's 'rule of nine' for the estimation of surface area, fluid replacement and urinary excretion. A useful guide is that the area covered by the patient's hand and closed fingers is 1% of his body surface.

Deep burns involving *total skin loss*, which may extend down to and involve bone. Deep burns will almost certainly require skin grafting to speed healing and prevent scarring.

Burns are further classified according to the area of skin loss, and a convenient method of doing so is Wallace's 'rule of nine' (Fig. 7). This division is helpful in assessing the area of skin loss, which is of value principally in determining the amount of intravenous fluid that should be given to a patient.

If a child has sustained a burn on more than 10% of his body surface or an adult has sustained a burn involving more than 20% of his body surface, then intravenous resuscitation must be carried out at once, plus all other forms of shock treatment. At this time treatment for shock is much more important than local treatment to the burnt tissue.

Usually a 50% full thickness (deep) burn is fatal, but this depends upon the patient's age and general condition; a fit teenager may survive when an ill, elderly patient would not.

If a nurse understands the *main complications* which arise as the result of a severe burn, she will be in a better position to understand the main principles of treatment.

Complications Arising from a Severe Burn

Mortality depends upon a variety of factors: the extent and depth of the burn, the health and age of the patient and the efficiency of early and long-term treatment.

Shock

If uncontrolled, shock results in death. This is first of all due to *pain*, i.e. *neurogenic shock*, because so many sensory nerve endings have been exposed, and is more marked in the very old and very young. This will rapidly merge into *oligaemic shock* due to the diminished volume of fluid in the vascular system caused by the continual seepage of fluid from the burnt surfaces. The permeability of the capillaries is increased greatly all over the body and not only in the burnt area. This causes much loss of plasma from the circulation. When haematocrit readings (Fig. 8) are taken it is found that the concentration of cells in the blood is much above the average 45%. These readings are taken at regular intervals as a guide to intravenous therapy. When the circulating blood has

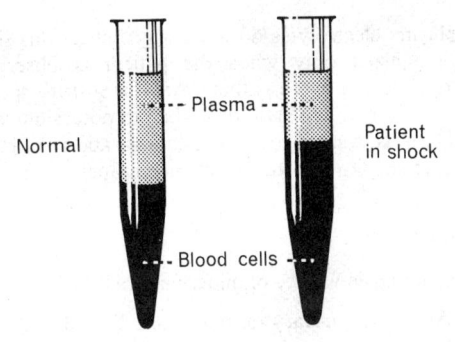

FIG. 8. Haematocrit findings. In a normal person the blood cells form about 45% of the blood volume (left-hand tube). In shock, fluid is lost from the circulation, resulting in a greater concentration of cells in the remaining plasma (right-hand tube).

been decreased by 15%, signs and symptoms of anoxia of the tissues develop. Some of the first tissues to be damaged are the kidneys and the production of urine is depressed or inhibited. Similar changes occur in heart, lungs, brain and liver.

Infection

Infection is a complication of all severe burns, and patients used often to die of septicaemia. A wide area of skin loss, one of the main body defences, leaves the tissues wide open to all forms of infection, including tetanus, and gas gangrene and continuing sepsis depresses the function of bone marrow and can cause various forms of *anaemia* as a late complication, and *amyloid disease* can result from chronic suppuration. In this condition waxy lardacious material is laid down in vital organs like liver, kidneys and intestine and interferes with their function.

Contractures

Contractures readily develop from the shrinking of scar tissue.

Electrolyte imbalance (the sick cell syndrome)

An electrolyte imbalance may develop owing to changes in the cellular membrane. Abnormality in the intracellular electrolytes occurs, potassium leaks out and sodium enters the cell. Measurements of plasma electrolytes do not always reflect this situation. It may be recognized only when the patient is observed to be confused, restless and overbreathing. A 24-hour urine specimen will show that the normal 2:1 ratio of sodium to potassium is reversed. This condition is treated by the administration of insulin and glucose, which help to restore the cell membranes to normal.

Renal failure

Renal failure has a variety of underlying causes.

Shock. An hourly urinary output of less than 35 ml is a serious sign. If this continues for more than two hours, a central venous pressure line will be introduced and the patient will be given intravenous fluids until the reading is increased to 15 cmH_2O. This in turn will increase the urine output if the low volume is due to oligaemia. If not, action will be taken to raise the blood pressure by means of drugs.

Uraemia. This condition may develop after the initial shock has been overcome and when the patient is producing several hundred millilitres of urine per 24 hours, with a specific gravity of 1010. The blood urea will be elevated and this, together with the presence of haemoglobin and casts in the urine, will confirm the diagnosis of uraemia. The patient will be given a high-calorie, low-protein diet and fluid will be restricted. If the burns are not too extensive, peritoneal dialysis will be performed.

Toxaemia. The causes of this condition are not fully understood, but it is present in all cases of severe burns. Chemicals released into the circulation from the site of the burn are particularly damaging to liver and kidney cells. Nephritis can develop and the urine becomes loaded with albumen and casts. Jaundice may occur and the patient may die of liver necrosis. It may also be the cause of severe duodenal ulceration and haematemesis, which sometimes occur as a later complication.

Treatment of Patients Suffering from Burns

At no stage must a nurse forget that the patient may be frightened, in pain, apprehensive of the future, afraid of losing his looks (men are every bit as vain as women) and afraid for his future employment. A nurse must never be so busy fetching and carrying that she

BURNS AND SCALDS

is unable to stop to comfort and reassure her patient. Many patients sustain psychological harm as a result of burns and so it is essential that the nurse encourages him to speak freely and if necessary to communicate any indications of this to the doctor. Fear aggravates shock and retards recovery. Morale is naturally low after a severe burn and energetic steps are required to rebuild it.

General Condition

In hospital the *general condition of the patient must be treated first of all*. The burnt area takes no priority and is not touched until the condition of shock is controlled by the following means.

Rest. The patient is reassured, if conscious, but handled and moved as little as possible.

Morphine and analgesics are given, frequently intravenously.

Intravenous fluids are administered without delay. Three-quarters of the volume of a patient's circulating plasma may be lost if there is delay. Blood and plasma or Dextran are the best fluids for intravenous infusion. Initially fluid is run in rapidly and the blood is alternated with bottles of Dextran. Blood pressure readings are recorded half-hourly. Haematocrit readings are repeated and usually an indwelling catheter is inserted for 48 hours so that urinary output can be easily and accurately measured. These readings enable the surgeon to control the amount and rate at which fluids are given.

Haemoconcentration indicates the amount of fluid required to restore the blood to normal. A 5% rise in haemoglobin means that the average adult will require 0·5 litre of intravenous fluid to restore the figure to the normal one of 15 g/dl. As the burnt patient is losing fluid so rapidly he will probably require more than this. Some surgeons give a bottle of blood early in treatment, despite haemoconcentration, as many red cells are known to have been destroyed. When neither blood nor plasma is available, Dextran may be used as a substitute and is often preferred. A specimen of blood for grouping should be taken before the Dextran is given.

Oxygen, given by polythene mask at 8 litres a minute, may help to relieve tissue anoxia, and reduces carbon dioxide retention. However, the cyanosis is mainly due to poor circulation and this is relieved by transfusion.

Building up calories

After the condition of shock has been controlled the next hazard is that the patient will not have enough building materials available in his circulation to repair the damaged area. Patients with severe burns will commonly vomit during the first 24 hours. After that it is important that they have a *high protein intake*. When they are able to eat, the nurse must take much trouble to see that they get plenty of the type of protein foods that they enjoy and can digest. Because many patients suffer from anorexia the surgeon may order a nasogastric polythene tube to be passed, through which a high calorie–protein feed, e.g. 1 litre Complan yielding 2000 calories, can be run in by drip at night. This will supply the patient's basic calorie requirements; he can then eat and drink whatever he can manage during the day. Unless active steps are taken to meet their calorie requirements, these patients rapidly become very emaciated and healing is delayed.

Local treatment of the burnt area

Initial cleansing. In minor burns cleansing may be done under morphine injections, but in more extensive burns, the patient should be taken to the theatre and given a general anaesthetic. The use of a general anaesthetic with a very badly shocked patient is dangerous, but recently an anaesthetic gas has been introduced which makes this procedure much safer. Clothing can now be removed and the surrounding skin carefully washed with a solution such as cetrimide 1% or a cetrimide/chlorhexidine solution (Savlon). All dead tissue and débris is removed, the blebs are pricked and the whole burnt surface gently irrigated with warm sterile saline. Eschars (dry sloughs) may have to be actually excised. Because of extensive inflammatory oedema, it is not always possible to tell at this stage whether there has been partial or total skin loss. A variety of methods is used in the local treatment of the burnt area, which indicates that the ideal treatment is yet to be found.

The aims of local treatment are always the same:

To control oedema. Pressure dressings are seldom very effective and the help of *gravity* must be enlisted. For example, a patient with burns of face, neck or chest should sit up once the initial state of shock has been controlled. A number of devices can be used to elevate a burnt arm or leg.

To avoid infection. Rigid asepsis at all stages is essential. In burns units the patients are treated in dressing rooms with air conditioning as in theatres. Antibiotics are used systemically and sometimes topically. Anti-gas-gangrene serum and antitetanus serum may be given. Skin grafting will not take on an infected surface.

To prevent contractures. As far as possible the necks, axillae and flexor surfaces of limbs are splinted in extension. A nurse will require ingenuity to keep the patient comfortable in awkward positions. Early skin grafting does much to prevent the development of contractures partly by cutting down the risk of infection.

Exposure treatment. This is probably the most popular treatment in use today. Antibiotic powders or sprays may, or may not, be used four-hourly during the first 24 hours and the burnt surface is exposed to the open air, or sometimes dried plasma is applied. An electric hair dryer may be used over the burnt surface to hasten the formation of a natural coagulum. Antibiotics are given systemically and skin grafting may be required later. The burnt area must be protected from injury by cradles and bed linen kept scrupulously clean by frequent changing since it will rapidly become contaminated by large amounts of serum exuding from the burnt area. The nurse must make every effort to prevent a crust from becoming cracked by movement and the formation of a circumferential crust must be reported at once, as this can impair circulation to and from the distal tissues. If the back or buttocks are burnt the patient should lie prone on a Wallace frame, but if the burn is circumferential then opposite sides can be exposed by the use of a special turning frame such as the 'Circ-o-lectric' frame. It is also possible to use a nursing aid which consists of a frame which has a nylon net stretched lightly over it. The net is covered with a layer of polyurethane foam (for comfort) and thus allows the involved area to be ventilated.

Ideally, in an attempt to prevent infection, the patient should be nursed at a temperature of 32°C as he will feel cold and in his own 'micro-climate', such as an isolation room or a linear air flow where he is surrounded by filtered air. The levitation bed is now being used where the air passes upwards and this supports the patient as well as providing a 'micro-climate'.

If the burns are superficial the crusts will separate in ten days to three weeks, leaving well-healed skin beneath. If the burns are deep, skin grafting may be required after the surgeon has removed the coagulum. Sepsis can occur beneath the coagulum and the nurse must observe the patient carefully for signs of septic toxaemia or local inflammation around the coagulum.

Treatment by this method really necessitates the patient being cared for in a special burns unit; improvisations in, say, the side ward of a general surgical ward are not really satisfactory. Unfortunately few surgical wards are sufficiently free of infection today.

Treatment by dressings. Dressings are used to provide a barrier to prevent bacteria alighting on the burn, to apply antibacterial substances to the area and to absorb exudate.

The dressing consists of *tulle gras* impregnated with an antiseptic, as this will not stick to the burn providing it is not allowed to dry out, covered with gamgee tissue and held in place by a firm pressure bandage, ideally a crêpe bandage. The whole dressing must be porous, otherwise tissues will become soggy and provide an ideal environment for the growth of bacteria. However, the dressing must be changed before the exudate soaks through it, as this will again encourage the entry of micro-organisms.

A variety of antibiotics may be used, such as neomycin, polymyxin, bacitracin, etc., but infection with *Pseudomonas* spp. is an ever-present danger and gentamicin is often used systemically or locally for this specific reason.

Initially the dressings are changed daily and later, after the discharge has subsided, every other day. After about 14 days the remaining loose or dead tissue is cut away; partial thickness burns should have healed by this time. Surgical excision of sloughs will be carried out after three weeks and this is usually necessary for full-thickness burns. In this case grafts may be applied at once, providing the raw surface looks healthy; otherwise dressings are continued until healthy granulation develops.

Skin grafting. Nowadays if the surgeon suspects that the burn involves the whole thickness of the skin, he will apply a closed dressing and graft a few days later if the patient's general condition permits. The graft will not take unless the area is clean; sometimes the surgeon will have to excise sloughs. In practice grafting is carried out either within the first 24 hours or after many days or perhaps even weeks. Swabs are taken from both donor and recipient areas before grafting. The sooner the operation is undertaken the less danger of sepsis and cross-infection. The graft will not take if the patient is anaemic or deficient in protein, therefore these matters are attended to prior to surgery. *Thiersch grafts* are commonly used if the burn is not too extensive. If extensive, 1 cm wide strip grafts will be used; also any spare graft can be stored and used later to repair an area where the graft has failed to take. *Whole thickness skin grafts* or *pedicle grafts* may be required for deep burns.

Where there is insufficient healthy skin to permit grafting, skin may be taken from a parent or relative, but this merely acts as a dressing and will be sloughed off in a matter of weeks. These grafts are termed autografts when taken from the patient's own body and homografts when taken from a relative's body.

Biological dressings, such as armour porcine (pig) skin, have proved to be very effective as a temporary dressing until human skin grafting can be carried out. It reduces fluid loss, protects vital exposed structures, reduces or prevents infection and reduces pain.

The porcine skin can be obtained perforated or plain and is first reconstituted in sterile saline for 30–45 minutes. Then the dermal surface is placed on the wound, adjusted to the body contours and left (if possible) uncovered until the wound starts to heal and the graft sloughs off.

Any bubbles must be gently expressed to the edge of the graft and if there is any suggestion of infection the porcine dressing is changed. These grafts are pre-sterilized by gamma radiation.

Nursing Care of Patients Suffering from Burns

The patient will require routine nursing care for a seriously ill patient. Much ingenuity will be required to keep the patient as comfortable as possible as such patients frequently have to be nursed in awkward positions. When an air-conditioned ward is not available the nurse must control ventilation and cleaning in order to provide a warm, dry, dust-free atmosphere. Boilable cotton blankets should be used and sunlight admitted when possible. Careful records must be kept, especially of fluid balance, blood pressure and temperature, as these will give indications of developing shock or sepsis.

Burns of the face require extra skilled nursing. They can produce severe psychological effects. If the eyelids have been burnt, there will be danger of corneal ulceration. When nose and mouth are involved, feeding may become a problem, but usually some form of

76 SURGICAL NURSING

tube feeding is possible and the mouth must be carefully cleaned. Occasionally a tracheostomy is required. Plastic surgery will be undertaken as early as possible.

Burns of the hands frequently heal well, but during healing the patient may not be able to use his hands at all and may find this almost intolerable. The nurse must use her imagination and anticipate his needs so that the patient does not always have to ask for what he wants.

Burns of the perineal area require special attention in order to keep the area clean. An indwelling catheter may be used or sterile normal saline irrigations, followed by careful drying, given after defaecation and micturition.

5

Tumours

A *tumour* (Latin: *tumor* = to swell) or *neoplasm* is a mass of new tissue which develops from the normal tissues of the body, but, unlike them, does not perform any useful function for the benefit of the body as a whole. It may develop in, and consist of, any type of tissue, e.g. muscle, fibrous or glandular tissue; it lives at the expense of the body tissues, obtaining nourishment from them, but doing nothing in return; it tends to increase in size, or at least to persist throughout life, although it may disappear spontaneously, e.g. simple papilloma of the skin (wart) or papilloma of the larynx. When growing very rapidly the tissue is liable to change in character, so that it no longer bears strict resemblance to the tissue from which it originates.

There are two main types of tumour:

1. Benign tumours (Latin: *bene* = well; *genus* = birth).
2. Malignant tumours (Latin: *malignare* = to act maliciously).

The *benign tumours* do not usually endanger life; they do not spread into the neighbouring tissues, nor by the blood stream and lymphatics, and do not give rise to secondary deposits. The *malignant tumours* always endanger life; they spread into the neighbouring tissues, by what is termed infiltration, and also spread by the blood vessels and lymphatics, giving rise to secondary deposits or metastases in many parts of the body.

Predisposing and Contributory Factors

The basic cause of tumour formation is not known, but research suggests certain factors which should be considered. Malignant

SURGICAL NURSING

disease is a universal form of illness, affecting all races, social classes, sexes, age groups and body systems.

Statistics show that different forms of malignancy are associated with race; carcinoma of the nasopharynx has a high incidence among the Chinese, but is comparatively rare among Europeans. Carcinoma of the bronchus is much more common in men than in women. So research is carried out to find the reason why.

It is appreciated that some malignant diseases have a specific association with the occupation of the patient or the environment in which he lives and works. There is a high incidence of rodent ulcers among fair-skinned sheep farmers in Australia, who spend a great deal of time in the bright sunlight, and tumours of the bladder are found among people whose work involves the use of aniline dyes. People who smoke heavily are ten times as likely to develop carcinomas of the lungs as non-smokers and the danger is clearly stated on cigarette packets and in advertisements.

Other theories, such as the 'virus' theory, are also supported by experiments and investigation. The virus has been seen in the malignant cells when examined under an electron microscope and, when injected into a mouse, the filtered extract of cancer cell from a human does cause a cancer to form.

Chronic irritation is also suspected, as there does appear to be a relationship between, for example, promiscuity and carcinoma of the cervix, and cancer and calculi are often found together in the same cavity.

BENIGN TUMOURS

Benign tumours may arise in any tissue of the body and are named according to the type of tissue of which they consist:

1. Papilloma, consisting of epithelium.
2. Myoma, consisting of muscle.
3. Osteoma, consisting of bone.
4. Fibroma, consisting of fibrous tissue.
5. Chondroma, consisting of cartilage.
6. Lipoma, consisting of fatty tissue.
7. Adenoma, consisting of gland tissue.
8. Neuroma, consisting of nerve tissue.

Two types of tissue may be present in one growth, e.g. fibromyomas consist of fibrous and muscular tissue, while adenomyomas consist of glandular tissue and muscle.

Characteristics of a Benign Tumour

1. It is enclosed in a capsule of fibrous tissue, built up by the surrounding tissues because of the irritation to which it gives rise; it can easily be shelled out completely from this capsule.

2. It does not tend to recur at the site since the whole growth can with certainty be removed, but fresh growths of similar type may arise subsequently in the same region, e.g. after removal of fibromyoma of uterus other fibromyomas may develop in it.

3. It does not infiltrate the surrounding tissues.

4. It does not spread by lymphatics and blood vessels.

5. It does not give rise to general symptoms as a rule, but as it increases in size (a) it may press on surrounding structures and obstruct them, e.g. adenoma of the thyroid may obstruct the trachea; (b) it may interfere with the normal functioning of an organ, e.g. fibromyomas of the uterus may affect menstruation, producing excessive loss; (c) it may become of enormous size and weight, disfiguring, exhausting and crippling the individual—this is seldom seen in developed countries today, because removal is generally undertaken in the early stages, but before Lord Lister made abdominal surgery safe, growths weighing 2 to 25 kg or more were not uncommon; (d) it may become malignant—certain types of growths are more liable to malignant changes than others, e.g. papillomas frequently become malignant but lipomas rarely.

Treatment

Benign tumours should be removed as a general rule, because they may become malignant or produce serious effects on the health of the individual.

MALIGNANT GROWTHS

Types of Malignant Growth

Malignant growths may arise in many parts of the body. They are divided into two varieties, according to the tissue in which they first occur:

1. Carcinoma.
2. Sarcoma.

SURGICAL NURSING

Carcinomas

Carcinomas are malignant growths arising in epithelial tissue. They are subdivided according to the type of epithelium.

1. *Squamous-celled* carcinomas develop in the squamous or pavement epithelium lining the mouth, oesophagus and vagina and in the outer skin. The term 'epithelioma' is applied to this variety.
2. *Columnar-celled* carcinomas develop in the columnar-celled epithelium lining the stomach, bowel and bronchial tubes.
3. *Cuboidal-celled* carcinomas develop in the cuboid epithelium of glands, e.g. in the breast.

The duct of the gland, being lined with a different type of epithelium, may give rise to a different variety of carcinoma.

Carcinoma spreads via the lymphatics to the lymphatic glands, and may thence be conveyed by the lymph stream into the circulation and affect any tissue of the body.

Carcinoma occurs chiefly after 50 years of age, but younger subjects are not immune. It occurs rarely between 20 and 30 years, and even more rarely cases have been recorded in patients under 20 years.

Sarcomas

Sarcomas are malignant growths arising in the connective tissue of the body, e.g. bone or cartilage. They are named according to the tissue of which they consist, for example, osteosarcoma occurs in bone and adenosarcoma occurs in gland tissue. Since these tissues are rich in blood vessels, the growth contains blood vessels and therefore spreads rapidly by the blood stream. As a result secondary growths in the lungs are the common result and lead to a fatal ending in a very short period of time.

Sarcoma, unlike carcinoma, is most common in younger persons between ten and twenty or under ten years of age; it may be seen in infants. It does also occur in old people, particularly where simple connective tissue tumours become malignant.

Malignant growths are termed:

1. *Scirrhous*, if hard, as when there is much fibrous tissue present.
2. *Encephaloid*, if soft, when there is much gland tissue present.

3. *Melanotic*, if they become pigmented and are black or dark brown in colour.

Characteristics of a Malignant Tumour

A malignant tumour has the following characteristics:

1. It is not enclosed in a complete capsule of fibrous tissue.
2. The number of cells undergoing mitosis within the tumour is greatly increased, so the tumour tends to grow much more rapidly than normal tissue.
3. The tumour spreads to other parts of the body. This can occur in the following ways:

a. Direct spread through the tissues. This is why extensive surgery is so often necessary.

b. Malignant cells can either be carried along in the flow of *lymph* or the tumour can actually grow along the inside of the lymphatic vessels.

c. The *blood* can also carry the malignant cells to other parts of the body and so metastases occur. This is commonly seen when the patient develops a secondary growth in the liver after cells have been carried in the portal circulation from one of the abdominal organs.

d. Accidental spread arises following excision of malignant tissue when cells have been liberated into the blood. This transplantation of cells can only take place into the patient's own body; the surgeon would not develop a neoplasm if he accidentally cut himself while operating on a patient.

e. Tumours can also spread by '*seeding*' down through a cavity or down along the endothelium. This is why patients with carcinoma of the kidney have a large part of the ureter excised, as it may also be involved.

Effect of Tumours

The effects of tumours are extremely variable, depending upon the area of the body involved.

1. *Obstruction* of a lumen may occur, either from within or from without. A tumour in the colon may cause an intestinal obstruction, and a tumour in the head of the pancreas will cause obstructive jaundice by pressing on the common bile duct.

2. *Irritation* of a serous membrane will cause increased production of serous fluid, so a pleural effusion or ascites may occur.

3. Tumours also *destroy tissue*. The lesions most commonly seen are ulceration, perforation, fistula formation and pathological fracture. The destruction often results in *haemorrhage*.

4. The blood vessels within the tumour may be abnormal, so *infection* may arise. This is because the body's normal inflammatory response cannot take place.

5. *Cachexia* is seen in most terminal patients. The cause is not really understood, but it is suspected that it is due to bacterial infection, interference with nutrition, loss of sleep, pain and recurrent haemorrhage.

6. *Anaemia* occurs in all cases and is due mainly to blood loss and malnutrition.

Malignant growths vary considerably in their malignancy, i.e. the rate at which they spread and threaten life. Sarcomas are highly malignant; rodent ulcers are comparatively benign, in that they merely spread into the neighbouring tissues but do not spread by the circulation and therefore do not cause secondary growths.

It should especially be noted that malignant growths do not give rise to pain in the early stages, though pain may occur later as a result of pressure on, or spread into, nerves. This fact often prevents the layman from seeking advice until it is too late. The nurse should advise every person complaining of suspicious symptoms to seek medical advice immediately, as the earlier the diagnosis is made and a definitive treatment started, the better will be the prognosis. Suspicious symptoms include:

1. A lump.
2. An ulcer, particularly one which is persistent and does not respond to simple treatment.
3. Bleeding from either an ulcer or a tumour.
4. Change in function of an organ, for example persistent constipation or diarrhoea, hoarseness or even blindness.
5. Persistent pain and tenderness.

Nurses should use their influence to persuade members of the general public to make use of any available facilities, such as cervical smears, so that in the event of an unsuspected case, an early diagnosis can be made, with a better chance of successful treatment.

Diagnosis of Malignant Tumours

Diagnosis may be made in two main ways:

1. Clinical diagnosis may be made by:
   a. The naked-eye appearance of the lesion.
   b. Palpation.
   c. Radiographic appearances.
   d. Examination of the blood or other body fluids.
   e. Positive radioactive isotope tracer tests.
2. Absolute diagnosis depends on histological or cytological examination of lesions.

Treatment of Malignant Tumours

Three basic methods are used in the treatment of malignant tumours:

1. Surgery.
2. Radiotherapy.
3. Drugs: either chemotherapeutic agents or hormones.

One basic method or any combination may be used.

Treatment may be curative or palliative. The choice of the most suitable and effective method of treatment for the malignant growth in an individual patient must be the subject of careful consultation between the various medical specialists.

Surgery

The aim of radical surgery is to remove the tumour completely and to leave no malignant cells behind. This often means removing the tumour and an area of apparently normal tissue surrounding it. Radical surgery should only be considered if:

1. The patient's condition allows.
2. The lesion is capable of being removed and not attached deeply or involving vital structures.
3. There is no evidence of widespread dissemination of malignant cells.
4. It will not cause considerable impairment.

The aim of surgery as a palliative measure is to relieve the patient of distressing symptoms, such as severe pain, offensive discharge, bleeding, ulceration or an unsightly mass. Extensive surgery to bring about remission of disease is less frequently performed as it can be so disappointing.

In some centres it is thought advisable to combine operative treatment and radiotherapy, sometimes using radiotherapy first so that there is less risk that the subsequent operation will release malignant cells into circulation, sometimes carrying out a local instead of radical excision of the part and then using radiotherapy both in the hope of preventing recurrence at the same site and to treat lymph glands draining the area.

Further information in regard to actual operations performed will be found elsewhere in relevant chapters.

Radiotherapy

This is the treatment of malignant tumours by ionizing radiation, which is effective as it kills sensitive malignant cells with limited damage to the surrounding healthy tissue. Radiosensitivity of tumours varies tremendously and is an important factor when method of treatment is being considered.

X-rays. These are produced from generators operated at varying electrical voltages. They may be superficial machines producing X-rays of low energy with voltage from 10 000 to 100 000 used for skin lesions as they will only penetrate tissue for a short distance. Then there are the deep X-ray machines producing energy with voltage from 200 000 to 300 000 (orthovoltage) used for less superficial lesions as the X-rays have a greater degree of penetration. These are now being replaced as X-ray machines called linear accelerators are becoming available. They produce energy with voltage of 4 to 8 million (supervoltage) which can treat very effectively deep-seated tumours with minimum damage to the surrounding healthy tissue. Dosage to which the patient is exposed is known as the roentgen (after the discoverer of X-rays). Dosage which is absorbed by the tissues is referred to as the rad. Dosage is very carefully calculated by the radiotherapist and physicist.

Gamma rays. These are produced during the breakdown or transformation of certain substances from an unstable to stable form. These substances may be in a natural state, e.g. radium, or artificially produced, e.g. cobalt. Substances which behave in this way—give out energy in the form of radiation—are known as radioactive isotopes. They are available in two forms: sealed and unsealed sources. Radium as a sealed source is used in the treatment of many malignant diseases.

1. It may be enclosed within small sealed containers, e.g. platinum, and inserted into thin hollow needles with a sharp point. These needles are then implanted directly into the lesion at selected points, e.g. for cancer of the tongue. Each needle has a silk or linen cord threaded through the eye by which it can easily be removed from the tissue for checking.

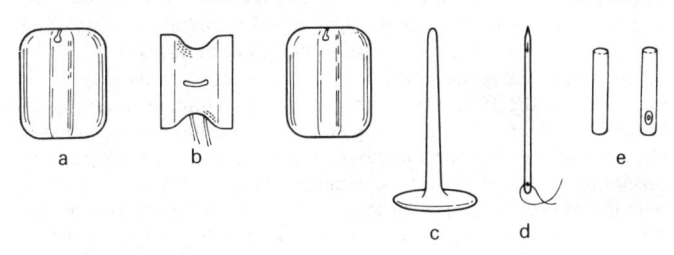

Fig. 9. Radium applicators for interstitial or intracavitary radiotherapy. (*a*) Vaginal ovoid. (*b*) Spacer. (*c*) Cervical tube. (*d*) Radium needle. (*e*) Radium tubes.

2. Radium needles and their containers may be fixed to moulds which can then be applied to the skin or elsewhere in the body, e.g. the palate, when the mould is structured like a denture.
3. Radium may be enclosed in containers and inserted into a body cavity, e.g. into the uterus and vagina for carcinoma of the cervix.
4. Radium can be applied in large amounts externally by means of a machine known as a radium bomb or teletherapy unit. These are no longer being used, having been replaced by machines which can accommodate more freely available radioactive isotopes, e.g. cobalt.

Whatever method is used it is vitally important for nurses to be aware of the hazards associated with the administration of radium and adhere strictly to instructions regarding dosage, duration of treatment, its removal and approved procedure as means of preventing contamination.

Radioactive isotopes. Artificially produced isotopes may be used for diagnosis as well as therapy for malignant and some non-malignant conditions. They include cobalt (as previously mentioned), iodine, phosphorus, gold, yttrium and many others. Some of these are absorbed normally by the body and are particularly useful in a radioactive form in treatment. They may be administered externally as sealed sources or internally as unsealed sources when stringent measures are taken to avoid contamination. Dosage is estimated in curies (named after the discoverers of radium) (1 curie (Ci); $1/1000 = 1$ mCr and $1/1\,000\,000 = 1$ μCi). The radioactivity of elements does not remain constant with time as atoms need to disintegrate to emit the radiations. The period during which half the atoms do this is known as the half-life of the element and is a constant for that isotope: that for radium is very long whereas others are radioactive for weeks, days or hours only.

Radioactive isotopes may be used in *diagnosis* as tracers to demonstrate the function of an organ, e.g. a minute quantity of radioactive iodine is taken orally so that the position of the gland is shown and reduced or increased activity can be determined by observing quantity of isotope retained. They can also be used to demonstrate the presence of lesions in the body by measuring the distribution of the administered isotope. Much research is being undertaken in furthering the use of this diagnostic technique.

It has already been noted that cobalt has replaced radium in needles and teletherapy units as a very *effective treatment* for malignant conditions. Others include phosphorus, which is taken up by the bone marrow and used in polycythaemia vera, thrombocythaemia and leukaemia. Gold can be used by injection either into a cavity, e.g. pleural effusion, or into the actual tumour, e.g. mouth lesions. Yttrium is used for pituitary ablation in advanced breast cancer.

Radiotherapy continues to develop in the light of research undertakings and nurses should be constantly on the alert to keep updated, thus giving the best possible service in this very important specialty.

Drugs

Drug treatment is usually only palliative.

Chemotherapeutic agents. One or more of these drugs may be administered systemically for advanced malignant disease with metastases as well as the leukaemias, Hodgkin's disease and other reticuloses. Long-term remissions have occurred, though results have been disappointing for advanced malignant conditions. Some of the cytotoxic drugs which can be used include methotrexate, cyclophosphamide and vinblastine. Cytotoxic drugs have a depressing effect on cells of the bone marrow with serious side effects, so very careful observations must be made of the blood count throughout the course of the treatment. Chemotherapeutic agents can also be given locally, either via a catheter inserted into the supplying artery or directly into a serous cavity, e.g. pleural effusion. This produces a high concentration of the drug to the part which would not be possible if given systemically.

Hormones. It seems that certain malignant tumours require certain hormones in their environment, i.e. are hormone-dependent; measures taken to alter the hormonal environment seem to have an adverse effect both on the tumour and on its metastases. Oestrogen suppresses the activity of prostate cancers, likewise testosterone is used for cancer of the breast with some response.

OTHER TUMOURS

Teratomas

These tumours have a different origin from the common tumour. They may be benign or malignant, and at one time it was believed that they represented an abnormal fetus, but this is not now accepted. They are found in the ovaries, testis, retroperitoneal tissue and at the base of the skull. On examination the benign type is usually cystic, with some solid areas which often contain tissue that can be recognized as teeth, hair or bone, and the malignant type is usually solid.

Teratomas should be treated by removal but this is not always possible.

NURSING CARE IN RADIOTHERAPY

In fulfilling her role effectively the nurse must not only meet the general basic nursing needs, but the very special needs of these patients with malignant conditions receiving radiotherapy.

Whatever the source of the radiation, treatment generally means repeated exposure over a period of six or more weeks, which is trying for the patient. Further, there is some general reaction after the treatments and these result in the patient feeling ill, weak and depressed, with possible nausea and vomiting. The effects are just as severe as a major operation, and the depression is likely to be much greater because of the more protracted and less dramatic nature of the treatment combined with the fact that the patient may realize his prognosis is not good. The nurse can therefore help the patient considerably by sympathetic encouragement and by ensuring that he mixes with other patients who have been successfully treated and whose symptoms are subsiding. She should see that he has suitable occupation and reading matter to help to pass the time and do everything that she can to ensure that his confidence is built up, so that he persists with the treatment until the specialist is satisfied that the maximum benefit has been obtained.

There is also always risk of unpleasant local reactions, which vary from a reddening of the skin to ulceration if there is overdosage. To prevent overdosage with teleradium, the radiation is directed through different areas of surface tissue at each application, the areas being generally outlined with a skin-marking pencil. Those marks must not be washed off. The reaction does not appear at once and the degree of reaction and time interval vary according to the idiosyncrasy of the individual patient. To lessen the local reaction, irradiated areas of skin must not be washed and should be treated with protective applications according to the instructions of the specialist carrying out the treatment. When the skin becomes red the application of starch powder or Johnson's baby powder is comforting to the patient and if no further skin reaction takes place this is all that will be necessary. The patient should be warned not to allow surgical plaster or Sellotape to touch the area, not to apply heat or expose it to the sun and not to let tight clothes rub the area. If the patient complains of burning pain and there is redness in addition to the dry desquamation, which is always present, the doctor will order calamine cream or lotion as a general rule. If in spite of this treatment moist desquamation follows, the doctor may suspend radiotherapy treatment for a few days and order the application of an oily preparation such as Serpasil cream. If the area should become infected an antibiotic cream will be prescribed. Ointments should be applied on the smooth side of white lint or on smooth old linen. Ulceration following radium treatment heals very slowly and is always avoided if possible, but some skins are very sensitive and give trouble. Skin grafting may be used to hasten the healing after treatment has been discontinued.

These patients should have a high-protein, high-calorie diet, with full vitamin content. They may need tempting to eat. A good fluid intake with glucose added to fruit drinks will help to lessen nausea and vomiting. Drinks like Lucozade are palatable and may tempt the patient to take more fluid.

There is no specific remedy for radiation sickness but certain drugs alleviate the condition, for example, pyridoxine hydrochloride, vitamin B6, 90–120 mg, given daily by mouth. Radium sickness resembles sea-sickness and drugs which prevent and relieve sea-sickness may, therefore, help, e.g. dimenhydrinate (Dramamine), 100 mg, three times a day. Where achlorhydria is present dilute hydrochloric acid, 0·6–1 ml, taken in water with meals may help. Dexamphetamine sulphate (Dexedrine), 5–10 mg twice daily, may be given early in the day to counteract the feeling of fatigue that the patient experiences in the early stage of the treatment. This should never be given after midday or it may produce insomnia. The patient also needs rest.

The symptoms of nausea, vomiting and lassitude usually subside once the treatment is completed. Leucopenia may also occur as the result of radiotherapy. This is especially serious when the fall in the white blood count is sudden. This fall may not occur until several weeks after the completion of treatment. Therefore the white blood count must be assessed regularly.

Precautions when Radioactive Substances are in Use

Nurses who are caring for patients who are receiving treatment by ionizing radiation must be familiar with the section of the code of practice which effects her work and well being. She must also read the local rules of her own hospital authority and sign a statement that she understands them.

The *Code of Practice for the Protection of Persons against Ionizing Radiations arising from Medical and Dental Use* was prepared by a panel of the Radioactive Substances Advisory Committee; the local rules of the hospital authority are based on the code and are created to ensure the health and safety of all hospital staff. The Advisory Committee have also produced a *Handbook for Nurses* which gives advice as to how they can make this form of nursing as safe to themselves as any other specialty.

When caring for patients receiving treatment from radioactive substances, the nurse must be very careful to guard against displacement of any surface applicator or loss of the substance and to protect as far as possible everyone who has dealings with the patient from radiation. To this end:

90 SURGICAL NURSING

1. The patient is kept in bed all the time that, say, radium applicators are in use; he is also encouraged to lie as still as possible to prevent minor displacements.

2. No bed linen or dressings from this patient are removed from the ward until the treatment is completed and the radium accounted for; if this is impracticable they must first be checked with a Geiger counter.

3. Radium must be removed from the patient punctually at the time ordered; it is touched only with long-handled forceps, transferred immediately into a special lead-walled container and taken at once to be locked in the radium safe.

4. Radium is signed for when passing from the custody of one person to that of another, in much the same way as registered postal packets.

5. Where several patients in a ward are being treated with a radioactive substance applied to, or inserted into, the body, they should never be nursed in adjacent beds and their beds usually carry some distinctive mark, e.g. the black on yellow radiation symbol, to warn staff not to loiter unnecessarily in close proximity to the source of radiation.

6. Staff caring for these patients wear film badges (Fig. 10) or some other suitable instrument which are developed weekly, and

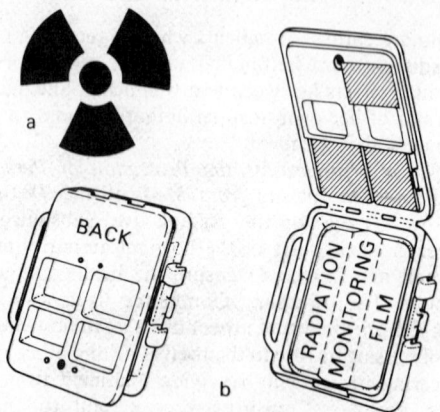

FIG. 10. Protection against radiation. (*a*) A black-on-yellow symbol used to indicate the presence of ionizing radiation. (*b*) A dosimeter badge worn by members of staff 'at risk'. The box contains film which, when developed, will indicate the amount of radiation to which the wearer has been exposed.

themselves have, e.g. monthly, both red and white blood-cell counts, so that if they are being exposed to dangerous amounts of radiation the fact can be detected and dealt with before serious harm is done.

Precautions when Radioactive Isotopes are in Use

1. The nurse must wear protective gloves and apron when attending to the patient. These do not protect her from radiation but from contamination by radioactive substances.

2. All urine passed must be collected in a special container for a number of days which will be stated on a special form by the physicist in charge of the patient. The period will depend on the radioactive life of the isotope being administered.

3. Other secretions and excretions, such as faeces or ascitic fluid, must be similarly treated.

4. After the prescribed period, during which the radioactivity falls, the excreta is normally disposed of in the usual manner and the containers washed and rinsed thoroughly.

5. Care is taken to ensure that treatment is not given when there is vomiting or incontinence liable to cause contamination of linen, etc., with a radioactive material. If accidental contamination does occur through spilling or leakage of, for example, ascitic fluid, the physicist must be informed at once and his advice sought. Contaminated bedding is bundled and put as far away from patients and staff as possible, e.g. on a balcony in winter, if there is room. It is the responsibility of the physicist to remove the contaminated articles and to monitor the area and reduce radio-activity by having it washed down, if necessary.

6. A marked bedpan and urinal must be kept for each of these patients.

When patients receive radioactive isotopes as an aid to diagnosis, nurses may note that these precautions are omitted; this is often because the dose of the isotope is so small that no appreciable radiations can be emitted from the patient or his excreta.

6

Preparation of the Patient for Operation

The Nursing Process

The nursing process is simply a means of planning individualized care for the patient in order to help meet his total psychological, physical and social needs, in both the long and short term.

On admission the routine procedure concerning identification and documentation is carried out, then the nurse will talk to and observe the patient in order to *identify his personal needs and problems*. These can be such things as intense embarrassment due to the close proximity of strangers in beds or a slight hearing defect that could interfere with communication, together with physical problems, i.e. discomfort due to incontinence or lack of mobility due to such things as osteoarthritis or rheumatoid arthritis.

Once the nurse has assessed the patient's needs she must consider what can be done about them and what the team's ultimate aim should be: in other words the *goals of care should be identified*. Identification of the goals is naturally followed by the production of *a plan of care*, this being produced in such a way that it is realistic and that all the staff, both during the day and at night, can follow it.

The method of recording and communicating this information varies a great deal as the basic philosophy is still being introduced into Europe and many of the original American and Canadian concepts are still being discussed. It is essential that these records are short, accurate, easily updated and available to all authorized personnel. This is essential if *continuity of care* is to be guaranteed. After a period of time the actual care given and its plan must be *evaluated to measure its effectiveness*, both from the aspect of good individualized care and to measure the reliability of communications. In this way all members will follow the patient care plan based upon the patient's own needs, not just the routine procedure carried out in different surgical conditions.

In many hospitals the nursing process extends into the operating theatres, the nurses visiting the patients prior to surgery, partially to introduce themselves and also to take the opportunity to identify and discuss any needs that are relevant to the operating and recovery rooms. These needs can be such things as hip lesions that prevent a patient being placed in a lithotomy position or prominent pelvic bones that demand the presence of a thicker than normal protection on the operating theatre table. If the theatre nurse is not aware of these problems she would not be prepared for the reception and care of the patient. Following discharge of the patient to the care of the community health team, the plan should be communicated to them, so that the pattern of successful care may be continued. The opposite should also occur (if appropriate), the community health nurse informing the hospital of needs that she has recognized together with the plan of care that she has found successful.

PREPARATION OF THE PATIENT

The patient should be admitted to hospital at least two days before operation, as this will allow all necessary documentation and information to be correlated. Further investigations can be carried out and the patient prepared both physically and psychologically for surgery. It also allows hardworking people to obtain some much-needed rest, which is often important for those living in a modern society, such as a married woman who works and still has to care for the home and family or single parent.

It is easy for the nurse in constant contact with operations to underestimate the effect of fear, and it is of the utmost importance that in manner, word and action she does everything possible to send the patient to the theatre in a confident and hopeful frame of mind. Research has been carried out in various centres into such things as postoperative pain and the elimination of fear: all nurses should read and take notice of these research findings. It is unlikely that the patient will sleep well on the first night in such strange surroundings, and it is very desirable that the patient should have a good night before his operation. However, the nurse should not suggest this to the patient as this could prevent him from sleeping and pre-operative rest is essential, especially as the patient may be disturbed during the postoperative night when the nurse is carrying out the necessary observations and treatment.

The surgeon will have explained to the patient the treatment he is going to carry out, but the patient may be afraid to ask questions, or fail to understand, and ask questions of the nurse. She should do everything she can to ease his mind by simple, accurate explanations, if she feels able to do so, making sure that she says nothing that will increase his anxiety. If she cannot relieve his worry herself, she should report it to sister or the surgeon. It is the surgeon's responsibility to make sure that the patient understands what will happen during surgery and he must witness the patient's signature on the consent form and then countersign it. This will be part of the preoperative 'check-list' which the nurse must make sure has been signed. If the patient is unable to sign the form the surgeon is responsible for the necessary signature: in certain circumstances, such as prior to a hysterectomy, the husband, wife, parent or guardian will also have to give written permission.

General Preparation

The general condition of the patient should be observed and should be improved as far as possible before operation. A light nourishing diet should be given, with extra feeds of milk if the patient appears undernourished, provided he can digest them. When a patient has had previous out-patient department appointments, any dietary problems will have been recognized and remedial 'therapy' will have been commenced prior to admission to hospital, but this must still be given careful consideration.

If required special intravenous preparations such as amino acids may be prescribed.

Both the urine and the blood chemistry should be checked to ensure that the water and electrolyte balance are normal at the time of operation. Sugar should be given in the form of barley sugar or glucose drinks to ensure a large sugar reserve in the liver, so that acidosis does not occur after the anaesthetic. If the patient is anaemic, blood transfusion will be employed in place of saline to correct this and transfusion must be given at least 24 hours prior to surgery because transfused cells have a reduced oxygen-carrying power and there is a risk of kidney damage if incompatibility is present between the donor blood and the recipient. For all but minor operations the blood should be grouped and cross-matched, in case transfusion is required during or after operation.

On the day of operation light solid food (if the preoperative preparation allows it) may be given up to five hours before operation so that the patient's blood sugar is not too low; fluids may be given up to three hours before operation if the anaesthetist permits. Great care must be taken with young or confused patients as they may obtain fluids or food for themselves. In certain conditions such as diabetes mellitus the doctor will prescribe the appropriate therapy. It is essential that the stomach should be empty at the time of operation, since the patient may vomit under the anaesthetic when the cough reflex is absent, resulting either in asphyxiation or in aspiration pneumonia from the sucking of organic material into the lungs; however, the use of the cuffed endotracheal tube reduces this risk.

The bowels should be well regulated, but violent purging must be avoided, as the consequent dehydration and electrolyte disturbance will greatly increase the shock of the operation. An empty bowel is most important in abdominal operations, but constipation must always be corrected beforehand, if necessary. In every case evacuation of the bowel is important to increase the comfort of the patient, as many factors during and after operation tend to cause constipation, for example, limited exercise and alterations in diet. Aperients such as bisacodyl (Dulcolax) or Normax should be carefully administered, so that the patient is not disturbed at night; quick-acting drugs should be given in the morning or early afternoon and slow-acting ones at night. The surgeon should be consulted with regard to his wishes about the aperient to be given; if the patient is in the habit of taking a particular aperient, it is common today to give a full dose of that particular one, or senna, cascara or vegetable laxative pills. In addition, or as an alternative when the bowels have been well regulated previously, a soap-and-water enema or disposable enema such as Fletcher's phosphate enema or Veripaque may be ordered the day before operation or the patient may be given suppositories, e.g. glycerine, Normax or one or two bisacodyl (Dulcolax). The latter is also available for oral administration. In selected cases rectal wash-outs may be ordered, especially when bowel surgery is to be performed. Careful bowel care is important for all patients since, when a patient is hospitalized, even if he has previously had regular and well controlled bowel actions, constipation tends to develop due to changes in diet, exercise and habits.

The patient should have a daily bath or a shower. The latter may be necessary if a patient finds a bath hard to manage, e.g. an elderly, physically handicapped or socially deprived patient. Breathing exercises should be taught by the physiotherapist as soon as possible and practised regularly and frequently, as should leg and other movements. The patient should also be encouraged to stop, or at least diminish, his smoking. Indeed, this is best discussed before admission so that the patient has had the opportunity to stop or reduce the habit while still in his normal environment. Hospitalization causes stress and is not the easiest time to give up smoking. Temperature, pulse and respiration should be recorded as ordered by the doctor and will depend on the patient's condition. The patient should be observed carefully for any signs of cold or cough, or other symptoms of disease. A specimen of urine should be obtained and tested for the presence of albumen, sugar and acetone. In this way unsuspected kidney disease and diabetes will be detected. In these conditions special care with regard to anaesthetics is required and in diabetes preliminary treatment is necessary to prevent coma; in addition, the sugar-laden state of the tissues will be favourable to infection. To ensure a good night's sleep before the operation the surgeon may order a sedative to be given if the patient appears to be worried or does not sleep well for any reason. This should be given with a hot drink and the patient should be carefully protected, as far as possible, from anything that may disturb his sleep, especially from unnecessary noise due to thoughtlessness on the nurse's part, resulting from her movement and talking in the ward and its annexes during the night, and from lights. The patient must be weighed, so that the anaesthetist can calculate the amount of anaesthetic drugs required.

Local Preparation

The skin at the site of the operation must be cleansed by bathing according to the wishes of the surgeon, with minute attention to detail. Some surgeons like an antiseptic preparation, such as Betadine, Savlon or Sterezac, added to the bath water. The site and an extensive area of the surrounding skin must be thoroughly cleansed and shaved of fine as well as coarse hair. Hair grows everywhere except the palms of hands, soles of feet and terminal phalanges, but shaving is usually omitted in the case of children and in the case of women when the face is to be the site of operation. If the patient is accidentally cut during shaving, the danger of infection is increased and the surgeon should be told before operation. Special attention must be paid to the umbilicus and the nails and hair, where dirt and germs are liable to collect. After this cleansing the patient puts on clean pyjamas or gown and is assisted into a bed made up with clean linen. *This is generally all the surgeon requires to be done in the ward.* Until fairly recently shaving was followed by further treatment carried out with aseptic precautions. This treatment consisted of cleaning the skin with methylated spirit or methylated ether, painting with an antiseptic, often coloured and in a spirit base, and covering with sterile towels. For orthopaedic operations this was repeated three times a day for two days preoperatively. Apart from being time-consuming for the nurse and uncomfortable for the patient this treatment is now thought by many surgeons to do more harm than good since the drastic degreasing removes the natural secretions which are claimed to have a bacteriostatic effect.

Immediate Preparation

A cotton operation gown, open down the back for easy removal, is usual and in some cases the patient also wears long operation stockings to prevent heat loss from the legs. However, this is rarely practised now as the patient is better protected by other means, e.g. the temperature of the environment. Duvets on the trolleys or the use of 'tinfoil' to wrap round the patient if there is a risk are particularly effective methods for use when the patient has to be wheeled along cold corridors or outside in the open air. All make-up must be removed so that the anaesthetist and nurses can judge the condition of the patient by the colour of the lips and cheeks. Hair should be covered by a paper cap, which may take the form of a triangular bandage; no pins or clips should be left in the hair because of the risk of injury. If the operation is such that the hair may become blood-stained, a waterproof cap may be put on to protect it. False teeth should be removed before the patient leaves the ward, likewise contact lenses if worn, and jewellery which may be damaged or lost or cause damage to the patient should be carefully locked away. A wedding ring should be covered by a strip of non-conductive strapping round the finger over the ring. It should be ensured that the patient is wearing some form of identity bracelet. Ideally a second bracelet should also be attached to the ankle prior to surgery because sometimes the anaesthetist removes the wrist bracelet when administering the anaesthetic drugs. The patient should be reassured in every way by the nurse during the final period of preparation.

Immediately before the patient leaves for the theatre, or before the administration of basal narcotics where these are ordered, the bladder should be emptied; if the bladder is full it may be emptied reflexly when the patient loses consciousness, or, much more serious, in abdominal cases it may be punctured accidentally and the peritoneal cavity contaminated with urine, which is extremely irritating and liable to result in peritonitis. Catheterization may be ordered, but because of the serious risks of infection, even when great care is taken, this procedure is not carried out today as a routine measure, but only if considered really essential for an individual patient. The nurse who has been responsible for the preparation and has gained the patient's confidence should go with him to the theatre and stay with him till he has lost consciousness. In some hospitals an escort nurse who is a member of the theatre staff will visit the patient the day before surgery, then will accompany the patient to and from theatre.

Preoperative Medication

Drugs are often ordered before the giving of anaesthetics, and must be administered accurately and punctually by the nurse.

Basal narcotics. These drugs depress the nervous system and therefore lessen the amount of anaesthetic required. All anaesthetics are toxic substances, so that the less the patient has the better. Nitrous oxide, or 'gas', is the least harmful and with oxygen and carbon dioxide is widely used today, but alone it does not produce sufficiently deep anaesthesia for abdominal surgery. Ether may be given in addition, but it is irritating to the air passages and unpleasant to take, so that it has been replaced to a large extent by thiopentone and muscle relaxants such as suxamethonium chloride or gallamine triethiodide.

Narcotic drugs which send the patient to sleep or make him very drowsy before he leaves the ward are usually given and are invaluable in lessening the fears of the patient, and so diminishing shock. The drugs employed include:

Omnopon 20 mg and scopolamine 0·4 mg by hypodermic injection

PREPARATION FOR OPERATION 99

Diazepam (Valium) 10 mg by mouth
Morphine 10 mg by hypodermic injection

The premedication dose is calculated by estimating the patient's body surface area from his height and weight. The resulting figure determines the dosage.

These drugs are given 30–60 minutes before the time of operation, as ordered: the actual time of giving must be written on the anaesthetic paper which goes to the theatre with the patient, so that the anaesthetist knows exactly the condition of the patient and can proceed with assurance in his work.

It should be remembered that if a patient is in a state of shock drugs given by hypodermic injection may not be absorbed, in which case premedication may have to be given intramuscularly, or intravenously by the doctor.

The patient will then become drowsy and may sleep. He should be kept under observation as he may try to get out of bed to obtain a drink. He may lose consciousness or have an idiosyncrasy for the drug and the depressing effect is so great that the respirations become dangerously slow.

Drugs to counteract the harmful effect of the anaesthetic. Though originally used, and considered to be of special value, when ether was the main anaesthetizing agent, atropine is still used, almost invariably, prior to the administration of any general anaesthetic (see sections on premedication). The patient must be warned that the mouth will become very dry and that fluids are not permitted to relieve this. The nurse must also realize that blurred vision, tachycardia and ataxia will also result.

Drugs to lessen the risk of infection. These are sometimes prescribed, a broad-spectrum antibiotic such as tetracycline usually being used so that the blood already contains the drug at the time of operation. Gentamicin may be ordered if the patient has a long-standing infection that has not responded to treatment. If gentamicin is used a specimen of blood is examined daily, the dose prescribed being adjusted according to its level in the blood. An average dose is 40 mg: this care is necessary as gentamicin is toxic. These drugs in no way lessen the need for the strictest aseptic precautions and some surgeons believe they are necessary only when infection is already present.

Hypotensive drugs. Drugs which lower the blood pressure may be ordered, either (*a*) for local effect to lessen bleeding at the site of operation, especially where the tissues are particularly vascular, e.g.

in brain operations, or (*b*) for general effect to help, to induce anaesthesia and hypothermia or artificial hibernation especially for operations on the heart and blood vessels. These drugs include chlorpromazine (10–25 mg) and promethazine hydrochloride (25–75 mg).

7

Anaesthesia

The nurse's most important function when working with the anaesthetist is to assist with the total management of the patient. Reassurance of the patient may be necessary, especially with children. Facts should not be over-emphasized, truth is essential and care must be taken to avoid possible psychological harm. In paediatrics, anaesthesia can be induced by means of a game: a child can be asked to take a deep breath in and blow up the balloon (which is part of the anaesthetic circuit). In many cases the face mask can be replaced by a cupped hand held near the face while a story is related.

Anaesthesia means loss of sensation and is usually synonymous with unconsciousness. In relation to surgery, anaesthesia permits operations to be performed. It can be divided into two main groups: local and general anaesthetics.

LOCAL ANAESTHETICS

These may be used in several ways.

Topical Anaesthetics

Topical application results in the blocking of sensory nerve endings. Cocaine is the best drug for this purpose. It can be applied to mucous membrane in the eyes, nose and throat to facilitate surgery. Some patients are sensitive to cocaine and collapse could occur. Cocaine must never be injected. It is more likely to cause addiction than any other local anaesthetic drug.

Local Infiltration

Local infiltration blocks the sensory nerves at the site of operation. Drugs such as procaine hydrochloride (Novocaine) 0·5–2% or lignocaine (xylocaine) are widely used for minor surgery.

Regional Anaesthesia

Regional anaesthesia or nerve blocking is produced by injecting a local anaesthetic around the sensory nerves that supply the operation site. The injection is made at some distance from the site of the operation. It is, therefore, a particularly useful procedure when there is local sepsis where it would be undesirable to infiltrate the affected tissues. Epidural blocks are commonly used for leg surgery and brachial plexus blocks for arm surgery.

Adrenaline is usually combined with local anaesthetics to constrict the blood vessels and reduce absorption of local anaesthetic into the general circulation. The local effect is enhanced and possible general toxic effects are reduced.

Complications of regional anaesthesia are tachycardia, vasomotor attacks and fits. If fits occur:

1. Maintain a clear airway.
2. Administer oxygen.
3. Administer anticonvulsant drugs, e.g. diazepam (Valium), phenytoin (Epanutin).

Spinal Anaesthesia

Spinal anaesthesia is a special form of nerve blocking whereby a suitable local anaesthetic solution is introduced into the subarachnoid space. Epidural anaesthesia is similar but the needle is introduced into the space between the dura and arachnoid mater (not into the subarachnoid space). Two types of solution are used:

1. Heavy solutions such as cinchocaine in 6% dextrose (Nupercaine); this solution is heavier than cerebrospinal fluid. The actions of such solutions are affected by patient posture and the anaesthetist can utilize position for the desired effect.
2. Light solutions have the same gravity as cerebrospinal fluid; the patient may be placed in the Trendelenburg

position after it has been introduced. Nupercaine (previously known as Percaine) is lighter than cerebrospinal fluid in weak solutions, and the patient's buttocks should be raised for at least five minutes after this injection.

With recent advances in general anaesthesia, spinal anaesthesia is being used less frequently. It is still used in developing countries where fewer doctors specialize in anaesthesia and the surgeon is responsible for both anaesthesia and surgery. In this situation low spinal anaesthesia may be used for operations on the urethra, perineum and anal canal; a light general anaesthetic may be administered at the same time.

There are two main advantages of spinal anaesthesia:

1. Muscle relaxation can be obtained to enable the surgeon to have access through the abdominal muscles.

2. It can be useful when there are respiratory complications, e.g. chronic bronchitis and emphysema.

Complications

Complications of spinal anaesthesia are:

Headache. About a third of the patients who have had spinal anaesthesia develop postoperative headache. This is difficult to treat, but the patient should lie flat and be given analgesics and intravenous fluids.

Nausea and vomiting. This is relieved by the same method as postoperative vomiting.

Backache. This can be minimized by seeing that the back is well supported.

Fainting. This may occur if the blood pressure remains low and the patient is allowed to sit up.

Infection and meningitis. To reduce this risk the anaesthetist wears a sterile gown and gloves and uses the no-touch technique.

Permanent paralysis of lower limbs. This tragic complication may occur and has resulted from sterilizing the outer surface of the ampoule in a solution of phenol. Traces of phenol seep through minute and invisible cracks or flaws in the glass into the anaesthetic solution. This method of sterilization must *never* be used. Ampoules are now sterilized by ethylene oxide. Since there is a temporary paralysis whilst a block is effective, the limbs must be supported and care must be taken not to overstretch joints. Following return to the ward the patient must be given nursing care as if he is a paraplegic until the effect of the drug has worn off.

Permanent paralysis of anal and urethral sphincters. This requires similar treatment to that for a paraplegic patient.

Respiratory paralysis. This is treated by the administration of oxygen and artificial ventilation and is possibly due to the drug reaching the medulla oblongata.

Burns. These can result from carelessly placed hot-water bottles while the lower limbs are anaesthetized and paralysed.

GENERAL ANAESTHETICS

General anaesthetics act by depressing the central nervous system. They do so in a progressive manner, affecting the cerebral cortex first and the medulla oblongata last; overdoses can result in death due to depression of the vital centres.

Stages of Anaesthesia

Most anaesthetists differentiate four stages of anaesthesia. However, stages one and two are passed through very rapidly due to the use of modern intravenous induction agents.

1. The first stage of analgesia lasts until the patient is unconscious.
2. The second stage lasts from the onset of unconsciousness until automatic breathing begins. At this stage the patient sometimes holds his breath or struggles.
3. The third stage lasts from the onset of automatic breathing until the respiratory centre is paralysed.
4. The fourth stage is the short interval between cessation of breathing and death.

The term induction is applied to the first two stages and the operation begins at a suitable plane of anaesthesia in the third stage.

Administration of General Anaesthesia

General anaesthesia may be administered by different routes:

1. By inhalation.
2. By intravenous injection.
3. Per rectum.
4. By intramuscular injection.

Inhalation anaesthetics

Inhalation anaesthetics can be divided into two groups:

1. Vapours of volatile liquids.
2. Gases.

Vapours. Ether, introduced in 1846 by Morton in America is a good safe anaesthetic. It has, however, the disadvantage of being inflammable and an irritant to the mucous membrane lining of the air passages and air sacs in the lungs with possible increase of post-operative pulmonary complications. A similar irritable effect on the gastric mucosa causes excess vomiting. A premedication of atropine sulphate 0·6 mg can reduce the over-secretion of respiratory mucus which result from the irritation.

Chloroform, introduced in 1847 by Simpson of Edinburgh into the United Kingdom, was widely used in midwifery. It is non-inflammatory and non-irritating to the respiratory tract and has a pleasant odour. It is effective as an analgesic, but unpredictable as an anaesthetic as it may damage the patient's liver or heart. The liver may be protected by generous intakes of glucose before anaesthesia.

Trichlorethylene (Trilene) is chemically related to chloroform but is distinguished by its blue colour. It is non-inflammable, safer than chloroform and is a useful analgesic in maternity work. It is a less potent anaesthetic than chloroform.

There are two *methods of administration:*

1. The open method is when the patient is allowed to breathe naturally through a cloth soaked in a volatile anaesthetic drug. The vapour will be carried into the lungs with inspired air. A Schimmellbusch mask is used for this and the anaesthetic agent is dropped onto the mask. This method is seldom seen in modern hospitals today; however, it has many advantages as it requires no

expensive apparatus and the patient's oxygen requirement is supplied from the air. It remains the ideal method where equipment and supplies are short.

2. The closed method is achieved by bubbling oxygen or a mixture of gases through a bottle containing a volatile liquid using a modern anaesthetic machine. The closed-circuit machine contains a canister of soda lime which allows expired carbon dioxide to be absorbed and the same gases are used again. Soda lime cannot be used if Trilene is the anaesthetic agent of choice as dangerous chemicals are produced which are very toxic to the patient.

Gases. The gases chiefly used for anaesthesia are nitrous oxide and cyclopropane. They are supplied in cylinders.

Nitrous oxide or 'laughing gas' was first used by Sir Humphrey Davy. It is a weak anaesthetic, non-irritant and relatively non-toxic, while both induction and recovery are rapid. This gas must be used with oxygen, as if used alone it will produce asphyxia.

Although *cyclopropane* is a very powerful anaesthetic, it is inflammable and explosive. It is non-irritant to the lungs, but can cause cardiac irregularity. It has the great advantage of producing muscular relaxation, but this is now achieved by other means.

The earliest machines for administration of gases consisted essentially of cylinders of nitrous oxide and oxygen, a mixing apparatus and a rubber tube to convey the gaseous mixture to a face mask. The complex modern machines are an elaboration of this simple type.

Endotracheal intubation is required. The tube is introduced via the nose or mouth through the glottis into the trachea. This tube is connected to the delivery tube from the anaesthetic machine so that gases are introduced directly into the respiratory system. A cuffed tube is usually used so that the anaesthetist can take complete control of the patient's ventilation. This is desirable in many surgical operations.

Intravenous anaesthetics

Thiopentone sodium (Pentothal) is the principal anaesthetic agent used to induce anaesthesia. It is one of the barbitone group and it is important that the anaesthetist ascertains if the patient has any known allergy to these drugs. It is supplied as a powder in a sealed glass ampoule and is mixed with an ampoule of sterile distilled water immediately before use. Precautions must be taken to avoid mistakes in mixing: any unused drug must be discarded.

Intravenous thiopentone has a rapid action and takes the patient to the third stage of anaesthesia in a matter of seconds. The unconsciousness it produces is of short duration, accounting for its prime use as an induction agent. Anaesthesia is then maintained by inhalation or other agents.

Thiopentone sodium has several disadvantages:

1. It is a respiratory and circulatory depressant and must be used with caution.

2. In the body, thiopentone has to be metabolized and broken down in the liver before excretion by the kidneys. Patients with liver complaints may be unable to break it down.

3. Thiopentone sodium tends to have a cumulative action, especially in the presence of other barbiturates. It is therefore unsafe to allow out-patients who have been given intravenous thiopentone sodium to return home unescorted.

Rectal anaesthetics

The dosage for rectal induction depends on body weight so accurate weighing of the patient is essential. The drugs are administered either in liquid form or as capsules which are punctured to allow readier absorption.

Intramuscular general anaesthetics

The only drug used in this field is ketamine (Ketalar). Ketamine is a drug which can induce and maintain anaesthesia. It can be given intravenously or intramuscularly. It can be used especially in circumstances outside the operating theatre, e.g. road traffic accidents. It has a major disadvantage in that it can cause emergence delirium in the non-premedicated patient, so that the patient *must* be allowed to wake up on his own and *not* be woken by the nurse.

MUSCLE RELAXANTS

These drugs are not anaesthetics and have no effect on consciousness or sensation. They produce the perfect muscular relaxation necessary for operations, thus enabling the surgeon to operate in ideal conditions. The main danger is that the respiratory muscles are affected, so artificial ventilation is used to prevent hypoxia developing. The paralysis is reversed with neostigmine, which is always given with atropine to prevent side effects. These include salivation, bronchial constriction, colic and a drop in the pulse rate.

The relaxants commonly used today are tubocurarine and pancuronium bromide (Pavulon) which are long-acting, lasting 30 to 40 minutes; gallamine (Flaxedil), lasting about 20 minutes; and suxamethonium (Scoline) lasting about two to three minutes. The last named short-acting drug is unaffected by neostigmine and has no antidote.

PREMEDICATION

The administration of any anaesthetic is usually facilitated by suitable premedication. The drugs used to prevent excessive secretions are atropine and hyoscine (scopolamine) which also have a sedative action. Drugs used for their sedative effect, to allay anxiety and to reduce restlessness, are the morphine group, barbiturates and tranquillizers, such as chlorpromazine (Largactil). Pethidine is also used as an analgesic in conjunction with the anaesthetic thiopentone.

More modern drugs have been introduced to act as premedication agents. These include diazepam (Valium) and lorazepam (Ativan). They have attained considerable popularity as they not only sedate the patients but also cause retrograde amnesia, so patients have no recall of the events taking place in the anaesthetic room.

Modern anaesthesia uses a combination of drugs with maximum safety to produce the best conditions for surgery. Intravenous thiopentone is usually used for induction. The patient is kept asleep by agents such as nitrous oxide in combination with sufficient oxygen. Muscle relaxants are given if complete relaxation is required. This will naturally involve respiratory paralysis so the anaesthetist will be responsible for artificial ventilation using a cuffed endotracheal tube and usually a ventilator. Drugs to deepen anaesthesia, such as halothane (Fluothane), methoxyflurane (Penthrane) or trichloroethylene (Trilene), may be added to the nitrous oxide and oxygen mixture. Intravenous analgesics, e.g. morphine and pethidine, are used and therefore sensory impulses are blocked. Seldom are fewer than four drugs used, making the administration of anaesthetics very complex.

HYPOTENSION

Hypotension is induced for some operations to reduce haemorrhage and thus allow a better surgical operating field. The principal indications for the use of hypotension are:

1. Neurosurgery, especially for highly vascular tumours.
2. Vascular surgery.
3. Plastic surgery. However, there is also a danger of leaving vessels untied, leading to bruising.
4. Fenestration operations, when blood oozing from the flap creates difficulties.
5. For operations where there is liable to be severe haemorrhage, e.g. external ethmoidectomy.
6. For patients with rare blood groups where transfusion would be impossible or where there is an inadequate supply of blood of a suitable group.

Methods of Producing Hypotension

The principal methods of producing hypotension are as follows:

Deep general anaesthesia. It has long been known that the nature of the anaesthetic influences the amount of bleeding. Ether and cyclopropane increase capillary oozing while deep anaesthesia using halothane reduces blood loss.

Posture. Normally the effect of gravity upon blood flow is controlled by the cardiovascular reflexes. These are reduced and then abolished by deepening anaesthesia. If, therefore, the patient is first anaesthetized and then correctly positioned the blood pressure will fall.

High spinal anaesthesia. This blocks the autonomic nerves in the subarachnoid space in the thoracic and upper lumbar region. This leads to the dilatation of the peripheral blood vessels and a consequent fall in blood pressure.

Hypotensive drugs. Methonium compounds are amongst the most satisfactory. These block the transmission of impulses across ganglia of the sympathetic nervous system and so produce vascular dilatation with a fall in blood pressure. These are dangerous drugs and can cause many complications. If the blood pressure falls too

110 SURGICAL NURSING

low the kidneys cannot function. To counteract these effects, vasopressor drugs, e.g. methedrine and noradrenaline, are held in readiness as antidotes. Trimetaphan (Arfonad) has a similar action and is short-acting, being metabolized in about 30 seconds. It is given by intravenous drip and is therefore easily controlled.

Dangers of Hypotension

The main dangers of induced hypotension are:

1. Cerebral and coronary thrombosis.
2. Permanent cerebral damage.
3. Primary cardiac failure.
4. Renal and hepatic ischaemia.
5. Reactionary haemorrhage.
6. Paralytic ileus.

Conditions which therefore contraindicate its use are:

1. Cerebrovascular disease, in certain cases.
2. Diseases affecting respiratory function.
3. Extremes of blood pressure, high or low.

HYPOTHERMIA AND ARTIFICIAL HIBERNATION

This is an extension of the method of tissue freezing which has been known for ages. The object is to lower the body temperature so that cellular metabolism is slowed down and oxygen requirements are reduced. Enzyme activity is also depressed. This makes possible certain operations on the brain and heart, such as repair of cerebral aneurysms and repair of septal defects. This treatment is also used in severe head injuries where the blood supply to the brain has been affected. It also helps to control reactionary cerebral oedema.

The maintenance of normal body temperature depends on the heat produced by metabolism and vasoconstriction of the peripheral vessels, when the body surface is exposed to the cold. Increasing muscle tone with shivering begins if further heat production is required. In hypothermia the patient is anaesthetized and drugs are given to inhibit normal temperature regulation. Those most commonly used are chlorpromazine 50 mg, pethidine 100 mg and promethazine (Phenergan) 50 mg given in divided doses. The doses may be varied considerably.

Methods of Cooling

Various methods are used to produce the required drop in temperature.

The surface of the body may be cooled. Cold sheets and icepacks may be used, but these tend to be messy. A cold bath may be used, although this involves moving the patient. A special coverlet may be used, constructed on the same principle as an electric blanket, only instead of electric wires it contains tubes through which iced water may be pumped. The advantage of this method is that, if necessary, warmed water can quickly be substituted for iced water.

The blood itself can be cooled. This may be done by drawing it off from, for example, the femoral artery, cooling it and returning it to the saphenous vein. Many anaesthetists regard this as too drastic.

Degree of Cooling

The temperature should not be taken below 28°C as the heart cannot withstand the effects of cooling as well as other tissues and ventricular fibrillation is likely to occur. Frequent temperature readings are taken from electronic thermometers in the oesophagus and rectum. The temperature must not be allowed to drop too rapidly and surface cooling must be stopped when the temperature is 30°C as a further drop of 1–2°C will occur. Nowadays it is realized that fairly rapid reheating is not harmful to the patient. When the temperature is raised to 32°C the patient will start shivering and warm up quite quickly. He should be wrapped in warm blankets, but hot-water bottles should be avoided as the skin, when cold, is extremely sensitive and burns could easily occur.

DANGERS OF ANAESTHETICS AND POST-ANAESTHETIC COMPLICATIONS

Respiratory obstruction. If the tongue falls back or vomit is sucked into the airway during unconsciousness, respiratory obstruction will occur. This is the greatest danger and is present in every case until the patient recovers consciousness. It should never cause death if the patient is well prepared and kept under

112 *SURGICAL NURSING*

observation until fully conscious. The greatest danger is after operations on the mouth, nose and throat, e.g. tonsillectomy, when there is bleeding. The condition should be prevented by keeping the patient well on to the side, in the Sims's semi-prone position if

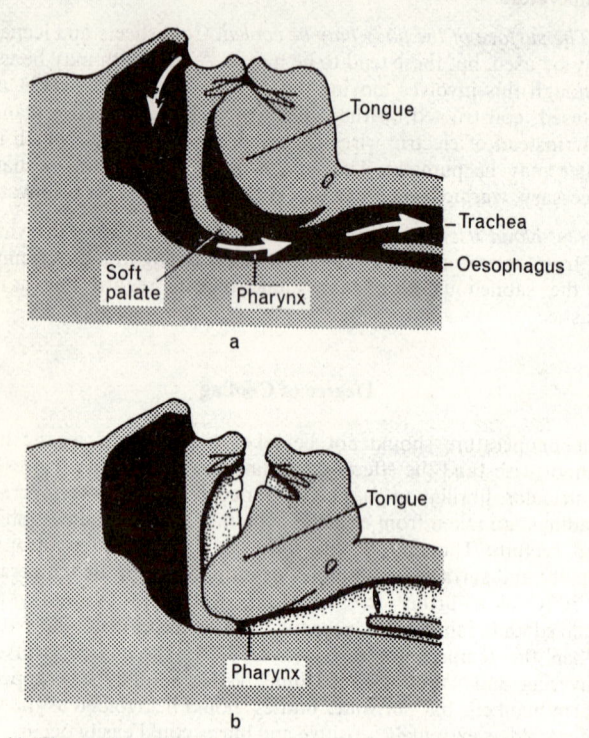

FIG. 11. The position of the tongue when the patient is lying on his back. (*a*) In a conscious patient the muscle tone maintains the position of the tongue, leaving a clear airway. (*b*) In the unconscious patient the tongue falls backward and occludes the airway.

possible. This keeps the tongue out of the pharynx, but if it drops back in spite of this, pressure in a forward direction exerted by the nurse's fingers behind the angle of the jaw will keep it forward. This lifts forward the tongue which is attached to the floor of the mouth. If by mischance fluid, e.g. blood or vomit, does get into the air passages and the patient goes black in the face, the nurse should send at once for medical aid and meantime raise the foot of the bed as high as possible to drain fluid back towards the nose and mouth by gravity. These can then be swabbed clear. Electric suction, if available, will help to clear the airway quickly. The nurse must see that no pillow ever obstructs the airway.

The patient must be fully monitored postoperatively by qualified staff as this significantly reduces the immediate postoperative mortality rate. The vital signs such as pulse, blood pressure, respiratory rate and colour are routine postoperative measurements and observations which are carried out and recorded. The administration of oxygen through various masks in the immediate postoperative period is mandatory. During this period there is a strong possibility, due to various influences, that the patient can become slightly hypoxic (the arterial oxygen content can become lower than normal). Routine oxygen therapy can prevent this condition developing. In some cases oxygen therapy should continue for some hours postoperatively and occasionally until the following day.

Aspiration bronchopneumonia. This is due to sucking of septic material like blood and vomit into the air passages. Asphyxia may be avoided, but pneumonia may develop later from blockage and infection of some smaller bronchial tubes. This can be prevented by careful pre- and postoperative nursing care and by use of electric suction to prevent harmful material ever getting into the air tubes; use of a cuffed endotracheal tube also prevents the aspiration of harmful material.

Cessation of respiration. If this occurs from overdosage of a depressant drug it is treated by using the antidote.

Pulmonary collapse. Collapse due to shallow breathing prevents expansion of the bases of the lungs, especially after high abdominal surgery when deep breathing is painful. Pulmonary collapse can be due to the inability of the patient to cough and sticky plugs of mucus can block small bronchial tubes and the patient may develop pneumonia.

Cardiac arrest. If this occurs oxygen is given and the airway must be maintained. Cardiac massage is commenced to maintain the circulation. The medical staff will intubate the patient and attach some form of artificial ventilation. Sodium bicarbonate is given by an intravenous infusion and an electrocardiogram is used to detect whether the heart stopped in systole or if ventricular fibrillations are present. Adrenaline is given if the heart stopped in systole and a defibrillator is applied if the ventricles are fibrillating.

Nerve damage. Lack of sufficient attention to the patient's position may result in nerve damage. Under anaesthesia the muscles are flaccid and all protective reflexes have disappeared; it is important, therefore, to see that the patient's limbs are in a good position and not subjected to stress and strain. For example, the ulnar nerve can be damaged on the edge of the operating table if the elbow is allowed to slip over the edge, or the brachial plexus can be damaged when the Trendelenburg position is used without adequately padded shoulder support, and these injuries can produce subsequent paralysis.

Emergency Resuscitation

The anaesthetic trolley must contain mouth gags, props and wedges, airways (of which there are many types), tongue forceps, bowl and cloth, stimulant tray with nikethamide, adrenaline and methedine, neostigmine and nalorphine (antidote to morphine and thiopentone) in addition to anaesthetic apparatus, according to the wishes of the anaesthetist. If these are ready for immediate use, the anaesthetist can deal promptly with emergencies as they arise. Oxygen and suitable apparatus for its administration must always be available.

8

Postoperative Care

ROUTINE POINTS IN AFTER-CARE

It is customary today for the patient to stay under the anaesthetist's personal supervision in a recovery room, which is part of the operating theatre department and is staffed by specially trained nurses. Otherwise the patient is returned to the ward where he should be quickly and carefully lifted into bed and covered with clean bedclothes.

The nurse should observe the pulse, blood pressure, temperature and respiration rate of the patient and keep a careful watch on the pulse in case shock or a reactionary haemorrhage occurs. The surgeon may request that a pulse chart be kept and also a chart of the blood pressure, at intervals according to the individual case. As well as these observations being made, the outer dressings and the bed clothing beneath the wound should be inspected at intervals to see whether there is any leakage of blood or serum.

The correct position for the patient in bed is described on p. 112.

Intravenous therapy

Intravenous therapy may be used following surgery to prevent dehydration occurring and to ensure that a normal electrolyte balance is maintained. Care must be taken not to over-infuse the patient; the doctor usually prescribes the type of fluid and the amount to be given over 24 hours. The nurse, however, is responsible for controlling the flow of fluid at the correct rate. This can be calculated by using the following formula:

$$(\text{Volume} \div \text{hours}) \div 4 = \text{drops per minute}$$

As an example, if 2000 ml are to be infused in 24 hours, the volume per hour is 2000 ÷ 24 = 83·3. Divided by 4 once again, this gives a rate of 21 drops per minute. The following table gives an easy reference to the number of drops per minute.

Amount (ml)	\multicolumn{12}{c}{Time (hours)}											
	1	2	3	4	5	6	7	8	9	10	11	12
100	25	12	8	6	5	4	4	3	—	—	—	—
200	50	25	18	12	10	8	7	6	5	5	4	4
300	75	37	25	19	15	13	11	9	8	8	7	6
400	100	50	33	24	20	17	14	13	11	10	9	8
500	125	62	42	31	25	21	18	16	14	12	11	10
600	150	75	50	37	30	25	21	19	17	15	14	12
700	175	87	58	43	35	29	25	22	19	18	16	15
800	200	100	66	50	40	33	28	25	22	20	18	17
900	225	112	75	56	45	37	32	28	25	22	20	19
1000	250	125	83	62	50	41	36	31	28	25	23	21

Body temperature

Care should be taken to maintain the patient's normal body heat, unless hypothermia has been employed or a lowered body temperature is desired to reduce oxygen requirements; overheating must be carefully avoided to prevent loss of body fluid by sweating. After hypothermia the patient is commonly, today, rewarmed before leaving the theatre or one sheet may cover the patient until he complains of cold, when one blanket at a time is added as required.

Pulse and blood pressure

The pulse and blood pressure must be carefully observed for signs of haemorrhage at suitable intervals according to the nature of the operation that has been performed. The pulse will normally be checked and recorded half-hourly at first and then at lengthening periods. Quarter-hourly observations are only made if there is a marked risk of haemorrhage, e.g. following a liver biopsy.

Mobilization

As soon as the patient's condition permits he is allowed to sit or lie in the position that is most comfortable, the nurse encouraging active exercise and early mobilization. Prolonged immobility increases the risk of certain postoperative complications such as deep venous thrombosis and joint stiffness in the elderly. Research indicates that some patients think that early mobilization is for the convenience of the nursing staff, so it is very important that the reason for this is discussed carefully with the patient so that he may cooperate fully in his own care.

Vomiting

Post-anaesthetic vomiting seldom occurs today. If it does, it should be treated by sips of water and the deep breathing exercises. If this fails, the anti-emetic drugs are usually successful, e.g. metoclopramide (Maxolon) 10 mg, chlorpromazine (Largactil) 10–25 mg or prochlorperazine (Stemetil) 5 mg. If vomiting continues, a nasogastric tube will be passed and the stomach contents aspirated continuously or intermittently. The nurse should remember that post-anaesthetic vomiting may be caused by the patient's reaction to morphine.

Flatulence

Flatulence is liable to follow abdominal operations, but is less common now movement and early ambulation are encouraged. It is extremely painful if severe and should be treated by strong peppermint water, 30 ml in hot water. External application of heat to the abdomen also gives relief, if it is practicable. Passing a flatus tube into the rectum may also help.

Pain

Pain is often considerable during the first 12–24 hours and should be relieved by the use of drugs as ordered by the surgeon. In the major operation morphine 10 mg or Omnopon 20 mg is generally considered desirable to ensure a good night after the operation. It also lessens the restlessness of the patient and the subsequent strain on sutures and ligatures. It is not good nursing to withhold it in these circumstances, since the patient's pain is temporary and the need for the drug will not recur. In certain cases there may be special reason for withholding morphine on account of its paralysing effect on the bowel. Pethidine may be ordered as an alternative (50–100 mg). Research is being carried out into the use of a pethidine gun, the patient administering his own intravenous dose to relieve pain. It is not possible for the patient to give an excess dose.

Diet

Except in gastric and intestinal operations, fluids may be given by mouth as soon as the patient recovers from the anaesthetic, and post-anaesthetic vomiting has been relieved. A very light diet, consisting of broths, baked custard, thin bread and butter, tea, etc., is given until the bowels have been opened. After the bowels have been opened the patient should by gradual steps return to a normal diet as quickly as possible.

Bowels

Hospitalization alone causes alteration in the patient's bowel habits so if a patient is discharged home early, e.g. on the second postoperative day, to the care of the community nurse, it is most likely that a bowel action will not have taken place and she will be so informed. In other cases if analgesia has been required at repeated intervals then glycerine suppositories will be administered on the third day as constipation is likely to develop.

Diet is not usually withheld until a bowel action takes place unless specifically ordered. Defaecation can be encouraged by allowing the patient to adopt a normal posture either by using a commode or by being taken to the toilet in a wheelchair.

Urinary retention

Retention of urine may occur after operation; therefore the nurse must keep a measurement of urine passed for 48 hours, especially in patients who have had abdominal operations. Should retention occur, it may be treated by one or more of the following:

1. Putting the patients into the most natural position possible in the circumstances. Men are particularly helped by being allowed to stand out of bed when this is permitted.
2. Applying warmth over the lower abdomen.
3. Giving hot drinks, e.g. hot sweet lemon or tea.
4. Bathing down the external parts with hot water.
5. Turning on the neighbouring taps so that the patient hears the sound of running water.

6. A simple enema in suitable cases.
7. The doctor may have to prescribe carbachol 1 ml by injection in selected cases.

In some cases, especially in gynaecological repair operations, hysterectomy or haemorrhoidectomy, there may be injury to the nerves controlling the bladder, so that retention cannot be relieved by these measures and catheterization is necessary. An indwelling catheter is used in these cases, controlled by a spigot, or continuous bladder drainage may be used.

A catheter should only be passed as a last resort, except when the patient is very ill and too weak to make the necessary effort.

Breathing exercises

Deep breathing is painful after abdominal operations, so that the patient tends not to use the lower lobes of the lungs; this may cause atelectasis (collapse of part of a lung) which is a complication most commonly seen if the patient is a heavy smoker. This collapse results from blocking of the bronchial tube supplying the part by a plug of mucus. To avoid these complications, the patient should be given deep breathing exercises by the physiotherapist (especially to breathe out fully) before the operation and should be encouraged to carry them out after it. The physiotherapist will visit the patient daily, but the nurse should encourage the patient to perform them at frequent intervals between her visits. In extreme cases, when the respiratory centre is depressed, the artificial ventilator, usually the positive pressure respirator, e.g. the Radcliffe or Bird apparatus, with tracheostomy, may be used to maintain satisfactory respiration for 12–24 hours.

Wound care

The risk of cross-infection is reduced if the wound dressing is not disturbed. If there is a wound drain which is allowing the escape of pus, blood and serum into the dressing, this must be changed as often as is necessary.

Trials are being conducted into the use of a special adhesive plastic film which is stuck over the wound and surrounding skin after operation instead of an orthodox dressing. This allows exchange of gases but not fluids so that cross-infection is prevented. This 'cover' is not removed until the wound is healed.

Ambulation

Most surgeons allow the patient to get up as early as possible, as this improves the circulation, lessening the risk of thrombosis. If the patient's condition is satisfactory he will be gradually assisted out of bed into a chair on the day following operation while his bed is being made. He may then be returned to bed, and assisted out again in the afternoon. The next day he will stay out of bed a little longer

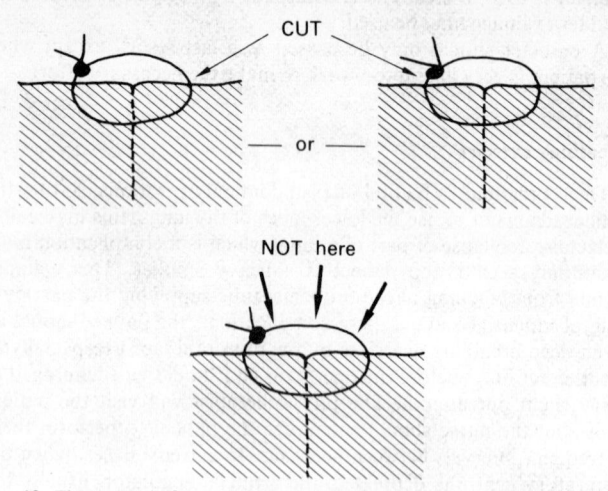

Fig. 12. The removal of sutures. Note that the thread or nylon should be cut close to the point where it enters or emerges from the skin, so that the least possible amount of thread which has lain on the skin has to be pulled through the subcutaneous tissue.

and walk a few steps. The degree of ambulation will then increase so that the patient will soon be walking round the ward; if necessary he will have his drainage bags attached to his dressing gown. It is important not to overtire the patient. Even when the patient is confined to bed (for example, a patient with heart disease) he is taught to exercise his muscles during this time, so that they are not too weak when he comes to use them again. The nurse should know what exercises he should be doing and encourage him to carry them out frequently. For the patient confined to bed for serious chest and heart conditions, reins tied to the foot of the bed help the patient to move during the postoperative days.

Removal of stitches

The stitches are removed when the wound has healed, usually between the seventh and tenth days. Clips are removed a little earlier and tension sutures two days after the skin sutures have been removed. Stitches may be taken out earlier on the face where the blood supply is very good and a minimum of scar tissue is desirable (third to fifth day). In some cases the surgeon inserts dissolvable

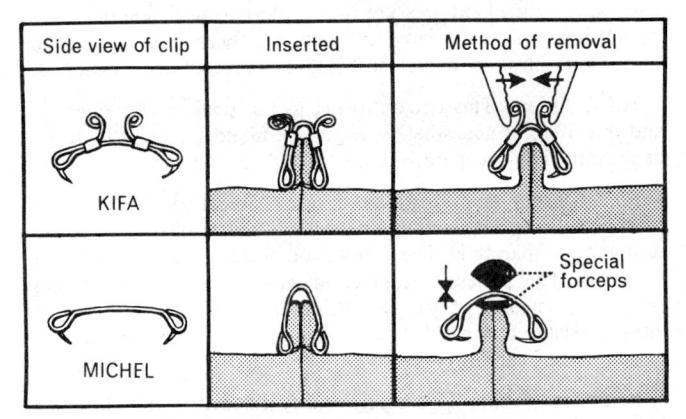

Side view of clip	Inserted	Method of removal
KIFA		
MICHEL		Special forceps

FIG. 13. The removal of two commonly used clips.

sutures that do not need removing. Alternatively, sutures may be inserted up to the level of the skin, then the skin is approximated with adhesive sutures. These are just taken off when the wound is healed. When the latter method is used the patient needs extra reassurance as the apparent absence of orthodox sutures causes anxiety.

COMPLICATIONS OF OPERATIONS

Respiratory obstruction may be due to the tongue falling back, or to vomit, blood or discharge from mouth or throat being sucked into the larynx on inspiration and obstructing the airway. This is prevented by keeping the head low and to one side during anaesthesia, keeping the jaw forward, using an airway.

Respiratory failure is due to the depressing effect of the anaesthetic and narcotic drugs on the respiratory centre. It is treated by giving respiratory stimulants, e.g. nikethamide, and artificial ventilation.

Shock and collapse. This is reduced and treated by the avoidance of movement, gentle handling (when handling is essential), the supine position with the foot of the bed elevated, the relief of pain by the administration of adequate analgesics, and the use of stimulants if the blood pressure is low. Blood transfusion or plasma transfusion will be ordered if there has been haemorrhage or haemoconcentration, and glucose/saline to prevent dehydration.

Heart failure. This occurs owing to the strain of the operation and the effect of anaesthetics, especially in elderly persons. It may be prevented by preoperative medical and nursing care.

Postoperative vomiting. This may be indicative of a variety of postoperative complications, such as acute dilatation of the stomach or paralytic ileus, both of which require immediate attention. The patient's stomach must be emptied and be kept empty by means of gastric aspiration; fluids must be given intravenously. During this time the serum electrolytes must be observed very carefully.

Retention of urine. This is particularly associated with abdominal and rectal operations (see p. 118).

Pain. This may be severe and is relieved by the administration of a narcotic or in mild pain an analgesic. This is repeated four-hourly if the surgeon feels it is necessary.

Haemorrhage. This is not a common complication, but the risk is higher after certain operations:

1. Tonsillectomy: primary and secondary haemorrhage.
2. Thyroidectomy: with the risk of tracheal pressure.
3. Prostatectomy: resulting in clot retention.
4. Cholecystectomy: when the patient is jaundiced.

Sepsis. This is prevented by strict attention to the principles of asepsis in the theatre and ward. Chemotherapy may be necessary in its prevention and treatment.

Chest complications. Modern anaesthesia, physiotherapy and early ambulation have reduced the risk of chest complications, but they may be encountered in elderly patients, heavy smokers and patients who do not breathe properly as a result of wound pain. Atelectasis is sometimes seen (see Thoracic Surgery, p. 176).

Flatulence is very troublesome after abdominal operations, especially when there has been much handling of the gut. (For treatment, see p. 117.)

Hiccough. This is painful and if persistent is a bad sign. It may be treated by inhalation of carbon dioxide or by giving chlorpromazine or morphine.

Rupture of the wound. The sutures may give way, especially in abdominal wounds where there is great strain from distension, cough or persistent vomiting. Sometimes this rupture occurs while the patient is lying quietly and when there is no strain being put on the wound. Earlier leakage of pinkish serum is sometimes a warning sign. The nurse must immediately inform the surgeon, cover the intestines with sterile towels wrung out in warm saline and covered by a firm binder or many-tailed bandage and prepare for the surgeon to resuture the wound in the theatre. Treatment for shock should be carried out as necessary.

Deep venous thrombosis. This is liable to occur and may be due to external pressure retarding the venous return from the legs or to diseases of the blood or blood vessels, as in polycythaemia and diabetes mellitus. It causes local pain and oedema of the foot and leg and is dangerous because a portion of the thrombus may break off and give rise to embolism. The patient may be given heparin, followed by an oral anticoagulant to prevent the extension of clots which have formed. A daily record of clotting time is kept to prevent this becoming dangerously long and the dosage is varied and the drug withheld as necessary in accordance with this. The patient must be confined to bed and must move carefully: gentle movement is encouraged to improve the circulation and lessen the likelihood of further clotting. Exercising the calf muscle is particularly important in promoting the return of venous blood from the lower limb. If the limb is very swollen it is raised on pillows, but this is seldom necessary because heparin acts quickly and usually prevents further clotting.

If part of the thrombus is carried away in the venous circulation it may pass through the right side of the heart and then lodge in a branch of one of the pulmonary arteries. This can cause sudden death, or severe chest pain and shock; this is known as pulmonary embolism. It is specially liable to occur after gynaecological operations, though it is much less common than in earlier years. Research by means of Dextran trials is being carried out into a method of detecting very early thrombus formation.

The patient is propped up and well supported with pillows to ease the dyspnoea. Fear is marked, so the patient is in great need of reassurance. Movement must be carried out with great care to prevent dislodging more emboli. Oxygen is administered; morphine will be ordered for the relief of pain and stimulants as necessary for shock and collapse. Heparin, in large dosage, is ordered immediately by intravenous injection or intramuscular injection to prevent further clot formation, followed possibly by phenindione; it is so effective that Trendelenburg's operation to open the pulmonary artery and remove the clot, which was occasionally successful, is no longer necessary. Operation has been undertaken in severe cases, the pulmonary artery being opened and the clot removed. There was great risk of recurrence in successful cases. The blood clotting time is checked daily and not allowed to become dangerously low, when anticoagulants are being given. Where there is a danger of repeated emboli the femoral veins or even the inferior vena cava may be ligated.

Postoperative psychosis. When this arises the patient must be guarded and psychiatric help obtained.

EARLY DISCHARGE OF SURGICAL PATIENTS TO THE COMMUNITY

An increasing number of surgical patients are being discharged home early following surgery. This can apply to all age groups and to patients who have had a wide variety of operations.

The community liaison sister is informed well in advance of the patient's discharge; she will then visit the patient's home with a social worker. They will make sure that social conditions are such that the patient can be nursed at home and if necessary the patient's bed will be moved downstairs; ideally this should be a single bed of a suitable nursing height. Nursing aids are obtained from the loans service, and the bed is prepared. If the patient is to be discharged in a wheelchair, it may be necessary to have ramps prepared.

When the patient arrives home the community nurse will try to visit the same day, to assess the patient's needs and the frequency of visits that will be necessary. She also informs the doctor that the patient has arrived. He will visit the patient, the required prescriptions will be given to the relatives and the treatment will be written down on the 'messages and directions' sheet. The nurse and the doctor will then communicate with each other by writing requests and changes in treatment on this sheet. This is kept in an official envelope in the patient's home. Nurses attached to group practices will also discuss any particular points with the doctor before leaving for their visits.

When working in the community the nurse must remember that when a patient comes to hospital, he comes as a guest, but when the nurse knocks at the door of the patient's house, she is his guest, so she says 'I am the District Nurse, may I come in?' This relationship is a professional one, but the hospital nurse will find that it is different from the one that she often has in hospital with her patients.

The community nurse carries a black bag with her, and this contains the 'basic tools of her trade'—instruments (four dissecting forceps, one probe, one pair of sinus forceps, and a spatula), catheters, enema kit, douche kit, blue stone or silver nitrate stick (to burn down overgranulated tissue) and one sterile dressing pack. This pack must be replaced from the patient's own stock of dressings so the nurse can sterilize it ready for when it is next unexpectedly required. However, the advent of CSSD is increasing the amount of material the nurse must carry with her, although it is making her task easier.

The patient who has been discharged early following surgery will require his dressing changing, so the equipment must be available. This can be in two forms:

1. *CSSD pack*, in which case everything is included except lotions and strapping. The latter two items have to be prescribed by the doctor and obtained from the chemist. Some patients are exempt from the prescription charge, e.g. if over 65 years, but many are not, so the nurse must be economical, as this equipment is the patient's property and an ill patient may be in financial difficulty and unable to afford to pay for too many prescriptions.

2. *Equipment sterilized by the nurse.* The nurse carries her own instruments but everything else has to be prescribed, wool, gauze, lotions, strappings, ointment, creams (each item having to be paid for separately).

The following method is used in the home to prepare and sterilize the required equipment for a wound dressing.

126 SURGICAL NURSING

Dressings. A half-size biscuit tin is cleaned and scrubbed out, and six individual dressing packs are made up, enclosed in kitchen paper and sealed with sticky tape. They are placed in the tin together with some spare sheets of paper which will be required as dressing towels. The tin is placed in the centre of an oven with the lid half on. They are then 'cooked' for one hour at regulo 1 (if it is a gas oven). At the end of this time the oven is turned off, and the lid of the biscuit tin is carefully banged shut. This is then sterile and is ready for use.

Instruments and receivers. A large saucepan is required which can comfortably hold one saucer and two cups with handles. The nurse must make sure that these are not cracked or chipped. These are placed in the saucepan and the instruments are held between the two cups. To facilitate removal from the boiling water the cups are placed with the mouths together and the handles uppermost. The water is then allowed to boil for ten minutes; when ready the cups are carefully lifted out of the water with the instruments between them, and they are manoeuvred so that all of the water escapes and the instruments are not contaminated. They are then carefully positioned on the sterile dressing towel which has been opened out on the inside of the sterile biscuit tin lid which has been placed on a table. The equipment is then ready.

When actually performing the dressing the usual hospital method for one nurse is used.

Hand preparation may involve problems as many houses do not have a bathroom where the nurse may wash her hands under running water. In fact the nurse must carry soap, nail brush and a towel in her black bag as these may not be available for her to use. In this case she has to ask for a kettle of hot water, a jug of cold water and a bowl so that she may prepare her hands.

On completing the procedure the soiled dressing must be burnt, but once again this may cause difficulties as facilities may not be available. The nurse may have to burn the dressing in the garden in a bucket; alternatively it can be placed in a plastic bag (provided by the service) and taken to a local clinic for incineration. If the dressing is very foul then it will be placed in the plastic bag and be removed by the public health cleansing department for disposal.

The nurse will perform the dressing procedure as often as is necessary and in some cases she will have to arrange for the patient to return to the hospital so that an observation check may be made by the surgeon; this is a common practice when the patient has had an operation on a pilonidal sinus.

POSTOPERATIVE CARE 127

Laundry problems in the home can cause many difficulties, so a laundry service is often available. In this case a supply of linen and plastic bags are delivered to the home, and a relative has to sign a form accepting responsibility for the listed items. After use these are placed in the plastic bag and are collected by the laundry man who gives a one-for-one replacement. Should the linen be contaminated it is cold-water sluiced, left standing in a bucket of disinfectant for a while, wrung out and placed in the plastic bag.

Inco pads are also provided when required, and these are placed in a plastic bag and are incinerated.

The doctor may decide that the patient is to have an enema, in which case he writes it down on the 'messages and directions' sheet, so that the nurse has a definite instruction. Many of the patients are elderly and a soap and water enema is ordered, not the disposable type. A receptacle must be provided as the toilet may be too far away. If the patient is confined to bed then a bed pan will be on hand and elderly patients often have a commode by the bed, but if these things are not available then the nurse may have to remove the seat from a dining room chair, and place a bucket beneath it. She will also have to ask the relatives to provide her with a jug and some green soap or Lux flakes.

Any drugs ordered will be prescribed by the doctor and are once again the patient's property. They will be kept in a safe place in the house out of reach of children and out of sight. The relative will be instructed about the oral drugs and will give them to the patient, but if injections are to be given then the nurse will do this, the only exception being the diabetic patient who will give his own injections after the nurse has made sure that he is able to do so. Visits can be arranged three times during the day and once at night. The injections are given with a sterile prepacked syringe and needle and these are destroyed after use so that there is no possibility of them being used again.

The nurse in the community who is caring for surgical patients who have been discharged early from hospital often has to give a tremendous amount of emotional support. While in hospital the patient may appear to be confident and self-assured, but on return to his own home he often becomes very unsure and even frightened. It may be distress due to the type of operation, e.g. a mastectomy, ileostomy or amputation of limb, in which case the nurse will have to give a tremendous amount of reassurance. Alternatively the patient may be afraid of his wound: 'Is it all right to be at home with stitches in?' or 'What happens if the wound bursts and there is

128 SURGICAL NURSING

no one here?' These fears are not very obvious in the hospitalized patient, but are very common in the community. So when a patient is discharged from hospital to the care of the community following surgery the nurse must put into practice her hospital training, but must be prepared to adapt it to the different situations in which she finds herself.

9

Surgery of the Head and Neck

CRANIAL SURGERY

As a result of recent advances in anaesthesia and aseptic and antiseptic surgery, together with specialization by surgeons in the field of cranial surgery, great advances have been made during the last twenty years and many cranial operations which would previously have been considered impossible are carried out today.

The fields of neurosurgery and neurosurgical nursing are highly specialized and details are outside the scope of this book.

Preparation for Cranial Operation

The head must be shaved. Complete shaving is often required and in this case the patient will be reassured about his or her appearance and information will be provided about the availability of wigs. The fitter will visit the patient and discuss this in more detail. If the tumour is cerebellar the surgeon may, in the case of a woman, allow the hair to be left across the forehead so that it may be worn to cover the head while the hair is growing, with only the upper part of the patient's head being shaved. Other surgeons only require shaving of the hair on the side or area where the operation will be carried out, provided the remaining hair is kept away effectively from the operation site. Both the patient and his relatives must be given a careful explanation about the care which will be given post-operatively and the reasons for it. In some circumstances the patient will be too ill to understand, but the relatives must still be informed.

The operation may be performed under local or general

anaesthetic and the patient must be prepared accordingly. Local anaesthesia makes it possible to prolong the operation with less danger to the patient, so that all bleeding may be controlled and location and dissection of the tumour satisfactorily completed. Local anaesthesia is obtained by infiltration of the tissues with 1% procaine with adrenaline and is generally used, with or without light general anaesthesia, in the form of gas and oxygen, to relieve the strain if the surgeon thinks that it is desirable. Plenty of glucose should be given and the patient's confidence must be won completely.

Hypothermia is also used, especially for cranial vascular surgery, such as when the patient has a cerebral aneurysm. Cooling the body reduces the metabolic rate, which diminishes the cellular need for oxygen. So when cerebral vascular surgery is performed the risk of cerebral anoxia is greatly reduced. The patient is anaesthetized and his body temperature is reduced to about 32°C. (If the temperature drops below 29°C cardiac arrhythmia will develop.)

The blood should be grouped before operation, as blood transfusion may be required during or after it. However, blood loss is lessened by the use of local anaesthetics, hypotensive drugs and diathermy to clot the blood in the vessels at the operation site. Electric suction is used during the operation to keep the field clear of blood so that the surgeon can see the structures clearly. Alginate preparations may also be used to check bleeding. Systemic chemotherapy may be ordered and the drug chosen must be active against the causal organism and must be of a type that will diffuse into the cerebrospinal fluid. If there is brain abscess, the pus is evacuated and the cavity injected with penicillin; the treatment can be repeated if necessary. In cases of injury the site may be treated with penicillin and lactose in powder form by insufflation, or as a solution. This does not injure the delicate nerve tissue, but the surgeon may prefer to use penicillin systemically to lessen the risks of allergic reaction. The surgeon may also request that other investigations be carried out before surgery, such as chest and skull radiographs, lumbar puncture, air encephalogram, air ventriculogram, carotid angiogram, electroencephalogram and brain scan.

After-care

The patient should be kept under careful observation. He is nursed flat until he has recovered from the anaesthetic, which may be

SURGERY OF THE HEAD AND NECK

before he returns from the theatre; after this he may be propped up to lessen the blood supply to the brain and so diminish bleeding or oedema within the cranium, if the surgeon orders. If haemorrhage has been severe, blood transfusions, either single or continuous, may be employed. Observations should be made as has been described for patients who have sustained head injuries. The nurse must especially note falling pulse and respiration rates, with a rise in blood pressure, which indicate a rising intracranial pressure.

Discharge may come through the dressing, but generally a suction drainage bottle, e.g. Redivac, is used to draw out and collect fluid from the tissues. The dressing must be packed and repacked as required during the first 24 hours and then dressed daily with strict asepsis.

One of the proprietary tubular bandages is usually the most effective way of securing the dressing, or failing that a crêpe bandage.

The pillow must have a waterproof cover. The bowels should be opened early and kept well regulated. Intravenous infusion of Ureaphil 80 g or mannitol 10 or 20% may also be used for this purpose. The nurse should report any undue oedema, especially about the eyelid, and the return of pulsation in the brain at the site where it is only covered by the scalp.

Fluid diet is given by straws, spouted feeder or spoon when the patient's swallowing reflex is restored; later a light semi-solid nourishing diet is given. If the patient becomes very drowsy it is important to make sure that he takes sufficient fluid, by mouth if possible, testing to find out whether the swallowing reflex is present, using a swab soaked in water. If the patient sucks and swallows, spoon feeding can be carried out with great care; the nurse must watch for each spoonful to be swallowed before giving another. If the swallowing reflex is abolished, tube-feeding will be necessary and the giving of intravenous infusions containing glucose. Morphine is avoided for these patients since it so easily masks the signs and symptoms of rising intracranial pressure. Codeine phosphate 60 mg will be prescribed for the relief of pain. Paraldehyde is given by intramuscular injection in a dosage of 2–8 ml. Cot sides and pillow tied to the head of the bed may be necessary. A mouth wedge and gag should remain at the bedside after recovery from anaesthesia, as fits may occur. Diazepam 10 mg by intramuscular injection will prevent these.

The stitches are removed on the sixth day after operation; a wig will be prescribed and is provided by the appliance officer as soon as the patient can tolerate it on her head following surgery.

The mouth and pressure areas will require careful attention.

Scalp Wounds

Scalp wounds from a blow on the head may be very extensive and bleed freely, but, even when a large flap is torn off, the wound will heal readily on account of the good blood supply. The surrounding skin must be washed and shaved, placing a swab in the wound so that the loose hair does not fall in. Haemorrhage is arrested and the wound washed with antiseptic, e.g. aqueous hibitane, followed by penicillin as an insufflation. The wound is then stitched up with drainage and dressed. Systemic chemotherapy may be ordered.

AFFECTIONS OF THE MOUTH

These include:

1. Abscesses; these may occur at the roots of the teeth, in the tongue, round the tonsil (quinsy), and behind the pharynx (retropharyngeal).
2. Cleft lip.
3. Cleft palate.
4. Carcinoma of tongue or jaw.

Abscesses

Abscesses must be drained, but there are two special risks: asphyxiation from oedema of the tongue in tongue abscess and danger of asphyxiation or septic pneumonia due to the aspiration of pus, especially in quinsy and retropharyngeal abscess. Retropharyngeal abscess occurs in weakly infants with severe upper respiratory tract or nasopharyngeal infection and in the adult with cervical caries. In the infant a general anaesthetic is necessary and the child is placed with the head hanging right back over the edge of the table or trolley and supported on a special rest, and is nursed in this position so that discharge is not sucked into the lungs with the inspired air.

SURGERY OF THE HEAD AND NECK

In the adult with tuberculosis, opening from without is advocated to prevent septic infection, and anti-tuberculosis drugs will be used.

Non-tuberculous abscesses are nowadays (when they occur, which is rarely) opened under general anaesthesia and the aspiration of pus is prevented partly by the use of a cuffed endotracheal tube and by the use of suction.

After-care. Antiseptic mouth washes are given hourly and before and after all feeds. Soft semi-solid feeds are most easily swallowed. Cavities may need to be irrigated with syringe and nozzle or Eustachian catheter.

Cleft Lip and Cleft Palate

Cleft lip and cleft palate are congenital deformities due to the failure of the various parts of the upper lip and the palate to fuse in the normal manner. Both may be present together. Cleft lip is generally operated on about the age of three months so that normal moulding of bones and face may occur during growth, and cleft palate about the age of one year so that normal speech may develop. The parts are very small and delicate at this age and operation may be delayed, but defective speech habits are difficult to overcome so that the earlier date has great advantages.

Cleft lip

Cleft lip may be unilateral or bilateral, and may extend right up into the nostril. The surgeon pares the edges and stitches them together. The wound may be painted with spirit or iodine, or Whitehead's varnish may be applied.

Preparation. In caring for children, the mother should be encouraged to be with her child and to be involved as much as is possible. It is essential for the mother–child relationship that they are together during this traumatic period of hospitalization. To increase security and the continuity of care it is also advisable that children are cared for by their own special nurses. The child should be admitted several days before operation, as these infants are often very fretful at first. The child should be observed for any signs of a cold, as operation should be delayed if this is present and a throat swab should be taken. The haemoglobin must be 12 g/dl before operation is undertaken. He is trained in spoon feeding, putting the feeds well to the back of the tongue.

SURGICAL NURSING

After-care. The arms must be splinted with corrugated cardboard splints, so that the child cannot touch the wound. Feeds should be preceded and ended by tap water. The wound, unless it has been sealed with Whitehead's varnish, is swabbed with sterile water. A Logan's bow prevents stretching of the scar. Crying is prevented as far as is practicable by good nursing and by the mother spending as much time as possible with the child, nursing him or walking about with him. Drugs may be given to keep the child quiet; chloral is particularly well tolerated by young children. The stitches are taken out on the third to fifth day. It should be ensured that no visitors with colds come to see the child.

Cleft palate

Cleft palate is treated similarly by paring the edges and suturing, after cutting on either side and raising up the mucous membrane so that the edges come together more readily.

Preparation. The child should be admitted well before operation, so that he becomes used to his surroundings and the nurses. This is especially important since the child is often old enough to be aware of his surroundings, yet not old enough to understand explanations. He should be trained in spoon-feeding and if the surgeon requires any irrigation after operation it should be practised, so that the child is not afraid. His general condition must be improved in every way and he must not be exposed to infection. A throat swab should be taken to ensure freedom from infection. The haemoglobin must be calculated and must be 12 g/dl before operation is undertaken.

After-care. The arms must be splinted, so that the child cannot put his fingers in his mouth, and no long toys or pencils allowed, which might be pushed into it. Soft solid feeds are given by spoon placed well back on the tongue, and preceded and followed by sterile water. Neither boiled sweets nor chocolate are usually allowed. Antiseptic syringing may be ordered. No swabbing must be attempted, as the strain on the stitches is always very severe and the wound is very liable to break down. Some surgeons do not attempt complete closure, but provide the child with a dental plate and obturator shaped to fill in the gap. The lips may be smeared with petroleum jelly as these children tend to dribble a good deal. Ephedrine nasal drops may be ordered to try to improve the airway by relieving the congestion of the mucous membrane. These babies

SURGERY OF THE HEAD AND NECK

are very liable to streptococcal infection and no nurse must go on duty with any signs of a cold or sore throat, when caring for such patients.

Carcinoma of the Tongue

Carcinoma of the tongue causes an ulcer on the tongue and generally occurs on the lateral aspect. Simple ulcers may arise from irritation by a broken tooth; these will heal in a few weeks if the tooth is extracted.

Investigations

Prior to planning treatment the doctor will request that the following investigations are carried out:

1. Biopsy to confirm the diagnosis.
2. Chest X-ray to exclude the possibility of pulmonary secondaries.
3. X-ray of the skull and mandible to detect/estimate the extent of bone invasion.

Treatment

Treatment depends upon the site and extent of the neoplasm. The primary lesion may be treated by means of:

1. Radiotherapy, in the form of either radium needles or supervoltage therapy.
2. Radical surgical excision, if radiotherapy is not the treatment of choice. This could be removal of the affected half of the tongue called hemiglossectomy or a mandibulectomy.
3. If surgery is not practicable then cancer chemotherapy by means of regional perfusion into the external carotid artery may be carried out. This is, however, only palliative.

If the lymph nodes are also involved then:

1. Enlarged mobile glands will be removed by block dissection (providing the primary lesion is treatable), *or*
2. If the glands are enlarged and fixed, palliative deep X-ray therapy is carried out.

RADIUM TREATMENT

All septic teeth must be removed and teeth scaled and filled as required. Many radiotherapists order a complete dental clearance as the teeth within the field of radiation receive a full dose. This will ultimately result in dental decay with the need for extraction at a later date.

Mouth-washes of Milton 2·5%, chloramine-T 0·5% or acriflavine 1 in 5000 are given two-hourly or four-hourly, according to the condition of the mouth, as the surgeon permits.

The patient should be trained to use a spouted feeder with rubber tubing attached. Some patients prefer drinking straws. The moustache must be either shaved or clipped as required by the surgeon. Prior to surgery it is very important that a careful explanation is given to the relatives about the patient's appearance and postoperative treatment. This must include instructions to talk to the patient in a manner that does not demand a verbal reply.

After-care. The patient is nursed in an upright position on recovery from the anaesthetic to lessen the risk of chest complications. Until the patient is conscious, the foot of the bed or trolley must be elevated so that saliva and discharges are not sucked into the trachea and lungs. A tongue ligature with Spencer Wells forceps may have been inserted to draw the tongue forward as required and must be left in till the patient is completely conscious. The strings of the radium needles are brought out and strapped to the cheek and must be checked ideally every two hours but at least morning and evening and before and after any local treatment.

These strings are often threaded through a piece of Paul's tubing so that the lips are not irritated by the presence of a rough surface.

Fluid feeds are given but the patient may be rather afraid of dislodging the needles or becoming nauseated. Also drinking is rather difficult and uncomfortable because of the swollen tissues, so the patient will be greatly assisted if a straw or piece of tubing is made available for him to suck the fluid through. Saline with 5% glucose may be ordered intravenously, if swallowing is difficult, to maintain the fluid and salt intake. The mouth is gently irrigated before and after feeds with normal saline or antiseptic solution, using either Higginson's syringe or irrigator, tubing, Eustachian catheter or soft rubber catheter. The radium must be checked before throwing away any used lotion. A second person should hold a light to assist the dresser. No sloughs must be forcibly separated, but left to come away.

Pain is severe, and is controlled by morphine 10–15 mg or pethidine 50–100 mg as required. The needles are removed from the sixth to tenth day according to dosage ordered; they are often sloughing out about the sixth day. The patient is discouraged from talking and a writing pad must be provided, so it is very important that the nurse anticipates the patient's needs and that the patient learns to communicate with the nurse in a non-verbal manner. These patients are usually elderly men and the skin over pressure areas quickly becomes red. Patients should be encouraged to change the position frequently (without fidgeting and producing friction). When interstitial radium is being used patients are confined to bed.

Teleradium cures the condition with less discomfort to the patient where it is possible to carry out this treatment. Radium or X-ray treatment to the glands of the neck will also be necessary. The radium in the form of needles may be applied by means of a sorbo-rubber collar to hold the radium the required distance from the skin. Alternatively excision of the glands followed by irradiation may be carried out.

Surgical treatment

Preparation is the same as it is for radium treatment.

After-care. The patient is placed flat with the head to one side to prevent asphyxiation by the tongue, blood or saliva, or better still in the semi-prone position. High blocks may be placed at the foot of the bed to lessen the risk of aspiration pneumonia or asphyxia. A ligature is generally passed through the tongue with Spencer Wells forceps attached, by which it can readily be pulled forward. Intravenous fluids will be prescribed until the patient is able to take adequate volumes of fluid by mouth. Suction apparatus should be at hand ready for immediate use.

When the patient recovers consciousness he is nursed sitting upright with the head well forward, so that saliva may drain out. He should be provided with gauze swabs to wipe the mouth. Feeds may be commenced as soon as the patient can swallow. The patient often swallows more easily the next day than between the third to fifth days and feeding by stomach tube may be necessary during this period. If so, nourishing fluids should be given as advised by the dietician. The mouth should be irrigated two-hourly before and after feeds with normal saline or antiseptic solution, till the patient is able to rinse the mouth out himself with mouth-washes. The stitches will frequently slough out, otherwise they are removed

138 SURGICAL NURSING

about the eighth day. The bowels should be opened early, as blood and discharge are liable to be swallowed in the period immediately after operation. Chemotherapy will be used to lessen the risk of sepsis and the chest complications that the operation is liable to cause. The patient should be provided with paper or a slate and pencil so that he can write his requests while speaking is painful and difficult or with a gadget such as the Jeffery Communicator. Speech therapy will help these patients when healing has occurred.

The patient should be nursed on Sorbo rubber or interior-sprung mattress and the pressure areas attended to as required. He should get up early, if possible on the second day, to lessen the risk of chest complications and development of bedsores. Following surgery of this type patients tend to become very depressed, so early ambulation and the company of the nurses and relatives can be beneficial.

Complications

The chief dangers are:

Asphyxiation, from the tongue or from blood and saliva blocking the airway.

Haemorrhage, particularly secondary haemorrhage, occurring as a rule seven to ten days after operation. Severe haemorrhage is usually preceded by two or three slight oozings. Any haemorrhage, once the initial bleeding has stopped, should therefore be reported immediately even if the bleeding was very slight and has stopped. This complication has become rare since the introduction of chemotherapy for these patients.

Chest complications are liable to occur, since the patients are elderly men and may inhale septic discharge during anaesthesia and while swallowing is painful and the tongue swollen and oedematous. These should be prevented rather than cured. If the patient becomes cyanosed, establish an airway, give oxygen and apply artificial respiration if necessary. Raising the foot of the bed high will help to drain blood and discharge from the air passages.

Carcinoma of the Jaw

Carcinoma of the jaw is initially treated by radiotherapy but surgery is performed if the condition does not improve or recurs. A hemi-mandibulectomy is performed. This operation is extensive and associated with considerable shock and mutilation, but cure can be effected if it is performed early. Preparation and after-care are similar to that of tongue treatments.

AFFECTIONS OF THE NECK

Excision of glands of the neck is undertaken particularly for malignant disease in the region of the mouth and neck. Block dissection of all the glands is necessary and the wound has a drainage tube for prevention of haematoma. Extensive skin preparation is required, extending beyond the midline back and front, upwards to the jaw line and ear and downwards to an imaginary line drawn horizontally through the axilla.

The dressing must be carefully watched for postoperative haemorrhage, which is the chief danger.

Irradiation is generally given at three-monthly intervals for two applications and the patient is kept under regular supervision. Alternatively, a full course of irradiation may be used instead of excision.

Tuberculous Glands

In tuberculosis the whole outlook has been changed since the introduction of the successful antituberculosis drugs, beginning with streptomycin in 1944, followed by *para*-aminosalicylic acid (PAS) and isoniazid. Patients requiring surgery invariably receive courses of these drugs in addition. Measures to improve the general health are as important as in the past; rest associated with controlled exercise as ordered by the surgeon, a liberal, varied diet, with extra milk, cream and butter if they are well tolerated, fresh air, especially country or sea air, and the relief of worry concerning family security and future employment are all desirable in these cases.

The cervical and mesenteric glands are most frequently affected by the tubercle bacillus, but rarely the inguinal or axillary glands are involved.

Tuberculosis of the cervical glands

At one time this condition was commonly diagnosed, especially among children, but it is now relatively rare in the UK except

140 SURGICAL NURSING

among Asian immigrants. A suspected diagnosis is confirmed by taking a radiograph of the neck, when the radiologist will recognize the typical appearance.

The cervical glands are infected through the tonsils. The affected glands become much enlarged, but the inflammation is chronic, and if seen early there is no redness or heat in the part.

Treatment. Enlarged nodes are excised and if an abscess is present the pus is evacuated. A search is also made to detect any caseating (cheese-like) glands; if they are found they are removed by means of curettage. Surgery is supported by anti-tuberculous chemotherapy.

Thyroid Gland

There are three conditions affecting the thyroid gland which may necessitate surgical interference:

1. Simple goitre.
2. Exophthalmic goitre.
3. New growths, simple or malignant.

Simple goitre

Simple goitre (parenchymatous goitre) is an enlargement of the gland without over-secretion. It occurs in certain districts, particularly in valleys far from the sea, where there is a lack of iodine in the water and food. In England, it was most common in Derbyshire, where it was known as 'Derbyshire neck', and to a lesser extent in the Thames valley. It occurs in the Himalayas, the Andes, the Rocky Mountains and in Switzerland. It can be prevented and cured by giving iodides which may be added to the salt supply of a district where the disease is common. Surgical treatment is only required when enlargement has been neglected and is causing inconvenience, is unsightly, or there are pressure symptoms resulting in respiratory obstruction.

Signs and symptoms of respiratory obstruction. Dyspnoea, restlessness, stridor, cough, and cyanosis or lividity.

Treatment consists of removal of as much of the gland as is necessary to relieve the symptoms.

Exophthalmic goitre

Exophthalmic goitre (or Graves's disease) is an enlargement of the gland associated with over-secretion or thyrotoxicosis. This is a much more serious condition and in addition to the enlargement of the gland, which may be comparatively slight, gives rise to the following symptoms:

1. Protrusion of the eyeballs (exophthalmos) and retraction of the eyelids.
2. Quick, weak pulse (120 beats per minute and over).
3. Palpitations.
4. Loss of weight, though the appetite is good.
5. Fine moist skin with soft fine hair.
6. Tremor.
7. Irritability and nervousness; the patient is very difficult and is often hysterical and restless, and does not sleep well.
8. The patient feels the heat excessively.

If the enlargement occurs below the sternum in the thorax acute dyspnoea may occur from pressure on the trachea, necessitating an emergency operation. This is not common, but can occur.

If it is untreated the condition becomes gradually worse, with periods of remission, until ultimately the patient becomes very wasted and weak and a fatal ending is ushered in by auricular fibrillation, diarrhoea or maniacal symptoms. Auricular fibrillation may be found in the older patient before the terminal stage of the disease.

Early diagnosis can be confirmed by testing the basal metabolic rate; this is definitely raised in all cases of thyrotoxicosis, though it is a difficult investigation to carry out with absolute accuracy. Where there are the facilities the uptake of a small dose of radioactive iodine can be measured; this provides a more reliable guide in doubtful cases.

TREATMENT

This consists of the following:

1. Antithyroid drugs.
2. Surgery.
3. Radioactive iodine.

Medical treatment using thiouracil overcomes the thyrotoxicosis but does not cure the condition and is therefore now largely used to

142 SURGICAL NURSING

detoxicate the patient in preparation for operative treatment. Carbimazole has the lowest incidence of toxic side-effects, so it is used to inhibit the production of thyroid hormones in the treatment of mild hyperthyroidism and in the preparation of patients for operative treatment or radioactive iodine therapy.

SURGERY

Preoperative care and investigations. It is of the utmost importance that the patient's confidence should be won and his fears allayed, and here the tactful nurse is of great value to the surgeon. The patient should be kept quiet and visitors should be limited and allowed only if they do not disturb the patient.

Before admission to hospital the general practitioner and the consultant will attempt to control the patient's condition by means of drugs, for example carbimazole 5–10 mg or propranolol 40 mg, both three times a day. As a result hospital preoperative care can be minimal. Psychological care is very important at all times, both before and after hospital admission. Routine observations and records include weight, height, temperature, pulse, respirations and blood pressure, as well as urine analysis. An electrocardiogram is performed and the chest is radiographed. The vocal cords are examined the day before surgery; as this can be a very uncomfortable procedure an anaesthetic spray or lozenges may be used. If this is the case the patient must not be allowed anything by mouth for three hours after the examination. Night sedation, such as nitrazepam 5–10 mg, is generally prescribed and the anaesthetist will visit the patient the evening before surgery when he (or the surgeon) will also prescribe the premedication.

Local skin preparation varies a great deal according to the practice of the particular hospital, but is usually limited to social cleanliness; if a man has a very hairy chest this will have to be shaved.

An attempt is generally made for the patient to be operated on at the beginning of the list.

Postoperative care. The patient is nursed flat with the head to one side till recovered from anaesthesia. The head must be supported so that extension of the neck is avoided. He is then nursed sitting up with head and neck well supported.

Analgesia is prescribed and administered as required (usually on the first postoperative night), e.g. pethidine 75–100 mg by intramuscular injection. At first, prior to a meal the patient will appreciate oral soluble aspirin or distalgesic to relieve the pain on swallowing.

Observations are carried out half-hourly at first, taking particular note of anything that could indicate the onset of complications, such as difficulty in breathing, pins and needles, blood oozing from the wound or excessive quantity of fluid in the drainage bottle.

Many patients are afraid of moving their heads so the nurse must be gentle and give reassurance as appropriate.

The surgeon may decide to continue medication for five days postoperatively, such as propranolol 40 mg three times a day.

The dressing and suction drain are watched for haemorrhage. Sometimes this dressing will be replaced with a 'plastic skin spray' such as Octoflex or Nobecutane. The drainage tube (soft rubber drains or Redivac vacuum drain) is removed in 24–48 hours according to the amount of discharge. The stitches are removed about the third or fourth day and clips also to lessen the scarring. It is common practice to remove alternate clips or stitches one day and the remainder on the day following. Some surgeons close the wound with vertical strips of adhesive dressing, such as Steristrips. These are removed on the fifth day. If the patient is conscious of the scar a necklace of sufficient size to hide it may be worn. Some surgeons ask the patient to choose one for the purpose before the operation and mark the line with a skin pencil to ensure a satisfactory result.

Diet should consist of nourishing fluids and soft semi-solids until the patient can swallow with confidence, as this is very painful on the first postoperative day. Prior to discharge the patient is told to rub a cream such as lanolin into the healed wound gently; this will make it supple and much less easy to see.

The vocal cords are examined again and the calcium levels may be measured.

Sometimes the patient may be discharged home as soon as the sutures have been removed and the surgeon is sure that complications are not developing or actually present. The general practitioner is informed and he 'takes over' the care of the patient.

Special dangers

Tetany. This is muscle spasm due to removal of or damage to the parathyroid glands which control calcium metabolism. It is relieved by the administration of intravenous calcium gluconate. The typical carpopedal spasms affect the hands and the feet. An early warning occurs if the patient complains of pins and needles; if the spasm

144 SURGICAL NURSING

develops the patient will be very frightened as he cannot move his hands.

Injury to the recurrent laryngeal nerve. This affects the voice and causes dyspnoea which may be so serious that tracheostomy is necessary.

Haemorrhage. Should a ligature slip, for example as a result of vomiting, haemorrhage may occur and obstruct breathing by outside pressure. The wound must be opened at once to allow blood to escape, although some surgeons say that this must not be done, but that the patient must be intubated at once and taken to the operating theatre so that the wound may be opened and the bleeding point sealed. Opening the wound can result in severe loss of blood. After the nurse has opened the wound to relieve the pressure the patient will be returned to the operating table. Bruising is often severe.

Shock. See p. 18.

Myxoedema may follow if too much of the gland has been removed. This is treated by giving thyroid extract, as required, for the remainder of the patient's life. The patient must be followed up carefully after operation for this reason.

Acute thyrotoxicosis. This is unusual; it is marked by steady rise in pulse rate and temperature, which may lead to auricular fibrillation and hyperpyrexia, delirium or excitability, with sweating, rapid breathing and flushed skin. It occurs with 24–48 hours of operation. Steps are taken to reduce pyrexia and intravenous propranolol 1 mg may be administered. If so, the doctor will ask for atropine to be available in case it is required.

Radioactive iodine may be used to treat certain patients with thyrotoxicosis if more conventional treatment is not desirable, the substance being given in fluid form and remaining active for eight days. Cells which absorb iodine will pick the radioactive material up and be destroyed by it. It is used only for patients over 50 years of age since there is some fear that it may stimulate the development of malignant changes some 20 years hence. No special precautions are necessary as a result of this treatment.

Stridor. This may be due to oedema of the vocal cords, the patient experiencing great difficulty in breathing and becoming very agitated; the sound of the stridor is unmistakable. The patient must not be left alone as he will be panic-stricken and struggling.

This usually responds to the intravenous injection of hydrocortisone 500 mg.

New growths

Simple growths in the form of adenomas are quite common; they give rise to swelling in the neck and may result in respiratory obstruction or over-secretion, causing secondary thyrotoxicosis. Thyrotoxicosis does not arise until the growth has been present for many years; it gives rise to symptoms similar to those of exophthalmic goitre, but is not so severe. As the patient is generally over 40 years of age, the heart is not so well able to endure the constant tachycardia.

Early operation is desirable if there are symptoms of thyrotoxicosis; the same special points are required as in Graves's disease, but the risks are not so great.

Malignant growths may occur, carcinomas arising in the glandular tissue or sarcomas in the connective tissue. They are rare and as in other glandular carcinomas secondary metastases occur very early in bone, and may be the cause of diagnosis.

Treatment is operative if the condition is diagnosed early, but in many cases extension by the blood stream to the bone or locally into the trachea or mediastinum make removal impossible. In inoperable cases radium or deep X-ray therapy may be used: radioactive iodine is used if the cells of the tumour are of the secretory type and make thyroxine; this may be the case both in the gland itself and in the metastases to which such a growth gives rise. The value of radioactive iodine is checked by means of a Geiger counter over the gland. If the counter shows an accumulation of radioactivity over the gland, the treatment will be effective.

Parathyroid Gland

This gland may produce excessive parathormone which could result in pathological fractures, renal calculi and a high serum calcium level; when this occurs it may be due to a simple non-malignant tumour and the treatment is removal of the involved structure.

The preoperative and postoperative care for parathyroidectomy is basically the same as for a thyroidectomy, the main difference being that one hour prior to surgery 500 ml of dextrose saline containing 5 mg/kg body weight of methylene blue must be given.

This is taken up by the tissues and the parathyroid glands are clearly visible to the surgeon.

Following surgery the patient appears cyanosed because of the dye in the tissues, but this resolves within a few hours. The patient must be warned that the urine will be green until the drug has been excreted.

Tracheostomy

Tracheostomy means the surgical formation of an opening into the trachea, and the name comes from two Greek words, *trakus* meaning rugged and *stoma* meaning mouth. It is becoming an increasingly common operation and nurses are liable to meet this type of patient in many wards.

Advantages of tracheostomy

1. *The reduction of the dead air space.* The exchange of gases takes place only through the alveoli. Air in the rest of the respiratory tract must therefore be regarded as dead air space. If this is reduced a less forceful exertion is required to ventilate the lungs effectively. This is especially helpful to weak patients with extensive damage of the chest wall.

2. *The easy aspiration of secretions*, when the patient is too weak to cough them up. A sucker can be used to keep the lungs dry effectively and so prevent pulmonary complications.

3. *The maintenance of the normal compliance of the lungs.* When the lungs are under-ventilated their compliance is reduced. This means that it takes more effort to expand them, just as it takes more effort to blow up a completely deflated balloon than one which is partly filled. In recumbency after operation the lower lobes of the lungs tend to be underventilated. Pulmonary oedema and atelectasis may further aggravate this condition. This is the reason why movement (passive if neccesary), deep breathing and coughing up secretions are such an important part of routine postoperative nursing care.

4. *To enable the patient to breathe* when the upper respiratory passages are obstructed.

SURGERY OF THE HEAD AND NECK

Principal indications for tracheostomy

1. Obstruction of the respiratory passages.
2. To assist respiration.
3. After failure of normal respiration.

Obstructions necessitating a tracheostomy may be due to:

1. *External compression* of the airway from such conditions as tumours, goitres or aneurysms.
2. *Internal blockage* of the airway from:

a. Tumours, especially of the larynx.

b. Inflammation. Many of the older reasons for tracheostomy have disappeared owing to immunization against diphtheria, chemotherapy and intubation. Nevertheless a diphtheritic membrane, Ludwig's angina, quinsy, burns, scalds and stings may still necessitate the operation.

c. Trauma. Cut throats, gunshot wounds and other injuries.

d. Paralysis as a result of anterior poliomyelitis, polyneuritis or damage to the recurrent laryngeal nerve after thyroidectomy. The vocal cords may be adducted and permit insufficient air entry.

e. Spasm due to anaesthetic or tetanus.

f. Foreign bodies.

g. Contracture of scar tissue, e.g. after swallowing corrosive poison.

h. Congenital lesions such as laryngeal papillomas.

To assist respiration in the following instances:

1. After severe fractures of the ribs when paradoxical respiration is present.
2. After a severe fracture of the jaw to make sure that breathing does not become obstructed and after maxillectomies.
3. In certain chronic chest conditions, such as chronic bronchitis, to reduce the dead space and to assist the patient to expel secretions from his respiratory passages. This also allows more efficient ventilation of the lungs to take place.
4. In neurological conditions when the larynx, pharynx or respiratory muscles are involved in weakness or paralysis, such as polyneuritis, bulbar poliomyelitis and myasthenia gravis.
5. In some cases after thoracic surgery if the patient is too ill or weak to cough up secretions from his chest.
6. Before operations on the upper respiratory tract if there is a grave risk of blood or secretions being aspirated into the lungs.

148 SURGICAL NURSING

After failure of normal respiration Tracheostomy is now used with a positive pressure or positive–negative pressure respirator when normal respiration fails.

1. There may be *central respiratory failure* when the respiratory centre in the medulla is affected by head injuries or narcotic poisoning.
2. There may be *interruption of the nervous pathways* from respiratory centre to respiratory muscles, as in anterior poliomyelitis, polyneuritis, high spinal injuries and myasthenia gravis.
3. There may be *failure of the respiratory muscles* as in myopathy and dermatomyositis, especially when bronchitis supervenes.

Signs of failing respiration are:

1. Dyspnoea, shallow rapid respirations.
2. Accessory muscles of respiration are brought into use. The nurse can easily see the patient using the alae nasi and sternomastoid muscles.
3. The pulse rate goes up.
4. The blood pressure falls.
5. The patient starts sweating, especially round the head.
6. Mental distress is extreme, the feeling of suffocation produces acute anxiety and the patient may become restless and maniacal. The cells of the cerebral cortex are the first affected by lack of oxygen and carbon dioxide retention may help to produce cerebral irrtation.
7. Cyanosis is a late sign. A nurse should never wait for this to develop.
8. Convulsions and collapse are terminal signs indicating that a fatal ending will follow.

In addition signs of laryngeal obstruction are:

1. Stridor.
2. A hard ringing cough.
3. Sucking in of the soft parts of the chest during inspiration, termed recession.

Tracheostomy is an elective or an emergency operation. Emergency conditions can usually be treated by laryngoscopy and the introduction of an endotracheal tube; the operation can then be performed with greater comfort for both patient and operator. When the operation is performed as an emergency on an obstructed patient, it is usually done without an anaesthetic as time is of

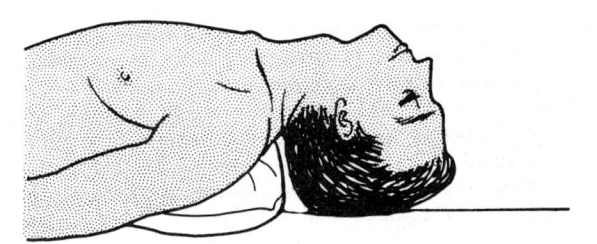

FIG. 14. The correct position of the patient for tracheostomy.

paramount importance. It is difficult as there is much bleeding owing to raised jugular venous pressure and the required position aggravates dyspnoea, thus harassing both patient and surgeon.

Position

A sandbag is placed high under the shoulders and the head hangs down over the end of the table and is held by an assistant, with the neck fully extended. This brings the trachea nearer to the surface and is described as Rose's position. The arms are constricted by a blanket or turkish towel.

Tracheostomy equipment

A tracheostomy set consists of:

1. *An outer tube* fitted with a shield to which tapes are attached to prevent the tube slipping in or out and these must be very carefully attached to the tube and tied round the neck.
2. *An inner tube* removable for cleansing purposes.
3. *A pilot or introducer* which fits into the outer tube. This prevents the edge of the tube from injuring the walls of the trachea as it is introduced.

There are many types of tracheostomy tubes:

The cuffed Radcliffe tracheostomy tube is used when positive pressure ventilation is required. It has a magnetic insert for the attachment of the tubing which leads to the ventilator and an inflatable cuff which allows the tube to fit snugly into the inner lumen of the trachea. The cuff is essential as it prevents the escape of air from the lungs around the tracheostomy tube and also

150 SURGICAL NURSING

prevents fluid entering the lower respiratory passages from the oropharynx. The cuff of the tube is released at set intervals to prevent pressure necrosis occurring in the walls of the trachea. When the cuff is reinflated care must be taken to use the specific volume of air. Before the cuff is deflated the oropharynx must be carefully cleared of fluid by means of suction. Neglect of this will result in fluid from the oropharynx passing down round the tube when the cuff is released and entering the lower respiratory passages.

The Negus tube (Fig. 15) is a very expensive silver tracheostomy tube which consists of the usual outer tube, inner tube and introducer, but also has an extra inner tube which has a valve in it. This is often called the 'speaking' tube, as its use allows the patient

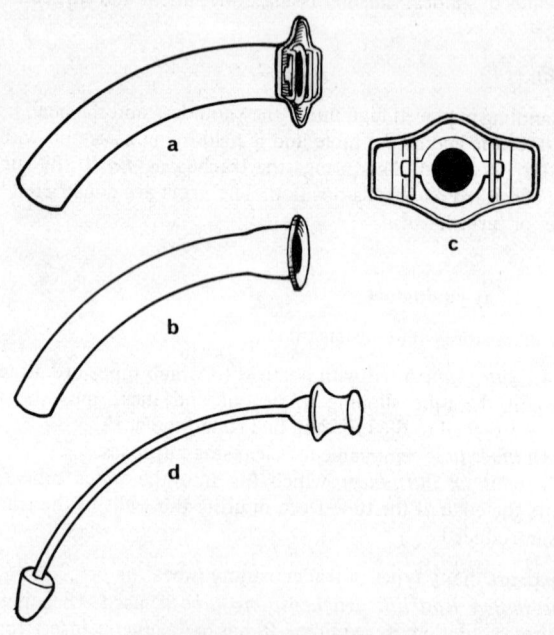

Fig. 15. The Negus tracheostomy tube.

to speak. The valve allows inhalation through the tube but expiration through the vocal cords, so that speech is made possible. During expiration the valve closes.

Parker's tube has a small clip to hold the inner tube in place similar to that of the Chevalier Jackson. The curve in the outer tube is less rounded than the Chevalier Jackson and to enable the inner tube to negotiate this rather acute angle of the outer tube there is a fenestration at its own point of greatest curvature.

The Chevalier Jackson tube consists of an outer tube, proportionately shorter and with a more rounded curve than that of the Durham tube, a pilot or introducer and an inner tube. There is a small clip on the shield of the outer tube and corresponding groove on the flange of the inner tube so that when the clip is turned the inner tube is secured and cannot be coughed out.

Durham's lobster-tailed tubes. The inner tube and pilot are jointed like a lobster's tail to allow them to pass round the acute

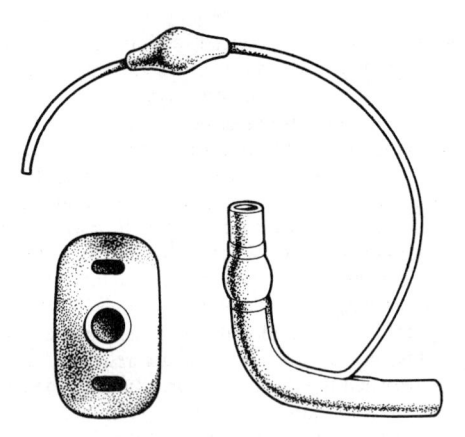

Fig. 16. A James' cuffed rubber tracheostomy tube.

curve in the outer tube. The shield of this tube is fixed with a screw so that its position along the outer tube can be adjusted by the surgeon to the individual patient. This lessens the danger of damage to the back wall of the trachea by pressure or scraping of the tube.

The last four tubes are hand-made of silver and are necessarily expensive. It is therefore vital to keep all parts of the set together as they are not interchangeable and to handle them gently while cleaning.

Later a silver tube may be replaced by a *Morant Baker rubber or plastic tube.*

Preoperative care in elective surgery

Psychological preparation of both patient and relatives is very important. They must be reassured that the artificial opening in the throat *will* make breathing much easier and a simple expalnation must be given about the equipment that will be seen around the bed following surgery. Many people are worried by the humidifier and the experienced nurse will show it to them and explain that it is basically like an electric kettle and it is used to moisten the air that is breathed in by the patient.

The physiotherapist will visit the patient and teach simple breathing exercises. At this time it is important to make sure that the patient knows that it is *not* necessary to breathe forcibly when a tracheostomy tube is in position as many patients tend to overventilate following surgery because they are afraid of the tube and feel that it is necessary to concentrate on their breathing. The patient can be greatly assured by having the opportunity to speak to a patient who has made a good recovery.

Normally the operation is performed under a general anaesthetic, but in some cases, such as when a neoplasm is present, the surgeon may wish to perform a tracheostomy under a local anaesthetic before the patient is given a general anaesthetic and is intubated. This is done if there is a risk that the growth may cause difficulty during intubation or if there is a risk of haemorrhage due to trauma to the growth. The incision is made in the midline below the Adam's apple; careful dissection is made and the trachea is not opened until the site is dry, otherwise blood and secretions may be aspirated into the trachea. The muscles of the neck are retracted and a hole is usually made between the third and fourth rings of the trachea. The isthmus of the thyroid gland can usually be moved up or down or divided. If the incision is made too high, there is danger that the obstruction might not be relieved and there is an increased risk of inflammation of the cricoid cartilage leading to stenosis. If the incision is made too low the innominate vessels may make the operation more difficult.

Equipment for after-care

1. Sterile set of tracheostomy tubes of the same size and type. Tapes already in position with pilot ready for emergency use.
2. Tracheal dilator.
3. Suction equipment ready for instant use.
4. Humidifier plugged in and primed with distilled water.

5. Pad and pencil so that the patient may make his needs known to the health care team.

6. Tissues for wiping away secretions.

7. Oxygen equipment. Oxygen is administered either via the humidifier or directly to the tracheostomy tube.

8. Container, such as a disposable bag, for the collection of soiled disposable articles.

Equipment for cleaning the inner tube:

1. Receiver.
2. Sodium bicarbonate powder.
3. Wire wool, to 'clean up' the tube.
4. Boiling water available.
5. Sterile distilled water.
6. Gloves to protect the nurse's hands.

Postoperative nursing care

The patient must be reassured that his 'voice box' has not been taken away and that he will be able to talk again, so an explanation must be given of why he cannot speak. If a Negus tube is in use the doctor will allow the use of the speaking tube as soon as the volume of secretions has lessened. Otherwise the patient must be taught to cover the entrance to the tube with his finger so that he can speak when breathing out.

Airway

The patient has probably already suffered the fear and distress of partial asphyxia and every effort must be made to ensure that he does not suffer in this way again. If the airway is unsatisfactory this may be due to any of the following.

A blockage in the inner tube. The inner tube must be removed frequently to prevent secretions building up in it. If this is done regularly it will not take long to keep the tube clean, and the patient is less likely to experience the fear caused by an obstruction to his tracheostomy tube. The inner tube is placed on a receiver, sodium bicarbonate powder is sprinkled on it and boiling water is poured over it. This causes the powder to effervesce and the secretions fall away easily and dissolve. The tube may then be rubbed with wire wool to remove any stubborn particles. The distilled water is used to rinse the tube and make sure that it is cool enough for reinsertion.

An obstruction below the level of the tube. The patient should be encouraged to cough, while steadying the tube against the neck. This is unlikely to be effective as the cough mechanism has been interfered with. A fine catheter, half the diameter of the inner lumen of the tracheostomy tube, is used for suction. When carrying out suction, either to clear the airway or prior to letting down the cuff of an East Radcliffe tube, great care must be taken not to damage the mucous membranes. A very effective technique is to use a Y-connection between the pressure tubing and the suction catheter. This allows the suction to be turned on prior to the introduction of the catheter and for suction to be created while withdrawing the catheter by closing off the open arm of the Y connection with the thumb. If the membranes are damaged bleeding will occur, a clot will form and mucus will 'stick' to it, so causing partial obstruction of the trachea. The catheter must be rinsed in sodium bicarbonate solution after use and a fresh sterile one must be used each time, using a no-touch technique and allowing suction to occur only as the tube is being withdrawn.

The physiotherapist will visit the patient frequently to encourage breathing exercises and if necessary to perform 'deep suction'.

It is essential that a cuffed tracheostomy tube is released for five minutes in every hour. If this is not done tracheal stenosis will result.

If the patient's airway appears to be obstructed and it cannot be cleared by means of suction, *medical aid must be obtained at once.* If the nurse suspects that the tracheostomy tube itself is the cause of the obstruction, it must be removed and tracheal dilators must be inserted to keep the trachea patent. The closed dilators are inserted into the trachea from the side, and the handles are then brought round towards the midline and up to a horizontal plane, so that the blades lie in the position previously occupied by the tube. Equipment must be available for the doctor to perform suction and if necessary carry out an examination with a laryngoscope so that he may detect any obstruction in the larynx. This must all be done quickly as the patient will asphyxiate rapidly. When the obstruction has been cleared a fresh sterile tracheostomy tube will be introduced by the doctor. However, obstruction is not likely to occur once the first routine tube change has been carried out by the doctor or specialist nurse.

OTHER POINTS IN NURSING CARE

Position. This will depend on the patient's condition. The upright position lessens the danger of chest complications. With an artificial positive pressure respirator in use, the flat position is usual, since it is likely that the patient will be unconscious.

Oxygen. This may be given by means of a mask over the tracheostomy tube or more commonly by means of the humidifier. In this way warm (about 40°C), moist air with an increased oxygen content is discharged into the air in the patient's immediate vicinity. The humidifier must be turned on before the patient's return from theatre in order to warm and moisten the air. Distilled water is used as the water in many areas is hard and this will rapidly 'fur up' the reservoir.

A steam tent may make respirations easier for some patients.

Communication. At first the patient must never be left without a bell and assurance that the nurse will always be where she can hear it, since he cannot call for help. He should be given a pad and pencil. The patient may be taught to place a finger over the tube when he wishes to talk, if a Negus speaking valve is not in use.

Dressings. These are renewed as necessary.

Feeding. This may present initial difficulties and the patient may have to be fed nasally. Normal feeding should be resumed as early as possible, the swallowing reflex being tested with sterile water. When the patient no longer chokes with this feeds are begun. He sometimes finds thickened fluids easier to manage than thin liquids.

Changing the outer tube. The doctor will change a silver tube after about five days, and a rubber tube during the first 24–48 hour postoperative period. After this an experienced trained nurse will change the inner tube.

Frequent mouthwashes will help to prevent septic material from being inhaled. Routine general nursing will be required.

Bathing. In many instances a patient with a tracheostomy may be 'up and about'. Such a patient should never be allowed to take a bath unattended; water should only be shallow. Should the patient slip when sitting in the bath the nurse must *immediately* pull out the plug as there is a very real risk of drowning.

CLOSURE AT THE END OF THE EMERGENCY

Decannulation is performed by inserting a cork with a wedge cut out of it into the tracheostomy tube. The size of the wedge is decreased until the patient is able to breathe easily when the tracheostomy tube is completely closed. The tube is then removed and the stoma will close. In this way the patient will gradually become accustomed to breathing normally through his own nose and will not be frightened by the sudden removal of the tracheostomy tube.

Alternatively a complete cork may be inserted (providing the patient is not too nervous) at intervals for 10 minutes every hour then two- or three-hourly until the patient is happy for it to be closed completely. Some patients (carefully selected) can tolerate the removal of the tube without corking, especially when they have been talking by covering the tube with a finger.

CARE FOLLOWING DISCHARGE

Patients and relatives care for the tubes and carry out the routine procedure as they were instructed in hospital. They are taught to change the whole tube so that if an obstruction occurs the necessary action can be taken. Usually they become very skilful and are able to handle the situation very well. Problems may arise in cold weather when the house is centrally heated as this may cause crusting which can be troublesome. They are advised to make sure that the air temperatures are not too high and that humidification is carried out by placing bowls of water near the radiators.

Complications

There may be:

Chest complications. These are more likely to arise if the patient has been a heavy smoker or if a chronic chest condition is present. Inhalation pneumonia could develop if foreign material entered the lower respiratory passages via the tracheostomy tube, or around it if a cuffed tube is deflated without the pharynx being cleared before the air has been released from the cuff.

Wound sepsis.

Surgical emphysema, i.e. air in the subcutaneous tissues due to obstruction and leakage round the tube. This causes rapidly spreading puffiness in the surrounding tissues which crackle like tissue paper when touched. The surgeon should be sent for and an attempt made to relieve the cause. The tube may not be fitting sufficiently snugly.

Stenosis of the stoma.

SURGERY OF THE HEAD AND NECK 157

LARYNGEAL OPERATIONS

Operations on the larynx include:

1. *Laryngeal fissure;* this is opening the larynx for removal of a localized malignant growth on the vocal cord.

2. *Lateral pharyngotomy*, which is performed in more severe cases to remove growths of the larynx, the pharynx being opened from the side of the neck to obtain access to the growth.

3. In very severe cases *total laryngectomy* is performed.

Some conditions are better treated either by introducing radium needles or by using a radium or cobalt bomb. Radiation may also be used after operation to prevent recurrences. Temporary tracheostomy may be performed, but this is avoided if possible because a tracheostomy carried out in the vicinity of a neoplasm may result in the grave possibility of tumour developing in the actual stoma of the tracheostomy.

Laryngeal Fissure

For laryngeal fissure the tracheostomy tube is left in for about 24 hours, using the suction apparatus freely to keep the air passages clear and lessen the risk of pneumonia. Systemic penicillin may be used today to prevent the onset of pneumonia and to treat it if it should occur. Other antibiotics may be used systemically for chest complications, in both prevention and cure. The patient is nursed sitting up and encouraged to cough. Nothing should be given by mouth for several hours, as the larynx is very insensitive; boiled water is used first, the patient leaning forward and taking small sips only. As the power of swallowing is regained, a varied, nourishing diet should be given. Thickened fluids are most easy to swallow, when food is first given by mouth. The patient should get up after two days and be ready to go home in seven to ten days.

Lateral Pharyngotomy

Lateral pharyngotomy should be preceded by removal of all teeth to lessen the risks of sepsis. A tracheostomy tube is inserted and a suction is employed to keep the air passage as clear as possible.

158 SURGICAL NURSING

Penicillin or other antibiotics, given systemically, protect the patient from chest complications. The tracheostomy tube is left in for about one week, as there is considerable inflammation. A feeding tube is introduced and left in position for about one week; it is then passed for feeds for another week. Care must be taken that it is not pulled out when the patient is regaining consciousness. Feeds of sterile water are given first, then nourishing fluids, 300–400 ml every four to six hours, preceded and followed by sterile water to cleanse the tube.

The wound is allowed to granulate up and must be dressed twice daily, more often if leakage or sloughing occurs. Oiled silk may be used to keep dressing from sticking and so lessen pain.

Total Laryngectomy

Preoperative preparation. The patient is generally in a dyspnoeic state and expectorates freely as a chest infection is usually present. Psychological care is again very important and is basically the same as that needed prior to a tracheostomy. The physiotherapist will teach the patient breathing exercises and the speech therapist will visit to introduce herself and to discuss the patient's future particularly the means of communicating with others in an effective manner. The surgeon may require a tomogram of the larynx to be performed because if there is infiltration into the surrounding tissues then a block dissection will also be necessary. A laryngectomy tube is very like a large Chevalier Jackson tracheostomy tube, but the set does not include an inner tube; this is because, since the stoma of the trachea has been brought up to the skin surface, the tube can safely be removed when it requires cleaning and there is rarely any difficulty about its reinsertion.

Postoperative care. The patient is nursed sitting up with the head well flexed to encourage sound healing. The chief danger is inhalation pneumonia and the suction pump, which is of great value, must be used frequently, together with humidification and oxygen as after a tracheostomy. Antibiotics are once again invaluable in the treatment of chest complications. The wound should be kept dry. Feeds are given, after the danger of vomiting has passed, by a feeding tube which is inserted at the time of operation and used for two weeks or more.

Sometimes a fistula develops due to saliva escaping out from the oesophagus through the wound onto the skin. This usually resolves

SURGERY OF THE HEAD AND NECK

when the patient takes solid food but plastic surgery may be necessary. The patient will be given some laryngectomy protectors, e.g. Buchanan, to wear round the neck. These are rather like a bib which is fastened round the neck, but has the appearance of a string vest. It has an upper layer of foam rubber and acts as a filter preventing foreign bodies from entering the stoma. The lower border is tucked into the clothes and looks very presentable. Some patients tend to develop a stenosis of the stoma so they are given a Portex tube which they insert into the stoma and wear at night; the same technique is used if viscous sputum is creating difficulties. Patients and their relatives rapidly become accustomed to the situation and within a short period following the patient's discharge develop a high degree of skill and confidence in carrying out laryngectomy care. They are all encouraged to regain a normal life as soon as possible.

The patient may be taught to swallow air and bring it up while changing the position of the lips, tongue and palate so that he can make sounds in spite of the loss of the vocal cords. With perseverance he will be able to make his wants known in this way; this method of talking is referred to as 'oesophageal speech' and the patient will need the help of a speech therapist, who should, if possible, visit him before operation. At present, new methods of speaking after laryngeal surgery are under investigation.

FOREIGN BODIES

Foreign bodies in the bronchial tree can be removed by bronchoscopy. The bronchoscope is a straight metal tube which is passed down the mouth and pharynx into the air passages under general anaesthesia, or after applying cocaine locally or other topical anaesthetic. It can be passed into the left or right bronchus and foreign objects can be picked out with special forceps, or suction can be used for the removal of a plug of thick secretion blocking a tube. The bronchoscope contains a light either at the near end with a mirror to reflect light down the tube or at the far end. If local anaesthesia is used, nothing should be given by mouth till sensation has returned, or the patient may choke; his first drink should be a spoonful of clear water.

10

Surgery of the Oesophagus

Common conditions affecting the oesophagus which may require surgical treatment are:

1. Obstruction due to carcinoma.
2. Hiatus hernia.
3. Obstruction due to spasm at the cardiac end of the oesophagus, termed cardiospasm.
4. Foreign bodies, such as false teeth, coins, safety-pins, children's toys or buttons.
5. Congenital lesions such as tracheo-oesophageal fistula.
6. Stricture due to scar contraction following burns by hot or caustic fluids such as strong acids or alkalis.
7. Obstruction from external pressure caused by such things as aortic aneurysm, bronchial carcinoma or enlarged mediastinal glands.
8. An oesophageal diverticulum or pouch.

Investigations

As in all other conditions an accurate history is important, also careful examination. The patient is watched actually taking food and fluids in order that the exact degree of dysphagia, or difficulty in swallowing, may be observed.

X-ray

A *barium swallow* gives valuable information in nearly all conditions. Special preparation is not essential, but the patient should have nothing to eat or drink for the preceding two hours. The patient, suitably dressed, is screened standing while actually swallowing the barium sulphate. This shows up strictures, dilatations, pouches and any abnormalities of peristalsis. In severe and chronic obstruction, when there has been ballooning of the oesophagus above the stricture, an oesophageal wash-out may be ordered prior to X-ray in order to free the oesophagus of stagnant food.

Oesophagoscopy

An oesophagoscope consists of a straight metal tube fitted with an electric bulb for lighting. Special forceps can be used with it for the removal of foreign bodies and an electric sucker must be at hand in order to prevent the aspiration of secretions into the lungs. The oesophagoscope has been described as the most dangerous foreign body that enters the oesophagus. For this reason it has to be handled with great care in order to avoid damage to the walls of the oesophagus. The patient is normally given a general anaesthetic and an intratracheal tube is passed. The patient's shoulders are brought to the end of the table and his occiput supported in a special head rest. Initially the head is slightly flexed on the neck and the neck on the trunk. The anaesthetist assists and the tube is carefully guided into the oesophagus. The head rest may then be lowered and the neck gently extended. At no time is any force used because of the danger of perforation.

Preparation. The patient is starved as for surgery and a premedication is given. Usually antibiotic cover is commenced, e.g. Ampliclox 250 mg twice daily and continued for five days. Nurses must make sure that the patient *really understands* why he must not eat or drink after the investigation.

After-care. On return from the X-ray department the patient is not allowed any fluids or food until a chest radiograph has been taken on the following morning. If the radiograph is satisfactory fluids are given and diet is recommenced. The antibiotic 'cover' is continued until the five-day course is completed. If perforation of the oesophagus has occurred, this will be recognized as the patient will complain of a very severe pain radiating round to the back of the chest and signs and symptoms of shock will be present. Rigidity of the upper abdominal muscles will also be seen. Surgical emphysema will develop in the supraclavicular region on the suprasternal notch. Crepitus in these situations is diagnostic of rupture into the respiratory passages. Air or fluid may appear in one or both pleural cavities.

If a perforation is diagnosed (following chest radiograph) a drain will be introduced into the pleural cavity to allow the lung to re-inflate. Oral fluids will be withheld and intravenous fluids will be administered to maintain the fluid and electrolytic balance. Chemotherapy will be continued and check radiographs will be taken. The surgeon will decide when fluids can be recommenced and this may be up to a period of ten days.

CARCINOMA OF THE OESOPHAGUS

Carcinoma of the oesophagus is not uncommon. It occurs chiefly in men between the ages of 50 and 70 years and is most commonly found in the middle and lower thirds of the oesophagus. This condition is also seen in females and is found in the postcricoid area of the oesophagus. There are few forms of malignant disease that cause greater misery and, although surgery still holds out poor hope of cure, it holds out good hope of palliation. These oesophageal operations have now largely superseded gastrostomy, the survival period after which was usually very short.

Signs and Symptoms

Dysphagia (*difficulty in swallowing*). The patient becomes aware of this gradually; first solids are difficult to swallow and as the tumour enlarges difficulty is experienced in swallowing fluids. Unfortunately dysphagia does not become obvious until late in the disease as the oesophagus is distensible so the food can get past the tumour. (In neglected cases, the patient cannot even swallow his own saliva. The patient can usually indicate with fair accuracy the level at which the fluids sticks.)

Weight loss. This becomes apparent when dysphagia occurs and is due to starvation.

Foul breath, due to arrest and decomposition of food in the oesophagus.

Cough, due to bronchial irritation.

Hiccough, due to phrenic irritation.

Boring pain between the scapulas is a late sign, indicating invasion of the surrounding tissues.

Hoarseness, also a late sign, indicating involvement of the recurrent laryngeal nerve, causing laryngeal palsy.

Surgical Treatment

Routine investigations are undertaken and in addition a bronchoscopy is always performed before operation to ascertain that the primary growth is not in the bronchus or that there is no infiltration, erosion or fistula formation.

The aim of the surgeon is to restore the ability to swallow. If removal of the growth is impossible, a short-circuit operation is devised. Multiple stage operations and antethoracic reconstructions are no longer attempted.

Growths in the upper third of the oesophagus and those behind the larynx are best treated by radiotherapy, especially as they are easily accessible and not buried in the thorax.

When the growth is in the middle third, the approach is usually by a right thoractotomy. When the growth is in the lower third, a thoracolumbar approach may be made. This gives freer access to the abdominal organs which may also be involved. The diaphragm can be divided and the stomach and intestine brought up into the thorax.

The treatment of choice is a *radical excision and restoration of continuity by oesophagogastrostomy*, the stomach first being mobilized and drawn up into the thorax as high up as may be necessary. Care is taken to see that the blood supply is preserved. The area excised usually includes the growth plus 3–4 cm of healthy oesophagus above it, below the fundus of the stomach and two-thirds of the lesser curvature and lymph drainage are excised. When the growth is high a loop of small intestine with a rich blood supply may have to be used in the thorax. When the growth is inoperable the oesophagus is mobilized and divided above the growth, the lower end is closed, and an anastomosis is carried out with the fundus of the stomach.

Preoperative care

Preoperatively the patient is given a high-calorie, high-protein diet for the preceding one to two weeks. This is because of the patient's general weight loss and poor level of nutrition. If a tube can be inserted past the tumour then the patient will be tube fed, otherwise the surgeon will have to insert an intravenous catheter into the patient's inferior vena cava and the patient will be fed parenterally using one of the intravenous solutions prepared for this purpose, such as Aminoplex 5 which is very useful as only one bottle is necessary, instead of the older combinations such as Intralipid, Vamin and dextrose/saline.

These operations have been made possible by the development of chemotherapy to combat sepsis, modern anaesthesia, transfusion and oxygen therapy.

Postoperative care

Postoperatively great care must be taken to get full expansion of the lung. The patient returns from the theatre with a drain in the pleural cavity attached to an underwater seal. Check X-rays are taken after operation and the drain removed 24–48 hours after operation, if the lung has expanded satisfactorily.

The patient, who has been trained before operation, is encouraged to cough and bring up his secretions two-hourly when awake. This will be painful, therefore he must be given analgesics and steam inhalations to loosen the secretions before the effort is made. He should be propped up comfortably with the sputum mug on the table in front of him and the nurse should support the operation site while he coughs. Antibiotics will be continued for about ten days.

Intravenous fluids are given and electrolytes in the blood are estimated. The balance is frequently disturbed after these operations. The oesophageal tube is aspirated and fluids are not given until the third day, then a test feed of sterile water is passed down it to make sure that the fluid flows on in the alimentary tract. If this is so then high-protein feeds are given and the intravenous infusion is discontinued. A barium swallow is carried out on the seventh to the tenth day and if the result is satisfactory then diet in a pureed form is commenced. The patient looks forward to drinking fluids naturally after removal of the oesophageal tube and eagerly anticipates being able to eat pureed food; this gives him enormous pleasure as it may not have been possible prior to surgery.

Complications of operation

Atelectasis. Bronchoscopy may be required to remove a plug of mucus which the patient is unable to cough up.

Atrial fibrillation may occur in frail elderly patients and be treated by digitalis.

Paralytic ileus is indicated by distension and absence of bowel sounds. This is treated by gastric aspiration and intravenous therapy. Some surgeons leave a Ryle's tube down after operation.

Pylorospasm after section of the vagi. This can be treated by a pastille of methacholine chloride sublingually. This is a parasympathetic stimulant.

Diarrhoea may be troublesome.

Leakage from the anastomosis is very serious and necessitates operation for repair, gastric aspiration, intravenous therapy and redrainage of the pleura.

Intubation

Although these operations are normally attempted today, occasionally only *palliative treatment* is possible in order to prevent starvation and pain.

Intubation is carried out through an oesophagoscope. A Mousseau-Barbin or a Celestin tube may be used. It has a wide mouth to prevent it slipping past the growth, but it sometimes does pass into the stomach and along the alimentary canal, causing no inconvenience.

Preoperative preparation

As the patient is unable to swallow food or fluids intravenous parenteral feeding has to be commenced. Mouth-washes are given to keep the mouth fresh; in addition an ample supply of tissues are provided as well as containers for the patient to dispose of his saliva. This is most distressing to the patient and the nurse must show great understanding. There is a danger of the patient inhaling saliva. Generally the preparation is the same as for routine surgery because an oesophagoscopy will have been carried out and the surgeon will know that the growth is not resectable.

Postoperative care

Once the patient's vital signs are stable he will be nursed sitting upright and intravenous fluids will be continued until bowel sounds are detected. Oral fluids will then be commenced and and a diet of pureed food will be introduced. 'Fizzy' drinks will be encouraged as these reduce the risk of the tube blocking. If it does block an attempt is made to clear it in the ward by giving diluted hydrogen peroxide (about half a tumbler) or other preparation: if this is unsuccessful an oesophagoscopy will have to be performed to overcome the obstruction. Following this large volumes of fluids are encouraged to flush it through. The patient will be discharged home to the care of relatives and the community health team. This operation is only palliative and it is unlikely that the patient will live for long.

Gastrostomy

Gastrostomy is the making of a permanent opening into the stomach through the abdominal wall so that the food may be introduced by catheter. This is also used as a temporary measure to allow local inflammation to subside.

HIATUS HERNIA

Following surgery, once the vital organs are normal, the patient will be nursed in an upright position. Fluids will be given intravenously and the oesophageal tube will be aspirated hourly. Once bowel sounds are heard oral fluids will be allowed and the oesophageal tube removed. A basal drain will have been inserted during surgery (because a thoracotomy has been performed) and this will be attached to an underwater drain in order to allow any drainage to escape. The chest will be X-rayed on the day following surgery and if the result is satisfactory the drain will be removed. Following this, routine care is given until the patient is home; recovery is usually uneventful.

CARDIOSPASM

Spasm of the muscle at the cardiac end of the oesophagus causes difficulty in swallowing and regurgitation of food; never having entered the stomach, this food will be unmixed with acid gastric juice. The oesophagus becomes very dilated above the site of stricture. This accounts for 20% of cases of intrinsic dysphagia. The onset is usually insidious, coming on early in adult life and affecting rather more women than men. The cause is unknown, but is thought to be associated with emotional disturbances. There is frequently such a history, but many of these patients appear very well balanced despite their distressing disability. At first only solids are held up and these will pass with the help of a drink when a sufficient head of pressure has been built up. Pain may occur early in the disease, but disappears later. Nutrition is impaired and vitamin deficiencies may occur. Pulmonary complications are caused by the spilling over of fragments from the oesophagus during sleep.

Treatment by mercury-filled bougies is seldom given today as they make any form of social life too difficult for the patient.

If diagnosed early oesophageal wash-outs may be ordered and a *Negus hydrostatic bag* introduced through an oesophagoscope. The bag is filled and exerts pressure so that the contracted circular muscles are evenly and fully dilated. This often gives permament relief.

For more advanced cases *Heller's operation* gives good results. A left posterolateral intercostal incision is made, the oesophagus is exposed and the longitudinal and circular muscle coats cut with a knife until the mucosa appears; but great care is taken not to injure this. The incision is extended over the lower 8 cm of the oesophagus and the upper 5 cm of the fundus. The chest is usually closed without drainage. Fluids are given for 24 hours, then soft solids, and soon the patient will be able to take a normal diet. In principle this operation is very similar to Rammstedt's operation used to relieve congenital pyloric stenois in babies.

FOREIGN BODIES

These are removed by means of direct vision using an oesophagoscope and special forceps or coin catchers. It may be necessary to break up the object, e.g. a set of false teeth, in order to prevent damage to the wall. Postoperatively the patient is given the same care as is practised following a diagnostic oesophagoscopy.

CONGENITAL LESIONS: TRACHEO-OESOPHAGEAL FISTULA

Both trachea and oesophagus are derived from the primitive foregut which divides into two tubes. Occasionally, in one in 2500 births, this division is incomplete. It is the commonest cause of blueness and choking in the newborn, after the fauces have been cleared out for the first time. The condition is incompatible with life, but can be

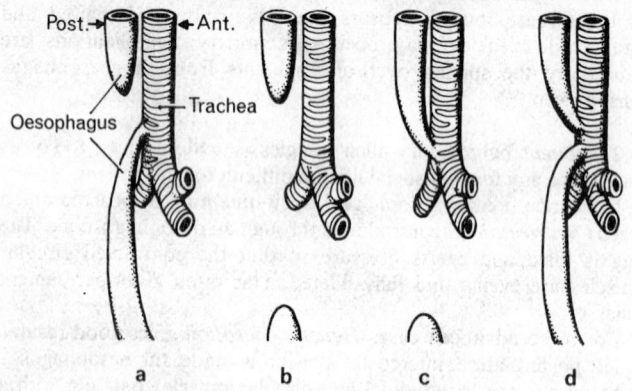

FIG. 17. Varieties of congenital tracheo-oesophageal fistula. Type *a* accounts for 80% of cases. The next commonest is type *b*, in which the gap between the oesophageal segments is so great that they cannot be brought together.

treated surgically. Success depends on prompt diagnosis. Each feed makes survival less likely. The commonest abnormality is that the upper end of the oesophagus makes a blind pouch which fills up and spills over into the trachea. The lower end of the oesophagus forms a fistula into the trachea.

Recurrence of cyanosis, frothing and choking once the fauces have been cleared should raise the question in the midwife's mind. The condition can be diagnosed by the doctor when he passes a soft, well-lubricated catheter into the mouth and down the gullet. If it stops 10 cm from the lips, atresia is almost certain.

No feeds should be given and the fauces kept aspirated. Subcutaneous fluids are given and antibiotics. Repair and closure of the fistula is usually possible. Postoperatively the baby is nursed in an oxygen tent. The main care is to keep the lungs dry by frequent suction of the fauces. If all goes well feeds can be started the third day after operation.

STRICTURE

Stricture due to scar contracture may be relieved by the passing of *bougies*, provided that the treatment is started early. As with passing the oesophagoscope care must be taken not to damage the oesophageal walls, which might result in sepsis in the mediastinum or surgical emphysema, if the trachea is involved.

In severe cases *temporary gastrostomy* may be necessary. This often permits inflammation to subside and makes the subsequent passage of bougies possible. In other cases the passage of a bougie from the gastrostomy opening may be easier than in the other direction.

OBSTRUCTION DUE TO EXTERNAL PRESSURE

Obstruction of this kind may be due to such things as aortic aneurysm, bronchial carcinoma, and enlarged mediastinal glands. If the obstruction is due to inoperable bronchial carcinoma, treatment by means of radiotherapy often results in the mass 'shrinking' in size and this relieves the pressure on the oesophagus.

DIVERTICULUM OF THE OESOPHAGUS

Oesophageal diverticulum usually occurs on the posterior wall. The pouch fills on swallowing, causing discomfort after a meal which is not relieved until the pouch is emptied by 'vomiting'. The condition can be treated by excision.

11

Thoracic Surgery

Enormous advances have been made in thoracic surgery in the last twenty years thanks to new techniques of anaesthesia which make it possible to open the thoracic cavity and yet maintain normal respiration and circulation. Advances in chemotherapy, transfusion and oxygen administration have also helped.

A lateral incision, thoracotomy, gives access to the lungs and pleura, the heart, the great vessels and the oesophagus.

Pulmonary condition now treated by surgery include:

1. Bronchial carcinoma.
2. Bronchiectasis.
3. Abscess of the lung.
4. Compound and complicated fractures of the ribs.
5. The presence of foreign bodies in the bronchial tree.
6. Pulmonary tuberculosis.
7. Sucking wounds of chest, which occur when air is sucked into the chest through a wound but cannot escape, and so collects under pressure and therefore displaces and disorganizes the action of heart and lungs.
8. Empyema.
9. Spontaneous pneumothorax.

Diagnosis

Some of the diagnostic procedures used are:

1. Chest X-ray, including mass miniature X-ray and tomography.

2. Bronchography.
3. Bronchoscopy.
4. Examination of sputum.
5. Examination of pleural fluid.
6. Erythrocyte sedimentation rate (ESR).
7. Respiratory function tests.

Preparation for Major Chest Operations

The preparation necessary is that for major operations anywhere in the body, but the following need special emphasis.

Respiratory function. This must be estimated before permanent collapse or removal of part of a lung. This is done by clinical observation of effort tolerance and by such tests as the forced expiratory volume in one second (FEV_1) and the vital capacity (VC). Using these tests the type of respiratory spasm can be identified. The degree of exhaustion caused by such effort as climbing stairs is a good indication of respiratory efficiency. The majority of patients with only limited respiratory disease have relatively little respiratory impairment, others suffer from severe disability especially where there is concurrent bronchitis or bronchiectasis. A nurse can give valuable help from her observation of the patient as he moves about during normal ward activities.

Breathing exercises. These improve respiratory efficiency. Although breathing is normally reflex in character the respiratory muscles are voluntary and can be brought under voluntary control. The patient is taught to breathe in fully and deeply and also to hold his breath while pulling his stomach in; he practises short sharp expiratory diaphragmatic movements that will be useful in helping to get rid of post-anaesthetic mucoid secretions. A futile persistent cough is discouraged and he is taught to cough only to bring up and expectorate secretions.

The patient is instructed on the importance of moving about the bed and especially mobility of limbs, in order to prevent circulatory disorders.

The skilled physiotherapist plays an important part in preparing the patient for operation and in his postoperative recovery. The nursing staff must reinforce her teaching and cooperate with her at all stages.

172 SURGICAL NURSING

Good posture. The patient is warned about faults that are liable to arise, such as scoliosis produced by leaning sideways towards the operated side and failing to keep the shoulders level, and is told how he can help to prevent them. Even very ill patients are able to cooperate in maintaining good posture and this also improves respiratory efficiency.

Shoulder, limb and abdominal exercises are also taught; the less muscle wasting that occurs the shorter the convalescence and the better the circulation, and these exercises must be taught in the preoperative period.

Oral sepsis and infection of the upper respiratory tract. This must be eliminated as far as possible.

Blood count and haemoglobin level. These should be estimated; anaemia will increase dyspnoea and must be treated prior to surgery. The blood is grouped and cross-matched.

Diet. A high-calorie diet should be given with adequate protein and 400 mg ascorbic acid a day to encourage healing. At least 2 litres of fluid should be taken daily. This will help to keep the secretions liquid so that they are easily coughed up.

Sputum. The character and quantity of sputum should be carefully observed so that it can be compared with the sputum produced postoperatively.

Drugs. Antibiotics such as ampicillin 250 mg or cloxacillin 250 mg may be prescribed and administered six-hourly. Sometimes other antibiotics are given instead depending upon sensitivity tests.

Other treatment. Many patients requiring chest surgery have neoplastic conditions and the nurse must therefore be prepared to give a great deal of psychological support to both the patients and their relatives.

Communication. All members of staff must reassure the patients and make sure that they really understand what is and what will be happening to them. This is most important, since the patient will already be anxious and confused by all the strange events and in many cases will have difficulty in 'taking things in'.

Preparations for the Patient's Return to the Ward

While the patient is in the theatre everything is prepared for the patient's return.

THORACIC SURGERY 173

The bed should be prepared freshly, with a back rest and five or six firm, but not hard, pillows. Two are placed horizontally and then two, with plastic covers, are placed vertically with a slight space in the near centre to accommodate the chest drain. There should be a softer pillow for the head, which must not be made to poke forward as this will give the patient a stiff neck which he is likely to attribute to a draught. An armchair arrangement of pillows must never be used, as this encourages deformity of the lumbar spine. A foot rest will help the patient to maintain a good position and reins attached to the foot of the bed will encourage early movement. A draw sheet and an air ring will be required. A cradle may be necessary. A transfusion pole, oxygen carrier and an underwater seal carrier should be attached to the bed if available.

Other accessories which should be prepared are an underwater seal bottle and two effective clamps. The Winchester bottle, tubing and rubber bung can be sterilized by superheated steam in an autoclave apparatus, by boiling or by dry heat. 500 ml of sterile normal saline or water are placed in the graduated bottle. If these are not used then the surface level is marked with strapping. This makes it easy to assess quickly the amount of discharge from the drain. The tube attached to the drain in the chest wall must penetrate below the surface of the fluid. The patient will return with either one or two drains, one from the apex of the pleural space to

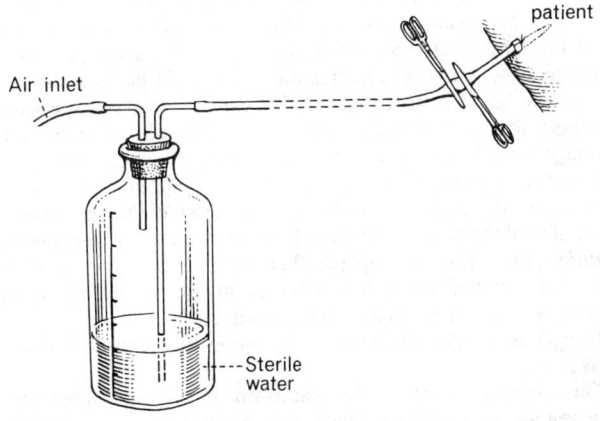

FIG. 18. A closed chest drainage bottle or water-seal drainage bottle. The long tube, ending below water level, must be attached to the patient.

allow for draining of air from the cut surface of the lung tissue and one from the base to collect any blood or serum. Both are attached to the underwater seal. There must be a sufficient length of tubing between the patient and the drainage bottle to permit reasonable movement of the patient without dragging on the stitches holding the chest drains in position; the walls of the tubing should be sufficiently rigid to prevent easy compression of the lumen, e.g. by the weight of bedclothes. The negative pressure within the chest makes the fluid rise in the tube and swing with respiration, rising higher on inspiration when negative pressure is greater and falling on expiration. If the open end is attached to a suction pump the swing will diminish or cease. The bottle must never be raised to the level of the patient's body or there is danger that fluid from the bottle may be aspirated into the pleural cavity. In order to work efficiently, the bung and all glass connections must fit securely. Two clamps must always be immediately available. These are clamped on the drain before the bottle and tubing are changed (after 24 hours). If an accident occurs, such as the bottle being knocked over and the cork dislodged, they must immediately be applied to prevent air aspiration. Disposable tops and tubes are also available, only the graduated bottle being re-usable, after sterilization. Draining is seldom required for more than 48 hours. Clotting in the tube can be prevented by regular 'milking'.

Care must be taken to prevent an air leak into the pleural cavity on removal of the drain. The intercostal drainage tubes are removed gradually, depending upon the doctor's orders, which are based upon the fluid levels seen when the chest is X-rayed. He usually states by how many centimetres the tube should be shortened and this could be from 1 to 5 cm. Following surgery, experienced members of the staff may gently rotate the tube to prevent the drainage hole being closed off as the lung expands and routine observation is made of the oscillation of the fluid in the tube of the underwater drainage bottle. This is done by digital pressure on either side of the drain wound until the skin suture has been tied and a *tulle gras* dressing applied. The *tulle gras* is removed the following day and the stitch at the drain site on the eighth day. Wound sutures are taken out on the tenth day.

Oxygen is usually administered by means of a well-fitting plastic mask.

The *sputum carton* will be placed on the patient's table within easy reach. The table is placed on the operated side so that the patient is encouraged to move that arm and shoulder from the first.

An *electric suction apparatus* must be available. Blocks may be required for the foot of the bed. Sphygmomanometer, stethoscope and pulse and respiration charts must be prepared.

Postoperative Nursing Care

The anaesthetist will not allow the patient to return to the ward until he is satisfied that consciousness has returned, as neither cardiac nor respiratory arrest can be treated efficiently during transport back to the ward. Before the patient leaves the theatre bronchoscopy is performed and blood and secretions are aspirated from the bronchial tree.

When the patient first returns to the ward, the pulse and respirations are taken quarter-hourly for the first three or four hours. The blood pressure is taken half-hourly for the first two hours or until it has reached a satisfactory level. An intravenous infusion will be running and this must be checked. Elderly emphysematous patients are usually given oxygen, as anoxia tends to produce mental disturbance and increase the difficulty of the postoperative period, otherwise oxygen is not normally required after consciousness has returned. The drainage must be watched for fluctuation, colour, consistency and quantity; the tube is milked as required and clamps are always available. More than 300 ml drainage in the first six hours should be reported.

Restoration of normal respiration. The principal aim postoperatively is to restore normal respiration, full aeration of the lung, and full mobility of the chest wall and so prevent atelectasis or collapse of the lung. This condition can be produced either by a plug of mucus becoming lodged in a bronchus, the air beyond being absorbed and the secretions stagnating, or by compression of the lung by air, blood and serum accumulating in the pleural space. This condition is most likely to arise within the first 48 hours. In order to prevent it the following measures are most important.

The patient must carry out *regular breathing exercises two-hourly* when awake and the nurses should be taught by the physiotherapist how to carry out the basic exercises. Postural drainage will help secretions to drain towards the hilum of the lungs where the cough reflex operates and away from the periphery which is insensitive. The physiotherapist, under medical supervision, shows the nurse the required position for postural drainage. This is usually lying on the good side with a pillow beneath the chest, the shoulder and hip being in contact with the bed. The patient is asked to breath out, cough and expectorate before he breathes in; this prevents plugs of mucus being inhaled further, which might occur if the patient took a deep breath in first. This will be painful, therefore *the wound must be supported* by the physiotherapist or nurse while coughing efforts are made and the drain must not be allowed to drag.

Shoulder exercises on the involved side are also encouraged.

Doctors often prescribe an expectorant such as carbocisteine 10 ml to be administered six-hourly. Steam inhalations containing tincture of benzoin also give a great deal of relief to the patient and are very useful if given prior to the visit of the physiotherapist.

Analgesics such as omnopon 10–15 mg or morphine 10–15 mg four-hourly are essential. Usually after three to four days two Distalgesic tablets may be prescribed instead. These must be timed in relation to periods of postural drainage; when sufficient to control pain, they tend to depress the cough reflex, therefore it must be impressed on the patient that he must make the effort to cough and expectorate, even though he does not feel the need to do so.

Patients in a very weak condition may have a *tracheostomy* performed so that suction can be applied to the respiratory tract if they are unable to bring up their own secretions.

Although this part of the treatment is vital, every effort should be made to see that the patient is not unduly exhausted, nor woken up. When the physiotherapist is supervising postural drainage the nurse should give whatever other nursing care is needed, e.g. to pressure areas, and thus prevent additional disturbances to the patient.

Atelectasis usually manifests itself by increased respiratory embarrassment. When it has been diagnosed the physiotherapist will encourage the patient to cough, then he will be nursed in a lateral position with the affected lung uppermost. One pillow will be placed beneath the chest wall and two beneath the head. This will encourage the collapsed area to re-expand. Percussion is not carried out after a thoracotomy and a bronchoscopy is only performed if these measures fail.

Haemorrhage or effusion. If the drainage is working satisfactorily *haemorrhage* and *effusion* should be immediately apparent and will be treated by morphine and transfusion if necessary. When the lung has re-expanded oscillation in the tube ceases, the drain can then be removed if the daily postoperative check X-ray is satisfactory. Should haemorrhage or effusion occur after removal of the drain, pulse and respiration will deteriorate due to mediastinal shift. This can usually be recognized by the altered position of the apex beat. Aspiration is necessary without delay and the reintroduction of a drain may be required.

Correct posture must be maintained from the first, but great tact should be used so that the patient does not feel that he is being nagged. He should sit, well-supported by pillows, in the centre of the bed, in the centre of his ring, both anterior superior iliac spines should be equally prominent, the shoulders level and in alignment with the hips, and the ears level and in alignment with shoulders. After the patient has sufficiently recovered, a mirror placed at the foot of the bed periodically is a great help. When the position has to be corrected the patient should be asked to move the good side; thus if the shoulder on the operated side is drooping he is asked to pull down the other one. Great care is taken to make sure the patient has a good posture and he may be taken to the gymnasium for exercises as he recovers.

Movements are generally encouraged, helped by the reins at the foot of the bed. Full dorsiflexion of the feet is important. Shoulder movements on the operated side must be practised and after the first few days the patient should be asked to hold his hands above his head while the bed is being tidied. Combing the back of the hair is also a good exercise. Walking is commenced as soon as the tubes are out and after two to three days the physiotherapist will encourage the patient to start walking up and down stairs. If the patient's general condition is satisfactory he may be allowed up out of bed into a chair on the second postoperative day. While this is being done care is taken to keep the drainage bottle below the level of the patient's chest and to make sure that drainage continues at all times. An added safety precaution is to make sure that all connections are secure to ensure that air does not enter the patient's chest by means of the drain.

The patient is supported by pillows in such a way as to avoid pressure on the tube and to minimize discomfort. It is only necessary to clamp the tube if there is a risk of air or water entering the thorax and with care and forethought this should not happen. Blockage of the tube is avoided by milking the tube and so causing semi-solid material to pass down into the bottle. The surgeon usually asks the nurse to connect low-pressure suction to the bottle and this helps to prevent the drain blocking.

After pneumonectomy the patient is nursed lying on the operated side with the head low until blood pressure has returned to normal. There is a clamped basal drain which is released for five minutes in every hour. Continuous drainage is not allowed as a certain amount of pressure must be present to prevent mediastinal shift occurring. During surgery a blood transfusion will have been administered and may still be in progress when the patient returns to the ward. A central venous pressure line may also be in position so that early signs of shock or over-transfusion can be noted.

Complications

Bronchopleural fistula was a common complication in the early days of thoracic surgery, especially after pneumonectomy. It was usually due to tuberculous invasion of the bronchial stump. It is much rarer today, but the patient should be told that if he suddenly coughs up much fluid sputum (it will be serum stained brown from changed blood) he must immediately lie on his operated side with the good side uppermost. This will prevent secretions from the dead space flooding the good bronchus. The fluid will have to be aspirated and the chest reopened to repair the fistula, unless it is a very small one. Surgeons today may use muscle grafts to try to prevent this complication.

Tension pneumothorax may occur as the result of leakage from the cut surface of the lung, thus allowing a sufficient pressure of air to build up in the pleural cavity and so collapse the underlying lung. This is usually prevented by the apical drain. Tension pneumothorax is another cause of mediastinal shift leading to circulatory and respiratory failure, cyanosis, faintness and mental confusion. A new apical drain must be inserted immediately. In an emergency an intramuscular needle and rubber tubing to an underwater seal will relieve the condition. Cardiac stimulants may be required. A bronchopleural fistula can also cause this condition if it acts as a valve allowing air to pass in but not out. Aspiration of fluid or air from the chest cavity and resuture of the bronchus will be necessary.

Paradoxical respiration readily occurs after thoracoplasty. The flail portion of the chest, from which the ribs, the firm structures of the chest wall, have been removed, is sucked in during inspiration and blown out during expiration. This means that air, instead of passing in and out, is passing from the lung on one side to the other lung, the patient gets insufficient oxygen, and disease is disseminated. Firm pressure over the flail area and encouragement of diaphragmatic breathing will help to correct it. As atelectasis can accompany paradoxical respirations coughing up secretions must continue.

Irregularities of the pulse may develop, especially in the elderly, and require treatment by quinidine or digitalis.

Bronchial spasm may occur after lobectomy or thoracoplasty, but will usually respond to 0·5 ml adrenaline 1:1000 hypodermically.

PULMONARY TUBERCULOSIS

Antituberculosis drugs like streptomycin, *para*-aminosalicylic acid and isoniazid have transformed the treatment and prognosis in pulmonary tuberculosis in recent years and represent one of the great medical advances in history. Today any type of surgery for pulmonary tuberculosis is extremely rare; many patients can be satisfactorily treated along medical lines in their own homes without admission to sanatoria (now usually referred to as chest hospitals).

Types of Operation

Chest operations for tuberculosis could be divided into two big groups:

Group A. Those in which localized disease was removed by *pulmonary resection*. Today these are the commonest operations, and their aim is usually to render a patient (who had a persistent cavity) non-infectious. In order of severity they are:

1. *Wedge resection* or local excision is the excision of a small superficial tuberculous lesion, usually a solid one, between clamps. The edges of the lung are then oversewn.
2. *Segmental resection* is the removal of a section or portion of a lobe by formal dissection of its pulmonary artery, vein and bronchus. This type of operation is most commonly used for apical lesions.

3. *Lobectomy* is the removal of the lobe of a lung.
4. *Pneumonectomy* is the removal of the whole lung.
5. *Pleuropneumonectomy* is the resection of the lung in the parietal pleura through the tissues outside them. It involves considerable blood loss and shock.

Group B. Those operations designed to *relax the diseased lung* so that it might heal by natural processes. However modern treatment has rendered these operations almost obsolete. They included:

1. Artificial pneumothorax.
2. Pneumoperitoneum.
3. Adhesion section.
4. Phrenic crush.
5. Thoracoplasty.

BRONCHIAL CARCINOMA

The great increase in the incidence of bronchial carcinoma has made it one of the major social problems of the time. It has replaced tuberculosis as the commonest serious lung disease, especially in men over 40 years old. It is now the commonest form of cancer in the country, and over 80% of the patients are men, but the proportion of women affected shows signs of rising. Between 1901 and 1910 the death rate per million living was 10·2; between 1950 and 1954 it was 335·6 and the increase continued. The incidence is higher in the cities than in the country, the death rate in London being twice that in rural districts. Everywhere the rise has closely followed the consumption of cigarettes, but the carcinogens they contain require some 20 years to have their effect. Numerous research surveys have been carried out, all producing strikingly similar results. Above the age of 45, the risk of contracting carcinoma of the bronchus increases in simple proportion to the amount of cigarettes smoked and the duration of the habit. Women are about 30 years behind men in smoking habits, which probably accounts for the smaller incidence among them so far.

Metastases

Carcinoma of the bronchus spreads via lymph channels, blood stream and air passages. By the lymph channels it spreads first to

THORACIC SURGERY 181

the mediastinal glands; by the pulmonary veins it passes most frequently to the brain and liver; by the air passages it is usually scattered distally.

Signs and Symptoms

Two out of three patients who come to the thoracic surgeon at present are inoperable. Delay in seeking advice and in making a diagnosis is all the more tragic, as with early diagnosis and a prompt operation many patients with cancer of the lung can be cured. Mass X-ray is proving valuable in picking up a number of early cases.

Cough is the first sign, but many of these patients have a 'winter' or 'smoker's' cough anyway. If a 'winter' cough persists into summer, or if the cough changes its nature, that is an unproductive cough suddenly becomes productive, or if sputum suddenly ceases, then future investigations and X-ray should be advised.

Haemoptysis may occur and is helpful in that it may bring the patient to the doctor in time for an operation to be successful.

Breathlessness will occur, but again many men of cancer age are already emphysematous.

Pain from the pleura as a result of segmental or lobar collapse is not necessarily a late symptom as in other forms of cancer.

Pleural effusion will probably be present.

Loss of weight is always serious.

Loss of appetite usually indicates the presence of secondary deposits in the liver.

A febrile illness may occur, which the patient calls a 'touch of 'flu'.

Treatment

Resection of the lung. Once the diagnosis is made resection of the lung, or a portion of it, is the treatment of choice. Nursing care is as described previously. Assessment must be made as to whether the patient can tolerate pneumonectomy, if that is required. A bronchial blocker gives a useful indication as to whether the patient will tolerate the operation.

Deep X-ray therapy has considerable palliative value, but it is not used routinely before or after operation, because so used it adds nothing to a patient's expectation of life and greatly adds to his discomfort. A full course will cause as much physical disturbance as surgery; it is therefore not a milder or more conservative substitute for surgery. It is valuable where there is pain due to invasion of the chest wall, or metastases in bone, where there is mediastinal obstruction, or difficulty in swallowing, or when the cough is exhausting. It is contraindicated when the growth has already disseminated, except in the conditions mentioned; when the growth is adenocarcinoma, which is insensitive to X-rays; when sepsis is present in the lung; or when the patient is too breathless from emphysema.

Palliation. As in all malignant disease something can be done to relieve symptoms and prolong a tolerable life. Patients can be taught to live with inoperable cancer. The surgeon will determine the best management of the patient; it is important that his teaching is supported by the nurses. Experienced doctors (and nurses) are unable to agree as to whether patients should be told the truth when they are suffering from carcinomatous conditions. This condition may be described as a partial obstruction or chronic infection for which excellent treatment is available. There is no drug so valuable as hope. Intractable pain may sometimes be treated by intercostal neurectomy, recurrent pleural effusion by radioactive gold and infection by antibiotics. Cortisone is sometimes valuable in the terminal phase. The patient shows subjective improvement and gains weight. Codeine and phenacetin are often the most effective analgesics and finally the Brompton 'cocktail' of morphine, cocaine and gin may greatly increase the patient's comfort. The dose varies considerably.

BRONCHIECTASIS

Bronchiectasis occurs commonly in infancy or youth, but it may not be manifest until later on when complicated by chronic bronchitis and emphysema. When the bronchus is obstructed from any cause, mucus secreted from the glands beyond the blockage is dammed up in the collapsed lobe or segment and passively distends the bronchi. When the obstruction is relieved the mucus escapes and the lung returns to normal. If the obstruction continues, the stagnant mucus soon becomes infected and turns to pus, the mucosa is ulcerated and the submucous layer inflamed. A fibrous reaction occurs with healing and the bronchial walls are weakened, eroded and distended. Once the damage is done it is permanent and the only cure is by surgical excision. All other forms of treatment are purely palliative. Clinical bronchiectasis is thus caused firstly by collapse and secondly by infection. *In children* it is usually caused by primary tuberculosis, producing enlargement of the hilar glands and so collapsing a bronchus. Enlargement of these glands also occurs during measles and whooping cough and bronchiectasis can complicate both of these diseases. Children with bronchiectasis are usually mouth-breathers, undersized and apathetic. They have a chronic productive cough and mucopurulent sputum; this is worst in the morning and makes their breath foul. Sinuses are frequently infected and a vicious circle is set up, the sinus condition lighting up that in the chest and *vice versa*. Metastatic cerebral abscesses can also occur.

In adults a neoplasm or a plug of mucus, possibly postoperatively, are common causes of bronchiectasis.

Diagnosis is made by bronchography.

Treatment

The treatment of choice is surgical excision if the disease is localized and the remainder of the lung healthy.

In patients over 40 years the condition is often complicated by chronic bronchitis and emphysema, so that they may be unable to tolerate the loss of any lung tissue even though diseased. If, however, the diseased portion is only a bag of pus, the redirection of the blood stream after operation will help them.

Palliative treatment. Postural drainage is given twice a day for 20 minutes. This means placing the patient in such a position that the secretions in the diseased portion of the lung can drain towards the hilum. The patient can then cough them up easily. Percussion by the physiotherapist helps to relax the bronchial muscles and assists drainage. Forced coughing also helps drainage by wringing out the lungs like a sponge. Sputum is measured or weighed. Infection of the upper respiratory tract and nasal deformity is treated. Antibiotics are used to treat acute exacerbations and aerosol inhalations are used.

Surgery is planned for the best time as regards weather and the patient's health. These patients are often better in spring and summer than in winter. They must have had a course of palliative treatment so that their general health has been improved and sputum reduced to a minimum.

Resection is carried out as in other lung conditions, the main complication being collapse of the remaining lobe segments on the operated side. Bronchoscopic aspiration must be carried out as soon as possible should this occur.

ABSCESS OF THE LUNG

Abscess is often caused by malignant obstruction or by the inhalation of material from a septic embolus while the patient is unconscious as the result of anaesthesia, trauma, drugs or alcohol and the cough reflex is depressed. It can occur during operations on the upper respiratory tract and patients with septic teeth are particularly liable to inhale flakes of infected tartar which subsequently lead to abscess formation. Inhalation of any foreign body capable of blocking an air tube can lead to formation of an abscess. In the USA accidental inhalation of a peanut, followed by abscess formation, is not uncommon. The amount of septic material determines the size of the bronchus blocked. It is usually a segmental or a subsegmental one. There is a latent period in which the abscess develops, then the patient may have a rigor and then a swinging pyrexia. He will probably have a pleural pain, look toxic, have a brown coated tongue and a foul taste in the mouth. The abscess usually ruptures into the bronchus and the patient coughs up foul stinking pus.

Complications

1. The abscess can rupture through the pleura and produce an empyema.
2. The abscess can spread by septic bronchial emboli and produce chronic suppurative pneumonitis.

Treatment

Antibiotics have transformed treatment. These abscesses now usually respond to conservative measures and open drainage is seldom necessary. The sputum is examined for causal organisms and their sensitivity, and a suitable antibiotic is ordered. *Bronchoscopy* is performed to determine involved segments of the bronchus, and slough and debris which may interefere with drainage are removed. *Postural drainage* is started as soon as the anatomical position of the abscess is known. Frequent X-rays are taken to assess progress. Cessation of drainage cells for another bronchoscopy. If conservative measures fail, *resection* of the involved lobe or segment may be necessary.

The condition of the teeth and upper respiratory passages should be checked. Frequent mouth-washes will be necessary and every effort should be made to improve the patient's general health.

COMPOUND COMPLICATED FRACTURES

Compound fractures are given normal wound toilet, but the techniques for thoracic surgery may be required. Haemothorax may have to be aspirated from the chest cavity and drainage established and secretions sucked out from the lungs by bronchoscope.

FOREIGN BODIES IN THE LUNGS

Foreign bodies, such as peanuts, small parts from toys, small screws, fish bones, chicken bones etc., usually enter the right bronchus, which is the larger and in a more direct line with the trachea. They can be removed by special forceps, through a bronchoscope. Occasionally open operation is necessary.

SPONTANEOUS PNEUMOTHORAX

This condition is treated by pleurodesis, carried out with a thoracoscope. Once it is in position, sterile iodized talc is puffed through it into the area involved. This causes a local reaction, rather like pleurisy, which sticks together the pleural layers.

12

Surgery of the Heart and Great Vessels

Surgery of the heart and great blood bessels is a field in which advances are being made all the time and operations frequently performed last year have been superseded by others, which give better results. On account of much publicity surrounding this branch of surgery many rather extravagant hopes are held by patients and their relatives as to what can be achieved. The heart and great vessels tolerate surgery well, but can seldom be restored to normal. There is, however, every reason to hope, as many conditions can be very greatly helped. These include:

1. Ischaemic heart disease increasing in frequency.
2. Valvular lesions due to acute rheumatism or calcium deposits.
3. Congenital defects. The incidence of these conditions may be reduced in the future due to the termination of abnormal pregnancies.
4. Constrictive pericarditis.
5. Wounds. These are unusual but may be due to stab injuries to the heart.

Success depends on good teamwork and the nurse can do much to create conditions which make this possible. The patient may be admitted to hospital some weeks prior to surgery. During this time investigations are made and the condition of the heart and the general health are, if possible, improved. The patient has the opportunity to get to know and acquire confidence in the various members of the team. The nurse should take every opportunity to observe the patient carefully and to build up his confidence. Her reports may help the surgeon to determine the most suitable form of

Echocardiography. Ultrasonic waves are 'bounced' on to the heart and they are picked up by a microphone. A graph is produced which helps to diagnose cardiac diseases such as septal defects.

Screening for sepsis is carried out as soon as the patient is admitted and may involve nasal tip swab, throat swab, mid-stream specimen of urine and sputum specimens being obtained for examination. Antibacterial nasal cream such as Naseptin is inserted into the nostrils as a prophylactic measure three times a day before surgery.

HYPOTHERMIA AND THE HEART–LUNG MACHINE

For many operations it is necessary to stop the action of the heart, therefore special measures have to be devised to make this possible. If the blood supply to the brain is stopped for more than two minutes, irreversible changes occur. This difficulty is overcome by hypothermia.

Body temperature is lowered, cellular metabolism slowed and oxygen requirement reduced; for example at 31°C the oxygen requirement of the tissues is 55% of normal. Enzyme activity is also depressed, and it is this that normally leads to damage and death of the cell in anoxia.

The procedure is relatively simple and safe, provided that the temperature does not go below 28°C. Both oesophageal and rectal temperatures are taken continually, using electronic thermometers: oesophageal because it gives a near approximation to the temperatures of heart and brain and rectal as it gives that of the more peripheral tissues. The temperature continues to drop two or three degrees after the cooling process has been discontinued. The main danger is that cooling alters the reaction of the blood, potassium is lost and the heart muscle becomes more irritable and ventricular fibrillation more likely to occur. In order to stop the heart for five to six minutes a temperature of 30°C is sufficiently low. The period of hypothermia should be as short as possible and the patient's temperature should be returned to normal as soon as possible. Most abnormalities of the pulmonary valve and most atrial septal defects can be repaired in this time. Hypothermia also produces hypotension and therefore a good bloodless field for operation.

Procedures demanding circulatory arrest for longer than eight minutes, for example closure of ventricular septal defects, require

190 SURGICAL NURSING

an artificial heart–lung machine: that is a machine that carries on the work of both heart and lungs while the action of the heart is stopped. The machine has been difficult to build as the area for the exchange of gases in lungs is equivalent to about 33 m². The blood in the machine has therefore to flow over a large number of plates during the process of oxygenation. Five litres of blood are required to prime the machine and 2 litres are held in readiness for

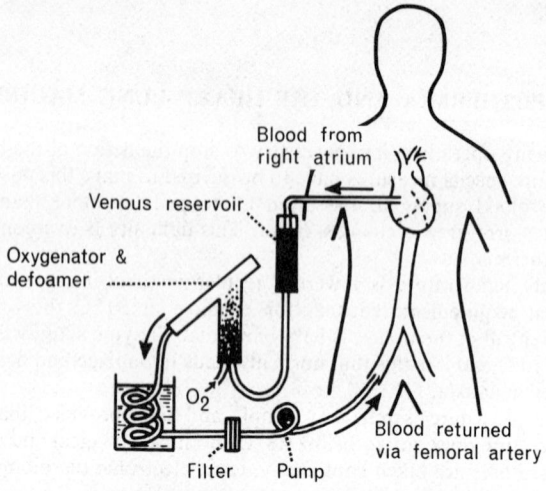

Fig. 19. The working of the heart–lung machine.

transfusion. All blood loss during the operation is very carefully measured. Plastic silicone tubing is used to carry the blood in the machine so as to avoid clotting and heparin is injected into the venae cavae before the cannulae are inserted into them. After passing through the machine the blood flows back through a cannula inserted into the femoral artery. Adequate pumping must be maintained, but it must be so gentle that the delicate erythrocytes are not damaged. From the femoral artery the blood flows backwards to the aortic semilunar valve supplying the various branches on the way. When the cannulae are in position the aorta can be clamped. This cuts off the supply to the coronary arteries. A solution of potassium citrate, 20 mg potassium citrate to 1 ml blood, is injected to stop the action of the heart. Usually about 20 ml is required. At the end of the operation the citrated blood is sucked out from the heart and the clamp is removed from the aorta. This allows normal blood to fill the coronary arteries. A heparin antagonist is used and calcium chloride can be used if necessary to reverse the effect of potassium citrate. If the heart does not start again once the normal blood supply is restored, the defibrillator is used. The pump is not normally used for more than twenty minutes.

It is also possible to reduce the patient's temperature to 15°C by using the heart–lung machine and chilling the blood outside the body. When the temperature has been reduced to 15°C the pump is switched off, artificial respiration ceases, and the surgeon can operate on a still, cold, empty heart. This method gives him a longer period in which to complete the operation.

ISCHAEMIC HEART DISEASE

Surgery is mainly carried out in the treatment of coronary artery disease which is localized to a part of the coronary tree. The extent of atherosclerosis is identified by means of a coronary angiogram. If it found that the extent of the lesion is suitable for surgery a section of the superficial saphenous vein is dissected from the patient's leg and is grafted onto the ascending aorta (bypassing the stenosis) and onto the coronary artery, so allowing adequate perfusion of the myocardium once again.

VALVULAR LESIONS

Rheumatic heart disease still accounts for an appreciable amount of cardiac invalidism. Rheumatic fever, chorea and certain streptococcal infections may set up a non-suppurative inflammation in the myocardium and endocardium causing the normal structures of the heart to be replaced by scar tissue. In the course of time scar tissue contracts, the mobility of the valves is impaired and the edges are fused together. The mitral valve is most frequently affected. There are four female patients to every male patient. Relief of this condition is one of the main triumphs in medicine of recent years, but success depends on the careful selection of patients.

Mitral Valvular Lesions

As the result of disease of the mitral valve two main conditions arise:

1. There is mitral obstruction or *stenosis* which means that insufficient blood can get through the mitral valve to supply the left ventricle and the systemic circulation.
2. There is *mitral incompetence* when the rigid cusps of the valve cannot prevent regurgitation during ventricular systole. Valvotomy is likely to be successful only where the first of these conditions predominates.

Sometimes two main graides of mitral stenosis are differentiated. The first consists of those patients who may be relieved by surgery because, although signs and symptoms may be severe, destruction of the cusps of the valves has only been mild; the second comprises those in which cusps, chordae tendineae, atrioventricular ring and even papillary muscles have been replaced by fibrous tissue. The cusps are enormously thickened and retracted so that they lie almost parallel with the ventricular walls; the chordae are destroyed and the cusps almost fused with the papillary muscles; so that even if the adherent commissure between the cusps can be divided they are prevented from functioning normally as they remain bound down to the ventricular wall.

Other patients have no disabilities associated with their physical signs, and should not be subjected to surgery, but are carefully 'followed up'. Where selection is careful excellent results are obtained in 60% of patients; 20% are improved and the remainder are left where they were, or worse. One of the main difficulties lies in the fact that the degree of destruction of the valves cannot be gauged accurately before the heart is opened.

Preoperative preparation

Preparation is as described for any major chest operation; nearly all patients require treatment with digitalis and, if heart failure is present, it is treated by rest, diuretics such as frusemide 40–160 mg depending upon the degree of cardiac failure, and salt limitation, for as long as these methods continue to produce improvement. This may be a period of several weeks. The patient is weighed daily.

Anaemia is corrected and antibiotics, such as ampicillin, are started 48 hours before operation and continued for a week to ten days subsequently. Anticoagulants and drugs affecting the blood pressure are stopped prior to surgery.

Before the consent form is signed the situation is fully explained to the patient. A perfect result cannot be guaranteed and after the operation a period of 'running-in' will be necessary before the maximum benefit is felt, as it takes some time for the heart to accommodate to the altered flow of blood.

Operation

The approach is through a left thoracotomy incision and through the left auricular appendage. A fingertip is passed into the valve orifice and an attempt is made to split first the posterior and then the anterior commissure as completely as possible. A Tubbs' dilator may also be used. This has to be done quickly as the finger arrests the blood flow and the pressure goes down to zero. An attempt is then made to separate the chordae tendineae if they are matted together and to restore their mobility.

Valvotomes of various patterns may be used. One of them consists of a flexible strip fitted to the index finger by a slotted finger ring, so that it can be advanced or withdrawn at will to permit further palpation. It terminates in a probe-pointed blade. The probe is inserted into the orifice and a little pressure on the blade cuts the commissure. At the end of the operation the valve orifice will generally accommodate two fingers.

Postoperative nursing care

While the patient is in the theatre everything is collected for postoperative care. On return from the theatre the nurse will observe the patient's general condition; the pulse rate, volume and regularity is noted and the peripheral pulses are felt in all four limbs because of the danger of emboli occurring. The colour and warmth of the skin is noted and the state of the airway. The position and efficiency of the drainage tube and the transfusion apparatus are checked. The amount of fluid allowed depends upon the patient's surface area. During the first three days it is administered partly by mouth and partly by intravenous infusion. Thereafter free fluids and then a light diet are offered. The patient is usually conscious and is asked to breathe deeply, to open his eyes, put out his tongue and move his limbs. This again checks the absence of emboli. It is a great help to have a nurse who knew the patient preoperatively to supervise this postoperative phase.

The position used depends on the state of respiration and the presence or absence of shock. Generally the position of maximum comfort is adopted, which is likely to be semi-recumbent or well propped up in the manner already described. Scoliosis with the concavity to the left is the deformity most liable to occur and must be prevented from the start. Most aspects of postoperative care are those of importance after any major chest operation.

An X-ray, using a portable apparatus, is often taken in the ward on the day of operation to check drainage and for a collapsed lobe. On the first day the patient is encouraged to swing his legs over the edge of the bed and if he tolerates this well he is gradually mobilized. The patient should be up in a chair by the third day and will commence walking on the fourth day. If the patient is progressing well and has a sternal wound the dressings are covered and a shower is allowed on the fourth day. He remains in hospital for 10 to 21 days and during this time exercise is carefully controlled, exercise tolerance noted and compared with the pre-operative record. When the operative result is good, the pulse quickly returns to normal after rest. Chest physiotherapy is very important as most patients have some degree of pulmonary congestion. So breathing exercises and coughing are essential.

Patients with sternal wounds, e.g. following valve replacement, have comparatively little discomfort, but those with thoracotomy wounds, e.g. used as the route of approach for valvotomies, patent ductus arteriosus and coarction of the aorta, do have discomfort as these are operations where bypass is not used (closed-heart operations), producing a higher level of pain due to the site of the wound.

Frusemide is continued, the dose depending upon the extent of fluid retention. Digoxin may also be administered: some surgeons order a smaller dose, e.g. 0·125 mg twice daily especially after valvular replacements. Potassium is given depending upon the dose of frusemide. Distalgesic or paracetamol are the analgesics administered.

Convalescence should be for not less than three weeks and the patient is advised to make haste slowly in his return to normal life.

Complications

The main postoperative complications are:

Cerebral embolism which may result in hemiplegia. Frequently this subsequently clears completely.

Aortic or popliteal embolism is indicated by sudden onset of pain and absence of peripheral pulses. The limb or limbs become cold, blue and mottled and sensation is lost. The treatment is by return to the theatre for embolectomy.

Pulmonary embolism. Anticoagulants and exercises will be given should any signs of thrombosis develop. This complication may be seen following vein grafts due to the excision of part of the superficial saphenous vein and following closed-heart operations due to a clot being dislodged from the heart. As a prophylactic measure against the risk of thrombus formation, patients who have had metal valves inserted will take warfarin for the rest of their lives. If the patients are not able to take warfarin then a metal valve is not inserted: a tissue valve is inserted instead.

Persistent postoperative pyrexia may be due to the reactivation of the rheumatic process, traumatic pericarditis or pleural effusion.

Tamponade, due to collection of fluid in the pericardium.

Atalectasis. In this case the patient is nursed in a lateral position with a pillow under the chest and the involved area uppermost. Two pillows are under the patient's head. This position encourages the area to re-expand.

Renal failure. All patients are carefully screened preoperatively to reduce the risk of this occurring. If there is any sign of this complication devleoping investigations are made and every attempt is taken to reduce the risk.

Aortic Valve Stenosis

This may be congenital or due to acute rheumatism, atherosclerosis or deposits of calcium. The condition can be treated by valvotomy or, if aortic incompetence, is present a Starr–Edwards prosthetic valve is sometimes inserted.

CONGENITAL DEFECTS OF THE HEART AND GREAT VESSELS

Ventricular Fibrillation

This occurs most readily in congenitally abnormal hearts and if the temperature is taken below 28°C. To restore normal coronary circulation the heart is stopped by a defibrillator; two electrodes, formed rather like sugar tongs and covered with moist sponges, are placed one on either side of the heart and an electric current of 110–130 volts is passed through for 0·1 second. After the shock, cardiac massage is given. If normal rhythm is not restored, the voltage can be increased by 30–40 volts, massage being given after each shock.

The evolution during fetal life, from a simple pulsating tube to a fully developed heart, is highly complex and many different defects can occur due to developmental failure at various stages. These are divided into two broad groups; the cyanotic defects when the patient looks blue, and acyanotic when the patient's colour is normal.

Cyanotic Defects

Fallot's tetralogy

This is the best known condition in this group. Tetra is derived from the Greek word meaning 'four', and the four defects usually seen in these hearts are pulmonary stenosis, dextroposition of the aorta, which arises from both ventricles, septal defects and, in consequence of these, hypertrophy of the right ventricle. These patients suffer from central cyanosis, as opposed to peripheral cyanosis seen in most types of heart failure and in cold weather, when the extremities become blue owing to vasoconstriction and stagnation of blood in those tissues.

SIGNS AND SYMPTOMS

These children are slow to put on weight. Their physical development is poor but they are seldom mentally retarded. They are frequently intelligent and spoilt. Untreated, about 50% die before they are seven years old; only about 10% reach adult life and they are ready victims of subacute bacterial endocarditis.

Central cyanosis. The blueness due to this condition occurs on surfaces that are themselves moist and warm such as the tongue, buccal mucosa and conjunctivae. The cyanosis tends to be progressive, and bouts of unconsciousness may occur due to cerebral anoxia.

SURGERY OF THE HEART 197

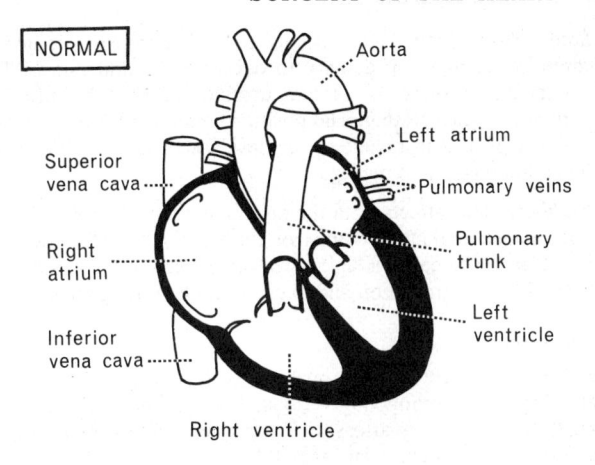

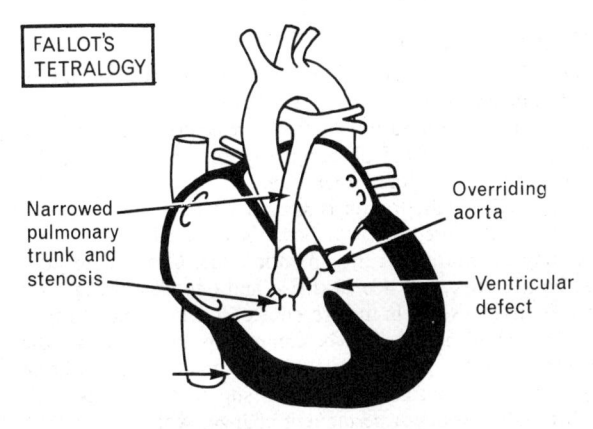

FIG. 20. The structure of the normal heart and the congenital defects which occur in Fallot's tetralogy.

Polycythaemia. This is nearly always found in association with cyanosis. The haemoglobin is raised but not in proportion to the increase in cells.

Breathlessness. This is marked and the patient is incapable of any effort, even crying, without distress.

198 SURGICAL NURSING

Squatting position. This will later be spontaneously adopted by children in the midst of activity to overcome breathlessness. This characteristic position is similar to that adopted by primitive eastern races when resting. The position enables them to withstand the effects of anoxia better, to increase the oxygen supply to the brain and diminish it to the legs.

Clubbing. This affects both the fingers and toes. It is a deformity of the nailbed making the ends of the fingers and toes look like Indian clubs. The cause is unknown, but is usually associated with abnormalities of circulation and oxygen supply to the tissues.

OPERATIVE TREATMENT

Since the advent of the heart–lung machine, Blalock's and Waterston's anastomotic operations, that is, anastomosis of the aorta to the pulmonary artery, in order to increase the blood supply through the lungs, have been carried out.

PREOPERATIVE PREPARATION

The child must be allowed to make friends with the staff and to become familiar with ward routine and be introduced to the oxygen tent, which will be used for the first few postoperative days. Some children are very afraid of being enclosed in an oxygen tent, in which case it is not used. Great attention is paid to fluid intake and output, because dehydration is very dangerous in the presence of polycythaemia, cerebral thrombosis is more likely to occur and there may be clotting at the operation site. Cross-matched blood must be available, but 4% dextrose and one-fifth strength normal saline are used, except in the presence of haemorrhage. Respiratory infection should, if possible, be cleared up and antibiotic therapy started 48 hours preoperatively. The main danger during the operation lies in cutting the oxygen supply to the heart muscle, which rapidly produces permanent changes which will prevent the restoration of normal rhythm postoperatively.

POSTOPERATIVE NURSING CARE

Nursing care varies considerably according to the condition of the child and the wishes of the surgeon. In the immediate postoperative period a doctor is always in attendance to direct postoperative care. The child is usually nursed by a special nurse in the recovery room or intensive care unit for at least 12 hours. Parents are always allowed to be present and the child must be kept as quiet as possible. These children are inclined to be restless and analgesics such as Omnopon and pethidine may be used initially in small doses, then oral drugs such as paracetamol elixir 5–15 ml depending upon the child's surface area. Pentazocine may also be used.

Position. The patient is usually nursed flat at first, but is later allowed one or two pillows as he wishes.

Oxygen therapy. This may be administered by means of an oxygen tent or mask. If a total correction of the Fallot's tetralogy has been performed then a ventilator will be used.

Physiotherapy. The child is encouraged to do deep breathing exercises and to cough. To do this it may be necessary to play games with the child as he may not understand what is meant by 'cough'. If a collapsed lobe has occurred then the child will be placed on his side in a cast, with the involved lobe uppermost. The position will encourage the lobe to re-expand.

Records. Quarter-hourly *pulse* and *blood pressure* readings are taken at first. Arrangements are made whereby the nurse can take the readings without disturbing the patient.

Fluid balance must be carefully recorded.

A nasogastric tube is introduced, and for the first 12 hours the patient is allowed nothing by mouth and the tube is aspirated hourly. 15 ml of water are then allowed hourly and this is gradually increased, if the patient does not vomit, until free fluids and then a light diet are allowed.

Intravenous fluids are also given for 24 hours or longer. A continuous drip infusion of 5% Dextrose or Hartmann's solution may be given into the inferior vena cava, through an incision in the groin, as well as an infusion into the arm or leg.

A urethral Foley's catheter drains into a closed sterile container and is released two- or four-hourly. An accurate urine measure and the taking of the specific gravity of the urine at frequent intervals is of great importance in helping to determine the correct administration of intravenous fluids. This catheter is introduced in theatre after the child has been anaesthetized.

Drainage tubes. Usually there are chest drains from the base of the cavity, a mediastinal drain which is just inside the wound and a pericardial drain to prevent a tamponade occurring. *The patient is turned two-hourly* in order to assist drainage and for the sake of pressure areas.

Antibiotics are continued for seven to ten days. Cephradine 250–500 mg or cephalexin 250–500 mg given six-hourly are often prescribed, but other antibiotics can be used such as ampicillin and cloxacillin. Healing tends to be slow and infection frequent as the circulation is defective.

As the child's condition improves the various tubes are removed and the child will feel much more comfortable. He will receive the routine care of a patient who has had a thoracotomy. Return to normal activity will depend on the condition of the heart.

Acyanotic Defects

In acyanotic defects there may be a shunt of blood from left to right and therefore an increased blood flow through the lungs. Children with these defects frequently enjoy good health during childhood, but they are liable to develop subacute bacterial endocarditis and usually die in early middle age from heart failure caused by the increased burden their defect throws on the heart muscle.

Patent ductus arteriosus

In intrauterine life the venous blood from the right heart short-circuits the unexpanded lungs to reach the aorta via the ductus arteriosus. When the lungs expand after birth the ductus normally closes very rapidly. Occasionally it remains open, more frequently in girls than boys, and forms an arteriovenous fistula between aorta and pulmonary artery. The blood flow is from the aorta where the pressure is high to the pulmonary artery where it is lower. This puts an added burden on the right heart which may go into failure later in life; or the pressure in the right side can be increased until the direction of the blood flow in the ductus is reversed. The condition can be successfully treated by ligature when the child is young and symptom-free. Prior to surgery the nurse should be able to feel a water-hammer pulse in many of these young patients.

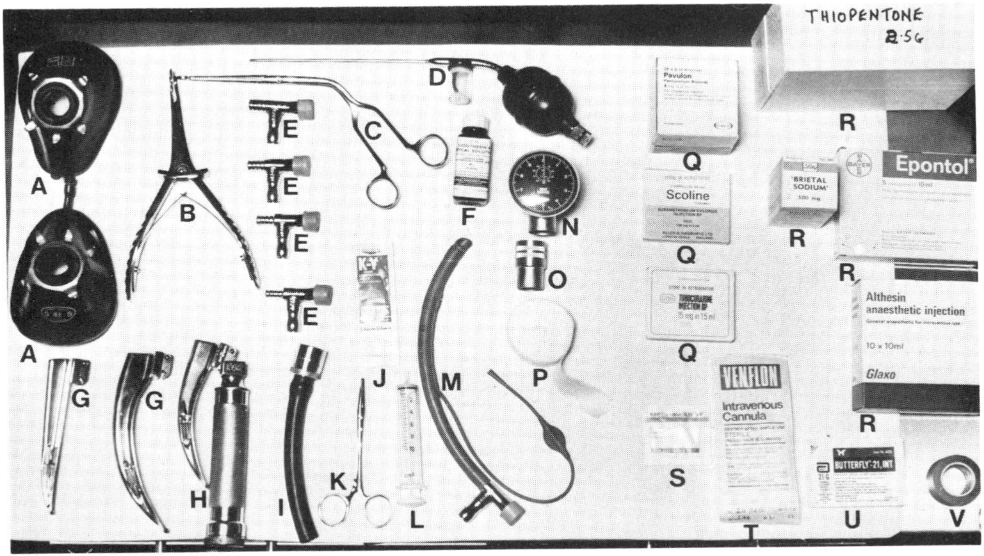

Plate 1. The basic equipment required for inducing general anaesthesia. A, McKesson anaesthetic face masks. B, Ferguson mouth-gag. C, Magill intubating forceps. D, Swerdlow anaesthetic throat spray. E, Magill suction union T-pieces to connect to the endotracheal tube. F, 4% topical lignocaine. G, Laryngoscope blades. H, Laryngoscope. I, Connection. J, KY jelly. K, Artery forceps. L, 10 ml syringe to inflate cuff of endotracheal tube. M, Cuffed endotracheal tube. N, Wright's respirometer. O, Connection for respirometer. P, Connection for spirometer. Q, Muscle relaxants: Pavulon, Scoline and tubocurarine. R, Induction agents: thiopentone, Brietal Sodium, Epontol and Althesin. S, Mediswab. T, Intravenous cannula. U, Butterfly to secure intravenous needle. V, Strapping. (*Department of Medical Illustration, University Hospital of Wales*)

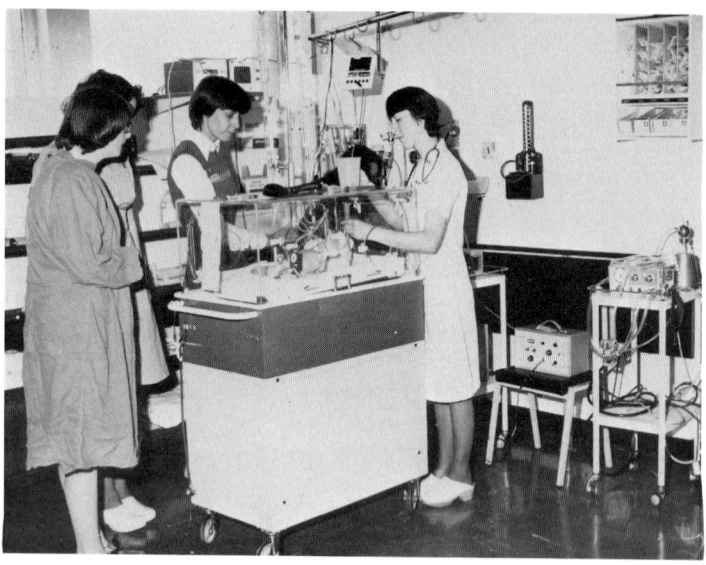

Plate 2. A neonate receiving intensive care before cardiac surgery.
(*Department of Medical Illustration, University Hospital of Wales*)

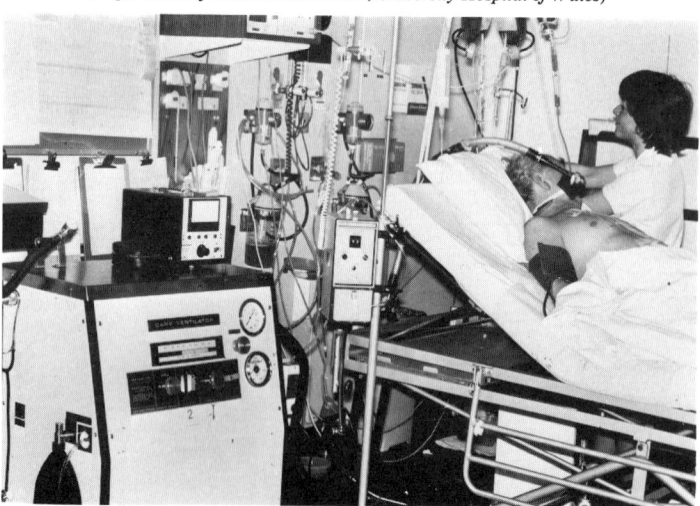

Plate 3. A patient receiving total care in one of the bed stations. He has had cardiac surgery and is being ventilated with a Cape ventilator attached to an endotracheal tube. A trained nurse is in constant attendance.
(*Department of Medical Illustration, University Hospital of Wales*)

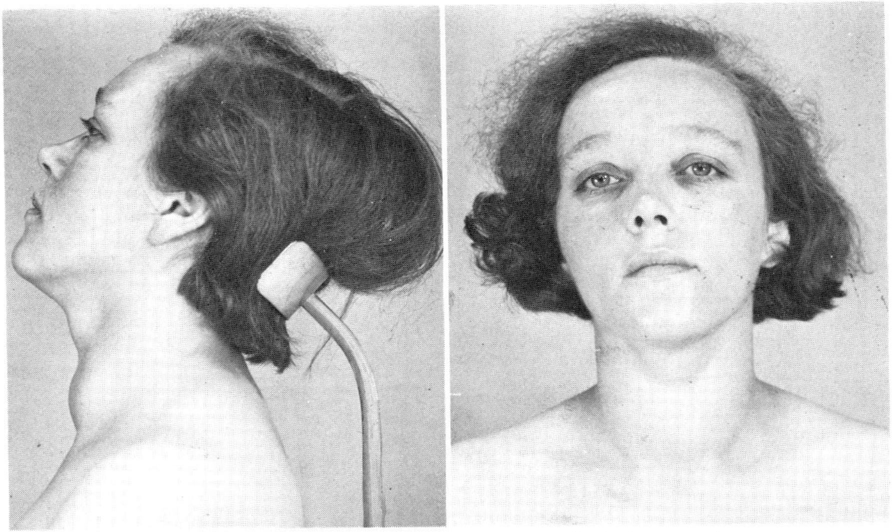

Plate 4. A case of simple goitre, showing slight swelling in the neck only.

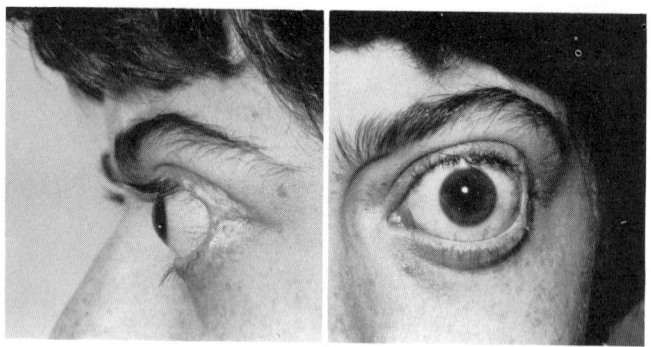

Plate 5. Exophthalmos, showing the protruding eyeballs and slight retraction of the lids seen in exophthalmic goitre.
(*St Bartholomew's Hospital*)

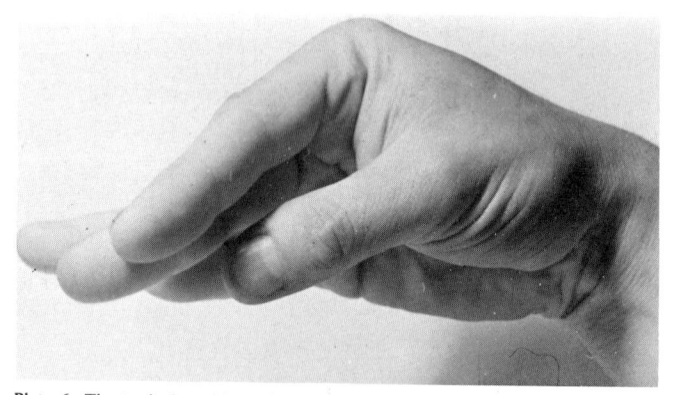

Plate 6. The typical position of the hand in tetany, produced by muscle spasm due to lack of calcium, i.e. carpopedal spasm.

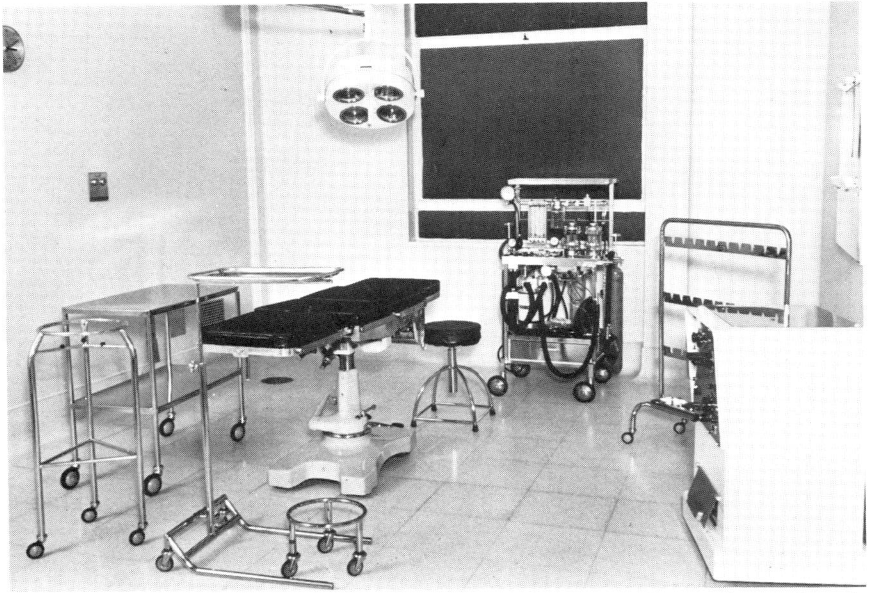

Plate 7. A day patient theatre for minor surgery. This enables the patient to return home on the same day to the care of the community health care team. The equipment is similar to that used in the main operating theatre. (*Department of Medical Illustration, University Hospital of Wales*)

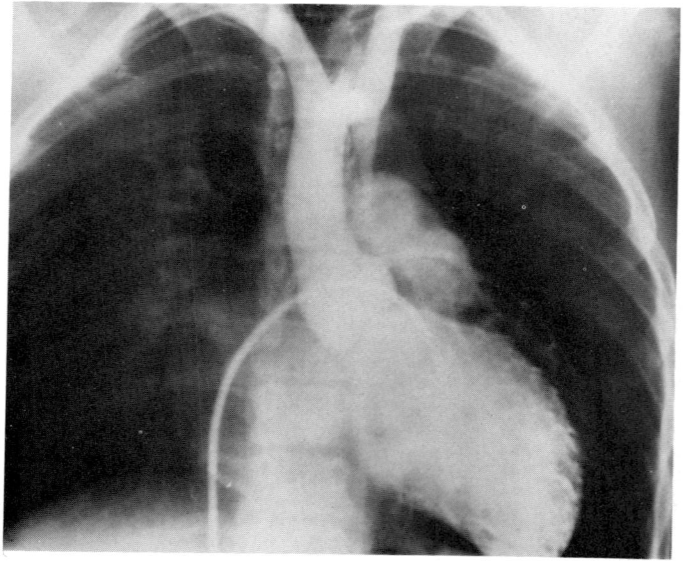

Plate 8. Cardiac catheterization. The catheter has passed from the right atrium, through the foramen ovale, to the left atrium, and then through the mitral valve into the left ventricle.
(*St Bartholomew's Hospital*)

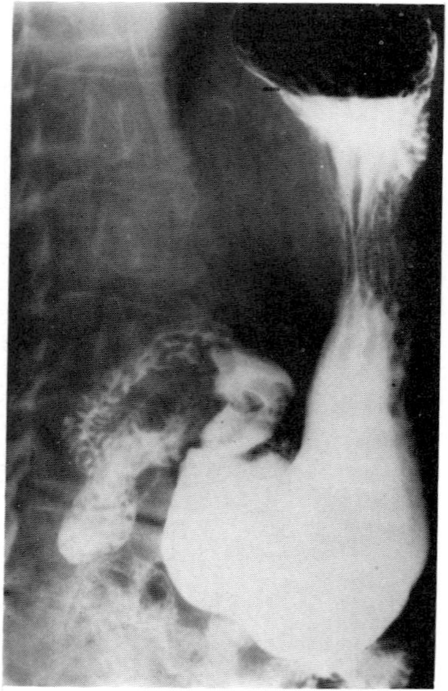

Plate 9. A barium meal is performed to aid the diagnosis of lesions in the digestive tract. This radiograph shows a normal stomach and small bowel.
(*Department of Medical Illustration University Hospital of Wales*)

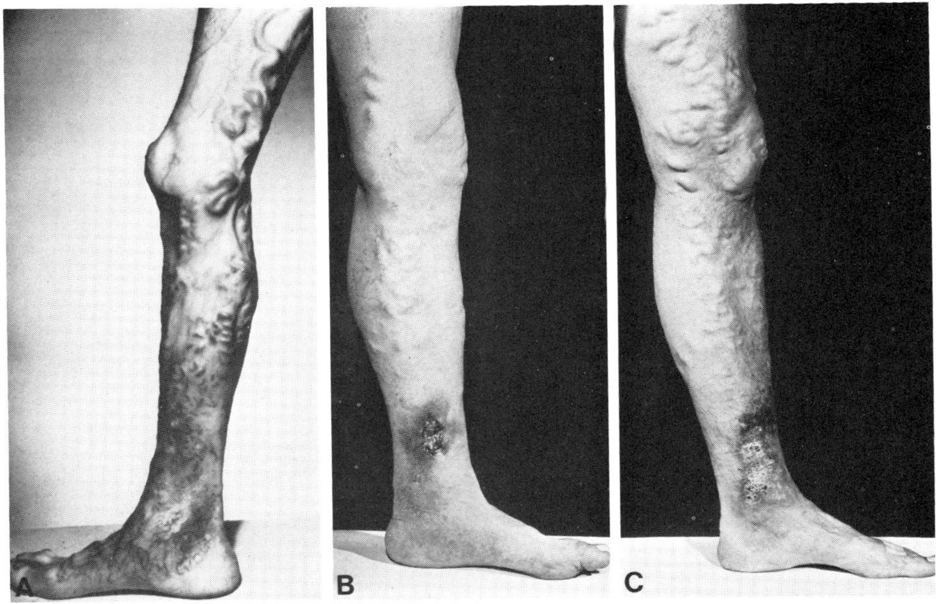

Plate 10. Varicose veins. A, These can be identified very clearly when photographed under infra-red light. B, C, Varicosed veins complicated by hypostatic dermatitis and ulceration. Ulcers develop on a site chronically affected by hypostatic dermatitis, due to failure of the circulatory return from the lower limbs. (*Department of Medical Illustration, Cardiff Royal Infirmary*)

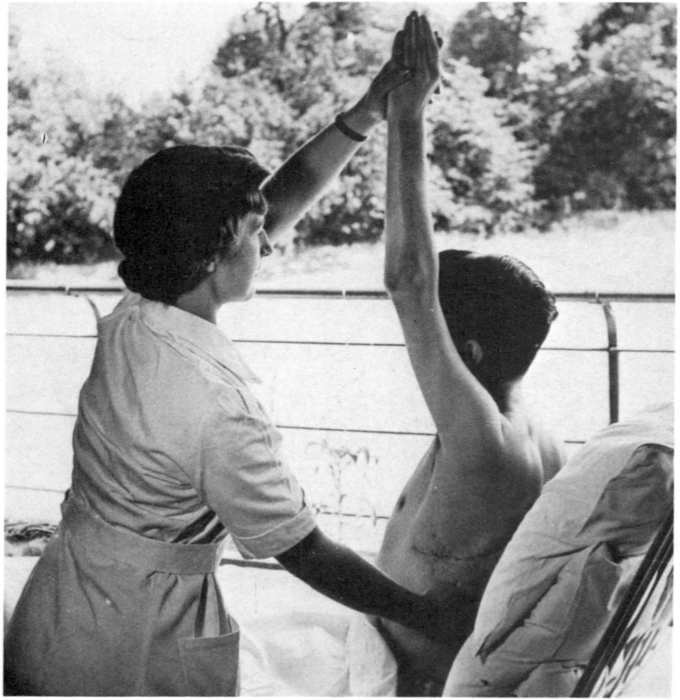

Plate 11. When the wound is healed, the physiotherapist continues the exercise to ensure a straight spine with no scoliosis and full movement of the shoulder.

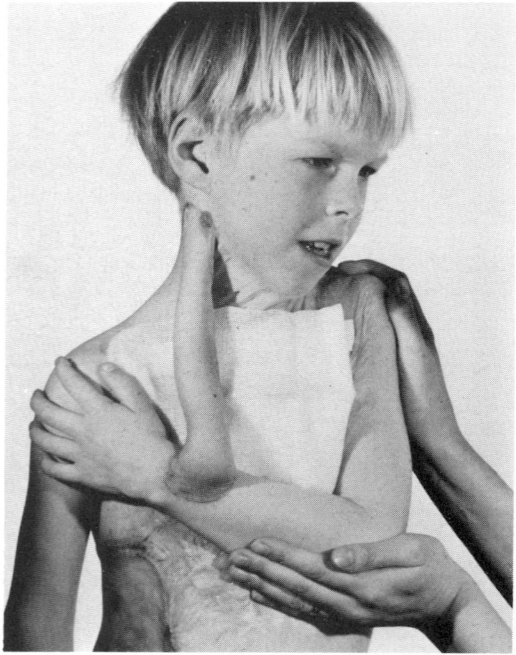

Plate 12. A pedicle graft. The skin has been taken from the abdomen and will eventually be used to replace the contracted tissue of the throat. Physiotherapy is important to maintain movement and muscle tone.

SURGERY OF THE HEART 201

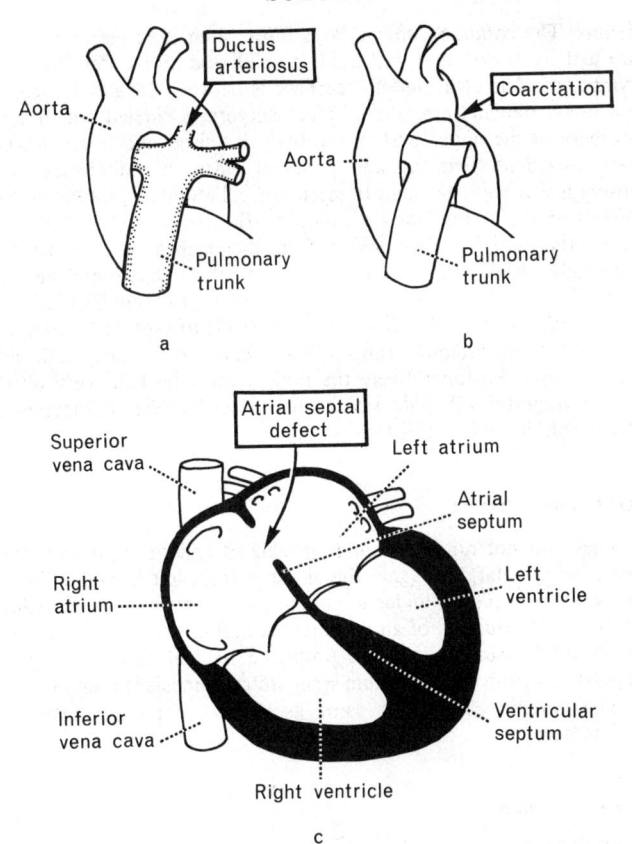

FIG. 21. Patent ductus arteriosus, coarctation of the aorta and atrial septal defect.

Coarctation of the aorta

Coarctation is a narrowing usually in the region of the ligamentum venosum which runs from the pulmonary artery to the aorta. It is thought to be due to a defect in the mechanism which closes the ductus arteriosus at birth. This either works too vigorously, involving the aorta as well as the ductus, or else it is misdirected as the lesion is sometimes associated with a patent ductus. The condition affects boys more often than girls and they are usually sturdy and well built in childhood and suffer from no symptoms. The ideal time for surgery is between 10 and 15 years, but many patients are adults before surgery is carried out. Blood pressure in the upper part of the body is raised and in the lower part depressed. Femoral and popliteal pulses are diminished or absent and there is evidence of increased collateral circulation in the vessels of the abdominal wall, particularly the intercostal arteries. Later the patients may suffer from headaches and giddiness, especially when they bend down; cerebral haemorrhage or intermittent claudication can occur. Aortography may be required to confirm the diagnosis. It is usually possible to excise the stricture and insert an arterial graft, if necessary, or to carry out an anastomosis. Postoperatively the patient must be kept very quiet as the hypertension puts stress on the suture line. Paracetamol elixir is often used for this reason.

Atrial septal defects

These do not normally cause trouble in childhood, despite the heart being enlarged. Again the shunt is from left to right. These can now be repaired under hypothermia, the main danger arising from the introduction of an air embolus during operation. This can cause results similar to those produced by emboli consisting of vegetations from the left atrium when mitral stenosis is present.

The nursing care is the same as that for a patient having a thoracotomy.

Valvular lesions

Valvular lesions occur for instance when a child is born with only two cusps to the aortic valve.

CONSTRICTIVE PERICARDITIS

This may be due to fibrosis of the pericardium which produces a condition of cardiac tamponade. In this condition the action of the heart, and particularly its filling capacity, is limited. The condition can also be produced by haemorrhage or effusion into the pericardium as the result of operation or injury, but if the condition is

SURGERY OF THE HEART 203

insidious in onset it is almost certainly due to tuberculous infection. At first an effusion may be present; later the fibrous tissue, laid down as a result of the chronic inflammatory process, may contract and calcify so that the heart is incased in a cuirass and its activity severely embarrassed. The first sign is often a fall in urinary output due to poor cardiac output; there will be raised jugular venous pressure, the liver will be enlarged and ascites and oedema will follow and the patient becomes very short of breath. The venous blood cannot be received back into the heart; therefore there is a poor cardiac output, low systolic and pulse pressure; because the

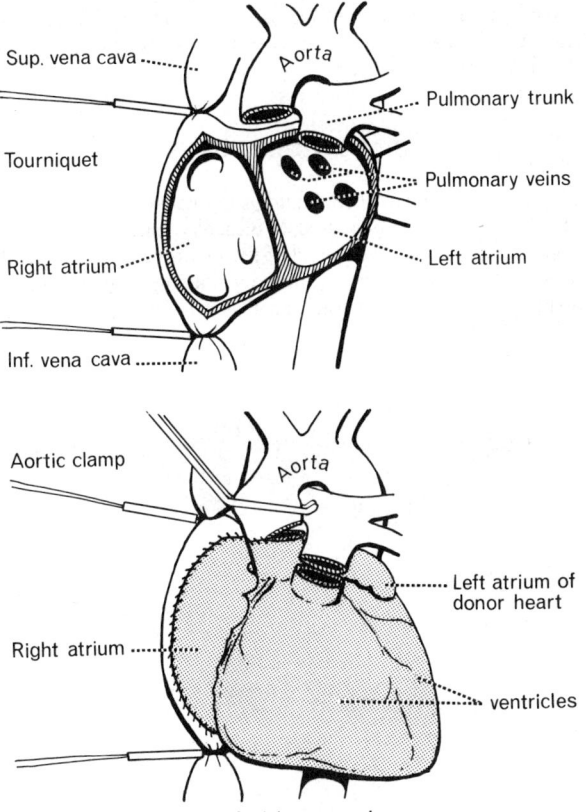

Fig. 22. A heart transplant.

size of the heart beat cannot be enlarged there is an abnormal increase in pulse rate on exertion and the pulse may be paradoxical, that is, decreasing on inspiration and increasing on expiration.

Treatment

Unless the condition is acute, no treatment is undertaken while tuberculosis is active. The patient receives anti-tuberculous treatment and when the condition is quiescent pericardectomy is performed through a left thoracic incision. The whole pericardium surrounding the ventricles is removed; it is not generally considered necessary to remove that round the veins and atria. The myocardium thus released can work more vigorously and the patient's condition is greatly improved.

HEART TRANSPLANT

This is carried out when heart failure is imminent and a donor heart is available. The technique used is basically removal of the total heart of the donor, by dividing all of the blood vessels, and grafting this to the atria of the recipient, his heart having been removed, but the atria remaining. This operation is illustrated in Fig. 22.

13

Vascular Surgery

ARTERIES

Arterial surgery is being used with increasing success in the treatment of disease and injury involving the large blood vessels, especially the aorta and the iliac and femoral arteries. The upper limb has a very rich collateral circulation and consequently arterial surgery is seldom required there. When it is necessary to clamp the aorta, hypothermia may have to be used.

Arterial conditions treated by surgery include:

Obliterative arterial disease. This at first produces intermittent claudication, or cramp in the calf muscles, after the patient has walked a certain distance. Later the patient will have rest pain and ultimately gangrene sets in, usually starting in the toes. Many of these patients have diabetes mellitus.

Aneurysm. Injury or disease of the arterial wall can produce a pulsating bulge which, if left untreated, will ultimately rupture.

Congenital lesions such a coarctation of the aorta.

Emboli. When these occur in a large vessel the patient suffers from agonizing pain and signs and symptoms of incipient gangrene appear. If the condition is diagnosed early, embolectomy can be successfully performed.

Injuries. Soft tissue trauma often results in damage to arteries which must be repaired surgically.

Arteriovenous fistulas. These are usually the result of an injury and may interfere with the normal circulation of a limb, but they may be congenital.

206 SURGICAL NURSING

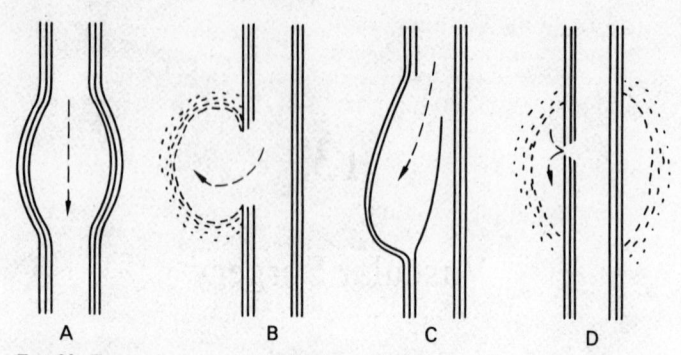

FIG. 23. Types of aneurysm. (A) Fusiform. (B) Saccular. (C) Dissecting, showing blood leaking *between* the layers of the vessel wall. (D) False, showing blood leaking *out* of the vessel to form a swelling enclosed in fibrous tissue.

Types of Surgical Operation

Arterial grafting

Obliterative arterial disease, when localized, and certain other conditions can now be satisfactorily treated by arterial grafting.

Types of grafts used are as follows:

1. Sometimes one of the *patient's own veins* ('reverse' saphenous) can be used. These survive as living tissues, but must be put in under tension, otherwise there is a danger of cork-screwing and clotting.
2. *Teflon* is also used and is capable of withstanding more heat than platinum. *Dacron* is now being used in preference to Teflon.
3. *Orlon* and *Terylene* have been used. The main disadvantage is that initially the blood tends to seep through the interstices; however, it soon clots and the graft is lined with a smooth layer like the endothelium of the artery.
4. *Polyvinyl alcohol sponge* has been used after moulding and sterilizing by boiling.
5. *Homografts* are now rarely used.

Arterial disobliteration

This may sometimes be undertaken as an alternative operation to grafting. It consists of disobliterating a portion of the interior of an artery. Two incisions are made into the artery and special instruments are used for removing organized blood clot and debris and syringing it through with heparin or normal saline. This operation may give very satisfactory results.

Sympathectomy

These operations have frequently been performed in order to produce vasodilatation of the peripheral vessels, but are only of value in the treatment of rest pain or Raynaud's disease. Some very satisfactory cures in the treatment of Raynaud's disease—a condition characterized by spasm of peripheral arteries—have resulted from the use of reserpine, given to inhibit the production of adrenaline and thyroxine which increases the metabolic rate. Many other drugs, such as tolazoline and papaverine, have also been tried. However, in severe cases, especially if ulceration is threatened or present, surgery often becomes necessary.

Amputation of a limb

This operation will be necessary if grafting or sympathectomy fails and in some cases is the immediate operation of choice. If possible a useful stump is created so that an artificial limb may be provided in order for the patient to regain a near normal life. Sometimes, especially in progressive arterial disease or in weak elderly patients, a wheelchair existence has to be accepted.

Preoperative Investigations Before Arterial Surgery

An *arteriogram* will be performed to demonstrate the level and severity of the lesion. The radiologist and surgeon will discuss the result and a decision will be made as to the type of surgery that will benefit the patient. Arterial reconstruction with a graft may be possible but if it is decided that the condition is too widespread then a sympathectomy only may be advised.

The *arterial pressures* in the leg will be measured with an oscillometer and the *arterial pulsations* and their strength (or absence) will be observed and recorded from the pedal, posterior tibial and popliteal arteries.

Specimens of *blood* are obtained for assessing the haemoglobin level, erythrocyte sedimentation rate, blood urea, serum cholesterol, triglycerides, LE cells and full blood picture and to carry out Wasserman and Khan tests. If the patient proves to be anaemic then this condition is rectified. Sometimes the patient is found to have polycythaemia and this also requires treatment by means of venesection.

If the patient's triglycerides are elevated than a cholesterol-free diet may be ordered. At the same time the fasting lipids are estimated to see if the patient has hyperlipidaemia and if this is so clofibrate 500 mg is given four times a day to reduce the cholesterol level.

An electrocardiogram will be performed to detect any cardiac lesion.

If the patient has an ischaemic limb and the site of arterial obstruction is clearly demonstrated by the arteriogram the surgeon may decide to attempt to save the limb or at least reduce the level of amputation by performing a bypass operation. If the limb is saved toes may still 'drop-off' and areas of gangrenous tissue may still need treatment and if a below-knee amputation still proves to be necessary then the patient will have much more useful stump when an artificial limb is provided and walking recommences.

Preoperative Nursing Care

The actual nursing care depends upon the patient's condition, such as an aortic aneurysm, ischaemia or gangrene, because the care required in ischaemia or gangrene is different from that required by a patient with an aortic aneurysm.

Obliterative arterial disease. The patient will be nursed in bed with a bed cradle taking the weight of the bed clothes from the ischaemic or gangrenous limb. In some cases the foot of the bed will be left open so that a fan may be used to direct cool air on to the limb. When this is done it is very important that the rest of the patient is kept warm. The ischaemic tissue is cooled to reduce cellular metabolism and so lower the cells' need for oxygen. If the surgeon considers that there is a chance that the limb can be saved then the patient has to remain in bed, only being allowed up in a chair for toilet purposes; alternatively if an amputation is to be carried out the patient may be allowed up and about in a chair. If rest pain only is present then the patient is allowed to walk about the ward.

The nurse will take swabs from the anterior nares, throat, both groins and each foot; these are then examined bacteriologically to identify the presence of pathogenic micro-organisms. A mid-stream specimen of urine and sputum specimen will also be obtained. The doctor will then prescribe an antibiotic to which the orgnism is sensitive.

If weeping or moist gangrene is present then some substance such as half-strength Eusol will be used either to swab a weeping area or in the form of Eusol soaks if the gangrene is moist. The toes must be separated with some non-sticking material such as Melolin.

Pressure to the heel must be avoided and the chiropodist will be requested to carry out specialist foot and nail care. Alcohol will be prescribed for the patient and all attempts must be made to help him follow the advice given prior to admission to hospital and to stop or reduce smoking.

Pain may be a marked symptom, especially if tissue ischaemia is present, and it will be necessary to administer pain-relieving drugs such as pethidine 50–100 mg either orally or by intramuscular injection, Omnopon, DF 118, distalgesic or dihydrocodeine 30–60 mg.

Reconstructive arterial surgery. Routine preoperative nursing care is carried, out, swabs are taken, antibiotics are administered as required, the skin is prepared and if the aorta is the vessel involved then a low-residue diet will be ordered and very careful bowel preparation will be carried out.

Postoperative Care

Following arterial reconstruction or bypass surgery. Oedema is very likely to develop so support is often given by means of a crêpe bandage and the foot of the bed is elevated. Initially observations are made every 15 minutes and these recorded observations will show improvement or any other change relating to the circulation through the involved vessel. These observations include pain, discoloration, temperature, sensation and function of the extremity, quality of the pulses and any bruising or oedema.

The patient will remain in bed for the first 48 hours and then be allowed up in a wheelchair. Sutures are removed after ten days and in some cases the surgeon instructs that the wound dressing is not disturbed until this time. Some patients are rather agitated following major aortic surgery and so it may be necessary to administer diazepam 5 mg three times a day. Initially many of these patients are cared for in an intensive care unit before returning to their ward as they require to be 'specialled'.

The hourly urine output is measured carefully as this is a very good indication of the patient's arterial blood pressure. If less than 30 ml is excreted per hour there is a risk that the graft will occlude. This may also suggest that renal ischaemia has developed, possibly because of the aorta being clamped during the grafting operation.

An intravenous pyelogram will be carried out on the seventh postoperative day so that any possible kidney damage can be identified.

The physiotherapist will visit the patient to encourage him to perform breathing exercises and to perform passive exercises to his leg for him. Care will be taken not to allow a sharp flexion to occur at the hip if the graft has been performed in the femoral artery, but the patient will be nursed in the position he finds most comfortable.

Small quantities of anticoagulants may be used during the operation, especially if the patient has a deep venous thrombosis. These are usually discontinued during the immediate postoperative period. Later they may be started again for patients with arterial disease. Prothrombin levels will be ascertained daily at first and later at weekly, or even three-weekly, intervals. After operations on the abdominal aorta, paralytic ileus may develop. Convalescence should always be gradual in order to ensure sound healing.

Following amputation. If this operation has been carried out the emphasis is on care of the stump, prevention of flexion deformity and preparation for an artificial limb. This involves a great deal of psychological care for both the patient and his family because the success of rehabilitation depends to a great extent upon their state of mind. Following surgery some patients become rather confused but this usually responds to the administration of vitamins such as parentrovite. Many patients who have had severe ischaemic pain are very relieved when the operation is over as the pain can be all-consuming; others are upset and feel abnormal, stating that life will never be the same.

Prior to discharge the nurse must make sure that active rehabilitation has been commenced and that all of the patient's social factors have been considered and remedial action taken where necessary. This will involve social workers, physiotherapists, health visitors, home nurses, general practitioners, relatives, the Department of Social Services and government training centres.

VEINS

Position and Function of the Leg Veins

Innermost lie the bones. These are surrounded by muscles, deep veins and arteries in a strong fascial envelope. Over this lies the skin, fat and superficial fascia, containing the superficial veins. These are the long saphenous vein, lying medially and communicating with the deep femoral vein in the groin, and the short saphenous vein, which runs on the lateral aspect of the lower limb and dips down to join the deep veins in the popliteal fossa. Besides these there is a third group of perforating veins which penetrate the deep fascia from the superficial to the deep veins. These are above the ankle, mid-calf and below the knee on the inside of the leg, and one above the ankle on the outside of the leg. The very powerful calf muscles play an extremely important part in the venous return from the leg where gravity seldom assists the return flow of blood. The calf muscle is sometimes called the peripheral heart as its contraction increases the pressure in the deep veins by 80–100 mmHg and because of the presence of valves in the veins the blood is pushed onwards towards the heart. As the calf relaxes there is a sharp fall in blood pressure in the deep veins and blood is aspirated into them from the superficial ones, via the perforating veins. Valves at the entrance of these veins into the deep ones prevent the return flow of blood when the muscle contracts again. Thus the superficial tissues are drained largely via the deep veins and the superficial veins are really vestigial structures of much less importance in man than the corresponding veins in some of the lower animals.

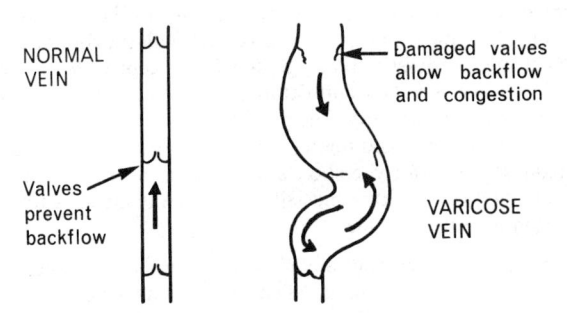

FIG. 24. A normal and a varicose vein.

Varicose Veins

Varicosity of the superficial veins is a common condition, in many cases due to a primary defect in the valves themselves. The condition is frequently hereditary. Occasionally varicose veins appear secondarily to increased intra-abdominal pressure, as, for instance, at the end of pregnancy or the development of an intra-abdominal tumour. Great saphenous incompetence is the commonest form; the whole vein dilates and becomes tortuous. Various tributaries also become vastly dilated and tortuous; these are the ones usually seen on the surface of the leg as varicose veins. The short saphenous vein is less frequently affected. Its main distribution is round the back of the leg.

Signs and symptoms

At first there may be no signs and symptoms associated with varicose veins and the cosmetic effect may be the main cause of anxiety to the patient. Later, if untreated, they will increase in size and extent.

Complications of varicose veins

Haemorrhage. If this occurs the patient must be placed in a recumbent position with the legs elevated and a pressure bandage should be applied.

Later, oedema of the ankles occurs as the result of chronic stagnation of the blood in that area. In the absence of heart failure, this is one of the commonest causes of oedema of the ankle.

Phlebitis. This may occur spontaneously or be secondary to trauma. The patient must be given bedrest with the foot of the bed elevated and a pressure bandage should be applied to the leg. If infection is present then antibiotics may be prescribed. Thrombophlebitis may also develop. The pain can be relieved by rest and the application of a lead and opium dressing. Infection is controlled by antibiotics. Fortunately emboli seldom arise from varicose veins. Pigmentation of the skin especially round the ankle appears as the condition becomes chronic.

Ulceration. This is especially likely to occur if the patient has had a deep vein thrombosis and is called a gravitational ulcer.

If the patient can be confined to bed the foot of the bed is

VASCULAR SURGERY 213

elevated and this abolishes the high venous pressure. Antibiotics are only given if a gross infection is present. If bedrest is not possible, e.g. for economic reasons, a tight elastic bandage is applied to empty the dilated veins; this allows oxygenated blood to reach the area and healing to take place. A saline dressing may be applied over the ulcerated area underneath the elastic bandage.

Treatment

Varicose veins can be treated conservatively by injection or operation.

Injection. Injecting a sclerosing agent into each vein produces an aseptic phlebitis and blocks the vein. It may be repeated two or three times, usually at fortnightly intervals. Unfortunately pressure of blood in the vein above frequently opens it again. For this reason some surgeons prefer surgery to conservative treatment, but others consider it to be an economic problem. Surgery results in the patient being unable to work for a period of about four weeks, plus the occupancy of a hospital bed. Conservative treatment only takes a few hours on a few occasions.

A variety of sclerosing agents are used, such as sodium tetradecyl sulphate with 2% benzyl alcohol, 0·5 ml being used for each injection.

Operation. Operative treatment may consist of ligaturing the main saphenous vein at the groin, where it joins the deep femoral vein, and also ligating above and below the knee and at the ankle, in order to interrupt the stagnant column of blood and produce an aseptic thrombosis in the intervening segments. Injections are sometimes combined with the operation of ligature. The skin of the whole leg must be prepared, including the suprapubic area and the groin. Any enlarged glands in the groin caused by phlebitis should always be reported as the operation will have to be postponed if any are present. The bed is usually elevated at the foot for the night prior to surgery in order to empty the veins as far as possible.

Stripping may be carried out instead of ligature at various levels. After ligating the vessel in the groin, a long flexible olive-tipped rod is passed from the groin to the lower end of the vein, or *vice versa*. The vein is tied to the knob at the end of the stripper and the rod is pulled out from the other end, stripping the vein through the subcutaneous tissues. The whole leg is bandaged with an elastic bandage as the vein is stripped out, in order to prevent excessive bruising.

Postoperative care

The patient returns from the theatre with a cradle over the limb and the foot of the bed elevated for 24 hours. The circulation in the foot is watched and any sign of deep vein thrombosis reported. This will be indicated by pain in the calf on dorsiflexion of the foot.

Stitches in the groin are usually removed on the fifth day after operation and the lower ones on the seventh day. The patient is allowed up after 24 hours and is encouraged to walk. He is not allowed to sit unless the leg is well elevated. He remains in hospital for a week to ten days and is taught to apply the Bisgaard's bandage himself, which he continues to wear for another fortnight.

If the patient can be discharged to the care of the community team he is usually transferred on the fourth day. The district nurse will remove the sutures on about the tenth day.

If the patient is considered unsuitable for the afore-mentioned forms of treatment then an elastic support stocking will be used to empty the dilated veins.

Varicose Ulcers

Varicose ulcers are caused by tissue hypoxia resulting from a poor venous return. The main principle of treatment is to support the tissues by means of pressure bandaging. A variety of bandages are available for this purpose.

1. *Bisgaard bandage.* This is an old favourite and is often used. It is applied from the metatarsal heads to the knee (including the heel). It is put on by the patient while still in bed in the morning and is not taken off until he returns to bed at night.

2. *John Bell and Croydon bandage.* This is skin-coloured so is favoured by women patients. The loop of the bandage is placed over the foot at the level of the base of the big toe and it is then applied in the same way as the Bisgaard bandage, care being taken to enclose all tissue in the area to be bandaged. The bandage is reapplied at midday if possible.

3. *Tubigrip.*

The dermatologist may also prescribe felt pads to be placed over the 'blow-out' areas and over obvious veins.

All attempts must be made to clean the ulcer and so a swab will be taken to identify any pathogenic organisms. If a gross infection is present the appropriate antibiotics will be prescribed. Alternatively an emulsion of Eusol and paraffin may be applied. The paraffin prevents the gauze sticking to the Eusol drying out.

The patient is given the following instructions:

1. Avoid standing still; take a few steps whenever possible.

2. Wear lace-up shoes, never slippers; if the feet get tired and hot change into another pair of lace-up shoes.

3. Do not sit with your legs crossed (this prevents venous return).

4. Do not sit with your legs up with pressure on the calf muscles, as this also reduces venous return.

5. Sit normally, but move your ankles up and down as though beating time to music.

6. Walk as much as you can.

7. Do not sit close to the fire. ⎫ These tend to engorge
8. Never bathe in the morning, only ⎬ the superficial vessels
at night. ⎭ with blood.

9. Raise the foot of the bed on 22 cm blocks.

Healing of the ulcer should be followed by surgery to the varicose veins. This is not undertaken until the ulcers are healed as they frequently cause enlargement of the inguinal glands, which can make the operation difficult, if not impossible.

The aims of *conservative treatment* of varicose ulcers are:

1. To control oedema and relieve venous stasis.
2. To restore joint mobility and keep the patient active and walking.
3. To soften the indurated areas.
4. To heal the areas of ulceration and eczema.
5. To instruct the patient in the care of the limb.

In order to achieve these aims the following methods are used:

Massage of the whole limb in an elevated position helps the circulation and softens the areas of induration. Local massage is also given to the indurated area around the edge of the ulcer.

The patient is encouraged to do *exercises* in the bandage. Toe and ankle movements are taught in order to increase joint mobility and to improve the pumping action of the calf muscle. Quadriceps drill is also taught. It may be necessary to treat the veins surgically to enable the ulcer to heal.

Post-thrombotic Syndrome

Post-thrombotic syndrome arises two to five years after thrombosis of the deep veins of the leg, occurring after childbirth or operation.

After the thrombus has formed in the vein it shrinks and there is a short period when there is great danger of emboli formation. After this the clot gradually becomes organized and adheres to the wall of the vein, which is recanalized. The valves, however, are destroyed, including those where the perforating veins enter the deep veins. Blood therefore tends to run from the deep veins where pressure is high to the superficial ones, where it is low. This leads to swelling, pain and chronic oedema of the ankle, prominent veins in the lower leg and finally gravitational ulcers. The condition frequently has little to do with incompetence of the superficial veins, but is due to thrombotic destruction of the valves in the deep veins. The condition must be treated by ligature of the perforating veins as they join the deep ones, thus preventing the outward rush of blood and its stagnation in the superficial tissues.

After the perforating veins have been controlled, healing of the ulcer may be accelerated by grafting.

14

Surgery of the Breast

CRACKED NIPPLES

Cracked nipple or fissure is a common complication of lactation, especially in cases where the nipple is flat or retracted. It can often be prevented by care in pregnancy, including drawing out of the nipple, and during lactation by washing and drying carefully before and after feeds. It causes severe pain, with the risk of infection, which may lead to acute mastitis and breast abscess. If severe, breast feeding must be discontinued and the breast emptied by breast pump; stilboestrol is ordered to dry up the secretion of milk; antiseptic is applied, e.g. tincture of benzoin or penicillin cream.

MASTITIS

Acute mastitis is the result of infection (often *Staphylococcus aureus*) entering through a break in the nipple and is generally associated with lactation. In the early stages it is treated by stopping breast feeding and by application of supporting bandages; local applications of heat and antibiotics may be ordered. Stilboestrol 10 mg daily for one week is ordered to dry up the secretion of milk if it is decided that discontinuation of breast feeding shall be permanent.

If the inflammation does not resolve and breast abscess follows, it may be treated by aspiration of pus or open drainage. Antibiotic treatment is given, e.g. the drug most suitable to the infection is determined by laboratory tests. If resolution occurs early breast feeding may be possible, but if it does not it is stopped early and the breast is emptied by a breast pump to avoid further congestion and pain.

218 SURGICAL NURSING

Mastitis may also occur in infants and at puberty and normally this condition resolves, unless septic infection is superimposed on the original inflammation, which is the result of endocrine stimulation in the infant from the mother's milk. As a rule no local treatment is needed, and any interference is likely to do more harm than good.

Chronic mastitis. During each menstrual cycle there is a slight enlargement of the breasts followed by regression. Sometimes this occurs unevenly instead of evenly throughout the whole breast and the areas of fibrosis which follow can be felt as lumps in the breast; such a lump can be as small as a pea. Since it is impossible to be quite sure that such a lump is not carcinoma it is common practice for these patients to be operated on (mammography being performed first). Initially a needle biopsy will be performed, then if malignancy is suspected the patient will be given a general anaesthetic and a specimen of the lump will be obtained in the operating theatre. A frozen section will be examined immediately and if the result demonstrates malignancy a simple mastectomy will be performed while the patient is still in the operating theatre. If malignancy is not present then the lump is excised. Occasionally enlargement of the rudimentary breast tissue present in the male occurs and is treated by excision.

NEW GROWTHS

Growths may be *simple* or benign, e.g. fibroadenoma of the breast or intraduct papilloma, or *malignant*, i.e. carcinoma or rarely sarcoma.

Simple growths cause a lump in the breast which is freely movable, and occur in younger women. Treatment consists of excision of the growth.

Malignant Growths

Carcinomas may be hard, when the growth is known as a scirrhous carcinoma, or a soft mass known as encephaloid carcinoma. These are both cuboidal carcinomas, but a squamous-celled carcinoma may occur, starting in the lactiferous ducts and giving rise to a blood-stained discharge from the nipple.

Signs and symptoms

There is a painless lump in the breast but some people do complain of a 'pricking' sensation. This becomes adherent to the skin and underlying tissue; the nipple may be retracted and there may be blood-stained discharge.

A woman complaining of any of these to a nurse should be advised to see a doctor immediately, as early treatment gives very satisfactory results. Some of these cases are still not seen till the growth is fungating or the glands in the armpit enlarged, when the chance of complete cure has been lost, and this situation has often arisen because the woman was afraid of hearing confirmation of the diagnosis she already suspected. Some patients are also afraid of being 'de-womanized' by removal of the breast. In view of the importance of early diagnosis, women should be shown how to examine their own breasts regularly for the possible existence of lumps.

Treatment

This depends upon the extent or staging of the neoplasia and may in advanced cases be preceded by radiotherapy. If the growth is small, a simple mastectomy will be performed immediately the diagnosis has been confirmed; if it is more extensive radiotherapy may be given then a simple extended (modified radical) mastectomy will be performed. A radical mastectomy is only carried out on rare occasions. If the condition is far advanced, especially in a premenopausal or early menopausal woman, an oophorectomy may be carried out to relieve the signs and symptoms, together with a mastectomy (especially if fungation has taken place). If the symptoms recur the surgeon may decide to perform an adrenalectomy. In very selected cases a hypophysectomy may be performed.

Hormone therapy with testosterone preparations, given by injection or by mouth, may be used in advanced cases with metastases in bone and other tissues. This may result in their disappearance, with complete relief from the pain they cause.

Cytotoxic therapy may be used to cause regression of the lesion if hormone therapy does not have an effect.

Preparation for mastectomy

The initial preparation for anaesthetic is required. If present anaemia must be corrected and as far as time allows the patient's condition built up by good diet with adequate protein and vitamin intake. Cessation of smoking and commencement of breathing exercises are important. Routine lung scans and skeletal surveys of skull, spine and pelvis are carried out to detect metastases. The areas which are to be involved in surgery are rendered as socially clean as is possible, first by bathing or washing, then by shaving. The patient is then given clean clothes for both herself and her bed.

After-care

When the patient returns to the ward from the operating theatre the nurse in charge must make sure that she knows which type of surgery has been performed and whether skin grafts have been taken or applied to the wound. If the patient is still unconscious routine care for the unconscious postoperative patient will be given and if she is conscious her condition will be evaluated before raising her to a sitting position. This will be done gradually and she will be well supported by pillows.

If blood loss has occurred during the operation it will be replaced by an intravenous transfusion, otherwise a dextrose/saline solution will be administered and this is usually continued for the first 24 hours. If the patient is not nauseated oral fluids are commenced and a light diet is introduced as soon as the patient feels ready to take it. Mobilization is commenced from the first day and ambulation is encouraged as soon as possible.

A suction drain is usually inserted into the chest wound to prevent the formation of a haematoma or the collection of tissue fluid which would cause the skin flaps to lift. The Redivac bottle is changed when required and the amount of drainage is recorded. When drainage ceases it is removed. Some surgeons favour the use of a pressure dressing on the wound to prevent fluid collecting but this can result in impairment of chest expansion.

If there is a risk of tension on the skin flaps when a large area of tissue has been removed then the surgeon may not insert skin sutures but will leave the wound open. A skin graft will be taken from the patient's thigh and this will be applied to the chest wound either at the time of operation or on the following day. This delay allows the wound area to become 'tacky', so that when the graft is in position it sticks to the area and so is much less likely to be washed off. In many cases this skin graft is then left exposed to the air as this prevents it being rubbed off by a dressing and allows direct observation of the area so that aspiration can be carried out immediately if blister formation should occur.

SURGERY OF THE BREAST

The nurse must remember that the donor area requires attention and should be aware of the fact that this may cause the patient a degree of discomfort.

Physiotherapy is given from the time of operation to encourage adequate chest expansion and to encourage the patient to increase her degree of arm movement gradually; neglect of this would result in a definite handicap.

The surgeon will request the appliance officer to visit the patient and to measure the patient and to evaluate which type of breast prosthesis will be most acceptable to the patient. This is usually done on the fifth postoperative day. The patient will then be given the opportunity to discuss the types and use of a prosthesis so that she may regain her confidence that she will look normal and feel comfortable.

Complications of mastectomy

1. *Limitation of movement* of the shoulder from scar contraction.
2. *Lung complications*, because deep breathing is painful, and in parts of the lung that are not well inflated mucus may plug a bronchial tube and lead to collapse. These complications are usually due to metastases.
3. *Local sepsis and sloughing*.
4. *Oedema of the arm*, which is usually due to metastases.
5. *Paralysis* may occur due to injury to the nerves during operation or their involvement in the growth. This may be only temporary if the nerve supply can be restored and the patient has special exercises to restore function and perseveres with treatment.
6. *Local recurrence* is not uncommon in advanced cases as a late complication. Hence the importance of a long follow-up period. These patients are likely to be seen one month after discharge; at three-monthly intervals for the first year; at six-monthly intervals for a further four years; and yearly for the rest of their lives.

Advanced carcinoma

The patient may have asked for help when her condition was too far advanced, in which case fungation may have occurred and metastases may be present in the lungs, liver, brain or bones.

If the neoplasm of breast has fungated then many surgeons will perform a simple mastectomy to relieve the patient's aesthetic distress and to reduce the risk of extensive infection or haemorrhage occurring. He will also perform a bilateral oophorectomy which in favourable cases brings about a remission lasting one year to eighteen months. When the tumour becomes active again he will consider performing a bilateral adrenalectomy which may give the patient another period of remission lasting about one year. Prior to this operation adequate steroid replacement therapy must be given. Postoperatively the patient is given hydrocortisone succinate intravenously, then cortisone acetate by intramuscular injection. By the third day the patient is able to take the cortisone orally. When the patient is discharged great care must be taken to impress upon her that she must take the cortisone every day for the rest of her life. She must also carry a card with her at all times stating that she must receive this drug and the daily dosage (usually 37·5 mg).

When patients have metastases in the bone pain may be intense, so radiotherapy is often ordered as it gives great relief.

Eventually, as the patient's condition deteriorates, terminal care is all that can be given.

HYPERTROPHY OF THE BREASTS

A general hypertrophy of both breasts is sometimes seen, even in young girls, and may cause great disfigurement and discomfort on account of the excessive weight. In severe cases, where the breasts hamper movement and cause discomfort, operation may be advised, as functionally they are of little use in lactation. This usually comes into the province of the plastic surgeon.

MALE BREAST LESIONS

These are rare, accounting for less than 1% of all breast cancer, but carcinoma, sarcoma, fibroadenoma and epithelial hyperplasia do occasionally occur. Prognosis is poor as the condition spreads rapidly to the regional lymphatic glands. Treatment is by means of a radical mastectomy with skin grafting and, in advanced cases orchidectomy, adrenalectomy and hypophysectomy are carried out.

15

Abdominal Surgery

Abdominal conditions requiring surgical treatment fall into three main groups:

1. Conditions which require surgical treatment for their cure but do not immediately threaten the patient's life.
2. Acute conditions which, unless the patient is operated on immediately, will prove fatal in a few days.
3. Laparotomy.

In the first group are patients who are suffering from mild forms of inflammation of the appendix or gall-bladder and patients who have developed a hernia or some form of chronic progressive intestinal obstruction. Other patients are also included in this category who have an acute condition involving organs such as the gall-bladder. These patients will have had conservative treatment during the acute phase and have been re-admitted for surgery two or three months later.

Patients in the second group are suffering from conditions which must be given urgent surgical treatment, such as acute intestinal obstructions, peritonitis, crush injuries and stab wounds to the abdomen when obvious damage has occurred. If surgical treatment is not given in these cases the prognosis is grave.

Certain patients are included in the last group when they have been given a provisional diagnosis but exploratory surgery is necessary to confirm the diagnosis. Treatment will be carried out at the same if it is necessary (or possible). These patients usually have a provisional diagnosis of carcinoma of one of the abdominal organs.

Preparation for Abdominal Operation

The preparation for abdominal operation is similar to that for operations generally, but all these cases are in the realm of major surgery and it is therefore specially important that the general condition of the patient should be good before operation. The

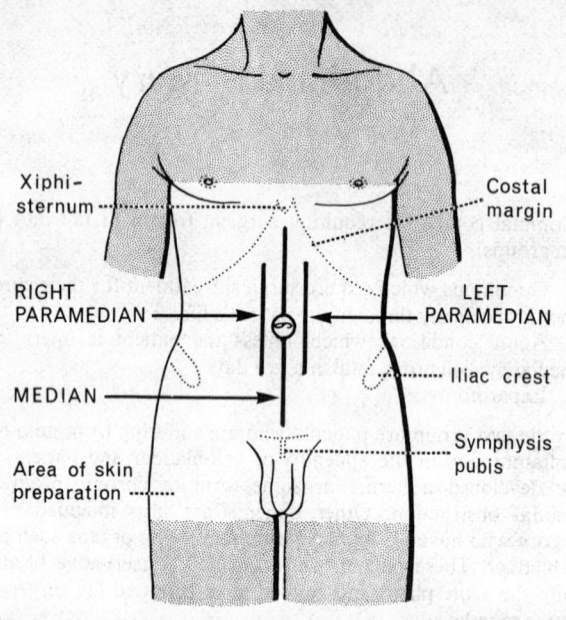

FIG. 25. Common incisions used for abdominal operations. Median and right or left paramedian incisions (high or low) are used for most laparotomies when the surgeon is unsure of the correct diagnosis. The area usually prepared (unshaded) extends from the nipple line to an imaginary line 7 cm down the thighs; it extends to each side as far as can be reached without turning the patient. As much of the pubic hair as possible is removed without separating the legs.

observations made by the nurse when the patient is admitted—temperature, pulse, respiration, blood pressure and urine analysis—must be repeated after a period of time as certain abnormalities may simply be caused by the stress associated with admission to hospital, such as tachycardia, hypertension and glycosuria.

The patient will be thoroughly examined by a surgeon and the anaesthetist. This will enable any other lesion to be identified, such as anaemia, heart failure, renal failure, chronic chest condition, or diabetes mellitus. If any of these conditions are recognized it may be necessary to postpone surgery until treatment can be given to improve the patient's general condition. If the patient has chronic bronchitis the specific antibiotic may be administered; the physiotherapist will encourage the patient to perform breathing exercises to allow adequate aeration of the lungs and if the patient smokes he will be asked to either stop smoking or at least reduce the number of cigarettes. This is very important as otherwise the risk of post-operative chest complications developing is high. To avoid communication errors, it is very important that the nursing staff knows what the doctor has told the patient, such as the type of anaesthesia to be used (general or epidural) or the possible extent of the operation. Usually the doctor will tell the nurse, but this will be written up in the patient's notes.

On admission some patients have been prescribed drugs by their general practitioner. The surgeon will have to decide if they may be continued or cancelled; for instance some doctors state that the contraceptive pill must *not* be taken within six weeks of an operation.

Attention to general hygiene will include a bath, shower or blanket bath before operation unless the patient is too ill. In all cases the abdominal wall is washed, paying special attention to the umbilicus in which dirt and organisms may collect, and the abdominal wall including the pubic hair is shaved. In emergency cases all this preparation may be left until the patient has been anaesthetized as handling the patient will only increase shock. Some surgeons like the abdominal wall to be painted with an antiseptic such as iodine or brilliant green before operation, but this is now uncommon.

Attention to oral hygiene is especially important as infected matter from septic teeth and gums will be present in the mouth and local sepsis may result; this is particularly so while the patient is taking little solid food by mouth, which checks the activity of the salivary glands and makes them prone to invasion by infection. Dental treatment may be necessary. If the patient has any capped teeth this must be mentioned to the anaesthetist: for this purpose a 'check list' is very useful.

Food or drink is not allowed by mouth for four hours before operation, or longer if the anaesthetist asks for this. If the operation is on the alimentary canal itself special instructions may be given; food may be withheld for a longer period and a stomach wash-out followed by leaving a Ryle's or Levien's tube in place and fixed by strapping over the nose or the zygomatic arch at the side of the face may be ordered. Some surgeons ask the nurses to cleanse the patient's bowel by giving fluids only for at least 24 hours pre-operatively and at the same time give 70 mg of sorbitol in 100 ml of water. This acts as a very strong aperient causing a rapid and extremely effective evacuation of the bowel contents about one hour after administration. A rectal washout is then performed to make sure the bowel is clean. When the operation involves the alimentary canal steps may be taken to render it free from micro-organisms, particularly in operations on the intestines. An antibiotic or sulphonamide which is not absorbed from the gut is used for this purpose, for example streptomycin, neomycin or phthalyl sulphathiazole by mouth. When these drugs are given the nurse must remember that they also destroy the normal organisms present in the mouth and intestines; parotitis and stomatitis may occur, so vitamin B is given orally to prevent conditions such as moniliasis (thrush) developing.

Heparin may also be administered prior to surgery and for two to three days following surgery to prevent deep venous thrombosis occurring. When this is used 5000 units are given subcutaneously with the premedication and three times a day until the patient is mobile again.

As for all other operations the patient's bladder must be empty before the anaesthetic is given; this is usually done immediately before the administration of the premedication drugs, the dose being calculated by the anaesthetist according to patient's height and weight. If the patient cannot micturate the bladder must be emptied by catheter or the surgeon informed that the bladder is not empty, since when full it rises up into the abdominal cavity and might be accidentally punctured allowing urine to escape into the abdominal cavity. Hence this point is of special importance. In all other respects the preparation has no special factors.

During abdominal operations the patient commonly lies flat on the operation table. If the pelvic organs are to be operated on then the Trendelenburg position, with the head low, the knees flexed over the lowest section of the table and the shoulders resting against special supports, is adopted. For operations on special organs such as the kidney, liver or gall-bladder the patient generally lies on one side and is held by special supports placed under him in suitable positions. Antiseptics such as Hibitane are applied to the skin before the incision is made, but once the abdominal cavity is opened no lotion other than sterile normal saline or Ringer's solution is allowed because the antiseptic solutions are irritating to the peritoneum and therefore liable to produce adhesions: these are bands of fibrous tissue binding the internal organs to one another or to the abdominal wall and are the result of inflammatory reaction in the covering peritoneum. Once the peritoneum is opened, the internal organs, if exposed, are covered with towels wrung out in warm, sterile normal saline solution, which are either changed, moistened with fresh warm saline, or enclosed in an intestinal bag. These prevent loss of heat and moisture from the peritoneal surface, as well as preventing abrasion of the delicate serous membrane.

Postoperative Care

Following abdominal surgery the patient care is the same as for any other operation. His immediate care consists of the routine necessary when a patient is unconscious and suffering from shock. As he regains consciousness and his blood pressure reaches its normal level he will be gradually placed in an upright position and will be encouraged to carry out breathing exercises. Mobilization will be commenced gradually but it must be emphasized that it is very important to encourage the patient to move round as freely as possible in bed and to cooperate with the health care team in becoming ambulant. Early ambulation reduces the risk of post-operative complications developing, but this is encouraged sensibly. If a patient is hypotensive or severely ill he must not be forced to sit out of bed in a chair. When the patient starts to walk the nurse must assist him to stand upright and must make sure that his footwear is safe, so enabling him to regain physical independence rapidly.

Initially the patient will be given intravenous fluids and the stomach will be kept empty by means of gentle suction. Then, as the volume of aspirate decreases the nasogastric tube will be removed: 30 ml of water will be given hourly. When the bowel sounds are heard or flatus is passed the volume of fluids will be increased to the level the patient chooses. On the following day soup will be given, followed by a gradual increase to a normal diet on the subsequent days. The diet will be decided by the surgeon and in most cases the patient will be allowed a light diet, which will progress to a normal diet as soon as he feels ready to eat it.

However in some cases, especially when the stomach or oesophagus has been operated upon, the surgeon will order a special diet which will be prepared by the dietician. In other cases the patient will be fed intravenously and special care will need to be taken to ensure that the patient's mouth remains clean and fresh. If the patient has to remain on intravenous therapy a central line will be introduced to replace the peripheral line so that parenteral nutrition may be given through it. Aminoplex, Intralipid, etc. will be used as these contain the required food values. The doctor will prescribe the type and volumes to be administered.

The wound need not be dressed until the stitches or clips are removed if the incision is closed without drainage, as is generally possible. If tension stitches have been inserted they are removed, as a general rule about the twelfth day. Clips which hold the skin edges together are removed on about the fifth to sixth day. Other stitches are removed on about the eighth or ninth day, although stitches in the back may be left longer as the circulation may be more restricted. Sometimes the dressing is removed on the first postoperative day and, if it is clean and dry, a 'plastic skin' is sprayed over the wound so that it can be observed without exposing the raw surface to the risk of infection. This method is not usually used if there are clips in the wound.

Wound drainage is often used following surgery. Vacuum, corrugated and round drains may be used. Sometimes a bag is placed over the end of the drain, because if fluid drains into the dressing there is an ideal breeding ground for infection. The bag collects the drainage fluid and holds it away from the skin. If the drain cannot be connected to the bag then a colostomy or similar bag is fixed to the surrounding skin.

Complications of Abdominal Surgery

Haemorrhage. This is not common but the nurse must be continually alert for either obvious bleeding or signs and symptoms which suggest that it is occurring.

Chest infections. A patient who had a productive cough before operation may develop a chest infection after it. His sputum will become purulent, his temperature will rise and other respiratory symptoms may be present. Infection is very likely to occur in heavy smokers, obese patients and those who are late to achieve mobilization.

Paralytic ileus is a normal physiological state for the first 24–48 hours following abdominal surgery and is due to the handling of the organs. It is also caused by irritation of the peritoneum, especially by blood which is very irritant to it. If the condition continues after this time then some other factor is involved, such as the loss of potassium by means of gastric aspiration. When this condition is diagnosed it is necessary to rest the bowel until bowel sounds can be heard again. This is done by feeding the patient intravenously with glucose/saline and performing gastric suction to stop the patient vomiting and to keep the stomach empty. The level of the serum electrolytes is measured daily; any deviation from the normal levels, especially of potassium, will be rectified at once. A record must be kept of all fluids given to the patient and of all fluids aspirated from or excreted by the patient. The mouth requires special care as it becomes dry and will taste very offensive to the patient.

Faecal fistula. This complication is sometimes seen when a patient has Crohn's disease and also following gastric surgery and following the closure of a colostomy when the distal segment of the colon was not patent. In this situation the patient may be given Vivonex or Flexical (a non-residue substance) as a diet which does not form residue as it is all absorbed. This rests the large bowel and prevents excoriation of the skin. The surgeon may have to close the fistula.

Femoral thrombosis. This may occur if the patient does not perform active leg exercises while in bed. The nurse must encourage him to tighten and relax all of his leg muscles, without flexing any joints, for a period of five minutes in every hour. For the same reason the patient is mobilized as soon as possible. The patient may, as has been previously mentioned, develop a pulmonary embolism.

Wound infection is recognized initially when the patient has a rise in temperature and complains of discomfort around the wound, which is red and swollen when the dressing has been removed. If a discharge is present a wound swab should be taken so that a culture may be made and sensitivity test may be performed. The appropriate antibiotic will then be prescribed if the doctor feels that it is necessary.

Burst abdominal wound. This is usually due to a weakness in the initial closure of the peritoneum. The tissues then divide, in layers, until the skin also separates to allow some of the abdominal organs to be visible, or to actually protrude. If this does happen the patient must be reassured, the surgeon sent for and the exposed bowel wrapped or covered with dressing towels soaked in warm, sterile, normal saline. It will be necessary for the patient to return to the operating theatre for re-closure of the abdominal wall.

Ventral hernia. A late result may be ventral hernia when the patient's condition is such that the muscular wall does not unite.

PERITONITIS

Peritonitis is inflammation of the peritoneum, the complicated serous membrane lining the abdominal cavity and covering most of its contents. It is due to infection and this may result from:

1. Rupture of any part of the alimentary canal, allowing the infected contents to escape into the peritoneal cavity. This may be the result of (*a*) disease, e.g. gastric, duodenal or typhoid ulcer, or perforated appendix (in addition to infection, rupture of, say, a gastric ulcer 'floods' the peritoneal cavity with the highly irritant acid gastric juice and the resultant effect is not unlike an extensive burn) or (*b*) trauma, e.g. a gunshot wound.

2. The spread of infection through the wall of a diseased organ, e.g. a gangrenous appendix, volvulus or strangulated hernia.

3. The introduction of micro-organisms from without through a wound, e.g. the battle casualty with gunshot, bayonet or bomb injury: in these cases the gut is also frequently perforated. In times of peace, gunshot wounds usually result from accidental firing of a gun carried by a careless sportsman.

4. A blood-borne infection such as infection by the pneumococcus or tubercle bacillus.

5. In a woman, infections can also enter via the open end of the uterine tube, but this is often blocked by adhesions in cases of infection, in which case either rupture of a tubal abscess or the passage of infection through the diseased wall may follow.

Peritonitis may be of various types. It may be acute or chronic, and the acute type may be generalized or localized. The acute types are serious and endanger life. The chronic form is associated with inflammation of the underlying organs, e.g. the appendix, intestine or Fallopian tube, and is a protective process tending to localize infection. It may give rise to adhesions which may result later in chronic or acute obstruction.

Acute Generalized or Diffuse Peritonitis

Acute generalized or diffuse peritonitis follows perforation of an ulcer or the spread of the local condition. At the onset the abdomen is rigid, because of the acute abdominal pain and there is great tenderness; the pulse is quick and wiry, the respirations thoracic, to reduce movement in the abdomen to a minimum and relieve the pain that it causes. There is vomiting, which becomes continuous and effortless and is finally bile-stained and foul, being described at this stage as 'faecal vomit' though in fact the vomited material does not consist of faeces, as the intestinal contents are regurgitated on account of the paralysis of the inflamed gut. The abdomen becomes more and more distended. No faeces or flatus are passed in the later stages. The pulse becomes quick and weak, the patient seriously ill with the typical 'abdominal appearance', the *Hippocratic facies*; the eyes are bright but sunken, the cheeks hollow and the expression drawn and anxious. (This was first described by Hippocrates, hence the name.) The temperature is generally raised at first, but later may be subnormal: the pulse is therefore the more important guide to the patient's progress.

Treatment

Immediate operation to drain the peritoneal cavity and deal with the cause is essential to save life. If the operation is performed early, the wound can be closed without drainage, otherwise drainage tubes are treated according to the surgeon's instructions. Penicillin, streptomycin and other antibiotics may be given systemically. Analgesics such as pethidine will be ordered to relieve pain. A Ryle's tube is passed and suction applied to relieve the vomiting. This will be continued till peristalsis can be heard by the stethoscope applied to the abdominal wall. A fluid intake and output chart will be kept and the electrolyte balance is estimated daily. Intravenous fluid will be ordered to prevent dehydration during the period of vomiting and syphoning off of gastric contents; the quality of normal saline given daily will depend on the electrolyte balance. Removal of digestive juice in large quantities very quickly upsets the electrolyte balance unless the appropriate precautions are taken. Good signs are a falling pulse rate, a falling temperature and improved appearance; gastric aspirate becomes less, flatus is passed, and the bowels are opened. Paralytic ileus will, and faecal fistula may, complicate these cases. The former may be fatal unless successfully treated by continuous aspiration, and drugs to rest the bowel. A faecal fistula usually heals satisfactorily, though it lengthens convalescence.

Acute Localized Peritonitis

Acute localized peritonitis results from an acute infective process within a cavity sealed off by adhesions, e.g. around an acutely inflamed appendix. Abscess formation may follow or the adhesions may break down, and the generalized condition will then result. In both cases surgical treatment to drain the infected matter from the cavity is essential unless a spontaneous cure occurs, without abscess formation. If an appendix mass has formed it is treated conservatively and an 'interval appendicectomy' is performed in three months' time.

16

Gastric and Duodenal Surgery

The chief gastric and duodenal conditions requiring surgical treatment are:

1. Gastric and duodenal ulcer, commonly classed together as peptic ulcer, and their complications such as pyloric stenosis.
2. Carcinoma of the stomach.
3. Hiatus hernia.

Rarely simple polyps may occur and cause vomiting of blood. These may be multiple.

Peptic ulcers and carcinoma give rise to indigestion but this may also be due to exhaustion, over-work and worry. In such cases the indigestion subsides if these causes are dealt with and the patient is given appetizing food, well cooked and nicely served, with rest and relief from worry.

Diagnosis

Various methods are used in diagnosing gastric and duodenal lesions; these include:

History. It is important that the patient's history is taken carefully. This may be difficult, for if the condition is a long-standing one the patient is likely to be very vague about its effects.

Manual examination with the patient in the dorsal position. This may reveal local pain and tenderness; a lump or dilatation may be felt, and slow emptying of the stomach may be detected.

Social habits. Smoking and stress have a particular bearing, especially in duodenal and gastric ulcers.

Examination of the stool for occult blood. This may reveal a positive result when there is no visual evidence of melaena; here it is the negative result that is of value as being indicative of the fact that there is no bleeding into the gastrointestinal tract; positive results could be due to very innocent causes.

Radiography. Straight X-ray will rarely be adequate and some contrast medium is required; this takes the form of various preparations of barium sulphate usually made up to a creamy consistency. For a 'barium swallow' the patient may only be required to take a few spoonfuls; he is then screened so that its passage down the oesophagus and into the stomach can be observed. For a 'barium meal' the patient is required to swallow much more of the barium preparation and is screened and has films taken over a period of hours—usually at least six but longer if information is required about the small and large intestine too. In preparing the patient it is very important to see that his stomach is empty of everything other than its own secretions. This examination may reveal the presence of ulcers, tumours, deformity due to scarring, rate of emptying and, during screening, the stomach movements.

Gastric acid test. This has now replaced many earlier methods of evaluating the acid content of the stomach. The patient is starved from supper-time on the previous day and on the morning of the examination a Ryle's tube is passed and the resting juice is aspirated from the stomach. The volume obtained and its pH are measured and recorded. An intramuscular injection of pentagastrin is administered and this will stimulate the production of hydrochloric acid in the patient's stomach. After one hour the stomach contents are aspirated and the volume and pH are again measured and recorded. If the volume and the pH of the gastric juice are above normal then a duodenal ulcer will be suspected; if they are below normal a gastric ulcer will be suspected. However, low levels are associated with achlorhydria from any cause.

Gastric cytology. This investigation is used to enable the detection of malignant cells in the stomach. The test is usually performed in the morning. The patient is given 1 litre of water to drink at 9 pm on the evening before the test and is not allowed anything at all orally overnight. At 9 am the next morning the patient is given another litre of water to drink, before the investigation is performed.

Blood investigations are carried out to detect any abnormality which would require rectification prior to surgery and to demonstrate typical blood pictures as found in patients who have suffered chronic blood loss.

Fibroscopy. The patient must be starved, as for any operation. One hour before the examination one amethocaine lozenge is given to the patient; he must allow this to dissolve in his mouth so that it anaesthetizes his mouth and throat. A second lozenge is given just before the examination is performed, and the premedication of atropine 0·6 mg is given according to the patient's age and general condition. The surgeon introduces the fibroscope while the patient lies on his left side without any pillows, and his eyes are covered with pads. The fibroscope is a long flexible instrument which enables the surgeon to have a clear view of the patient's oesophagus, stomach and pylorus via lens and light connected to the tube which consists of glass fibres. Following the examination the patient must not eat or drink for three hours.

Duodenoscopy. The patient is prepared as for a fibroscopy. The duodenoscope is passed and is used by the surgeon to inspect the duodenum. It can also be used for pancreatic and biliary studies.

Gastroscopy. The gastroscope is a tube of metal and rubber fitted with lens, eyepiece and hand bellows, by which the stomach can be inflated as required. It is possible to see the lining of the stomach and the action of the pylorus, but as with radiography, negative findings are not proof that there is no abnormality; possibly the greatest value of this investigation lies in being able to assess by repeated examination, whether an ulcer is healing. However since gastroscopy is very unpleasant for the patient this repetition cannot be lightly undertaken.

One or two amethocaine lozenges are given to the patient before the operation and Omnopon 20 mg is usually given first. The patient lies on the side with the head supported in a straight line on a suitable sandbag and held steady. The patient swallows the tube with the surgeon directing it, the head slightly forward. The head is then carried right back and the tube passed into the stomach. After removal a mouth-wash is given when ordered. Nothing should be given by mouth for some hours till the effect of the anaesthetic has passed off, or choking may result; then the patient can attempt to swallow a spoonful of clear water.

Ultra-sound. This procedure may be requested as an aid to diagnosis and is carried out in the X-ray department.

PEPTIC ULCERATION

Peptic ulcers consist of areas of erosion of a mucosal surface bathed with acid gastric juice. They are seen typically in the stomach (gastric ulcer), the upper end of the duodenum (duodenal ulcer), the lower end of the oesophagus if acid gastric juice is being regurgitated (so may therefore be associated with a hiatus hernia) and following surgery, on the line of anastomosis between the stomach and another organ (anastomotic ulcer).

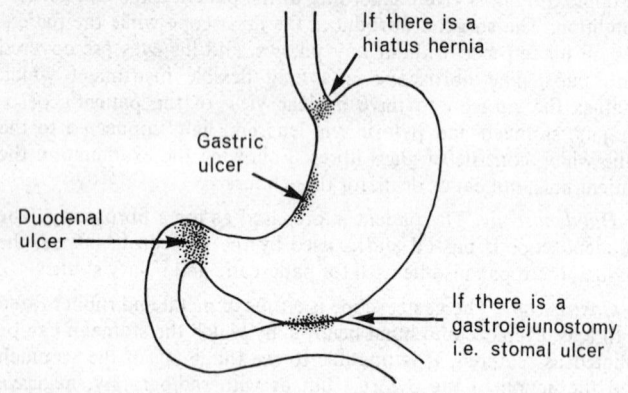

FIG. 26. Positions at which a peptic ulcer may occur.

In most instances they may be acute, subacute or chronic, the latter being the most commonly seen. Acute gastric ulcers are usually multiple, very small, producing transient effects and healing quickly. An acute duodenal ulcer may be seen as a complication, even in children, of severe burns and may draw attention to itself by means of a severe haemorrhage or by perforation.

Although distinction can be made, on signs and symptoms and on results of investigations, between gastric and duodenal ulceration such distinction is not of great importance.

Causes

The reason that peptic ulcers develop is unknown and many theories have been put forward over the years and then rejected. There is a greater degree of agreement as to what delays healing of an existent ulcer than in what in the first place caused it; these factors which retard healing include:

1. Overwork and worry.
2. Contact with acid gastric juice.
3. Irritant foods, e.g. those which are fried or those containing roughage or spices (now considered of less importance).
4. Smoking,
5. Excess alcohol.
6. Drugs such as steroids and aspirin.

Gastric ulcers are found on the lesser and never the greater curvature of the stomach; duodenal ulcers are found high up near the pylorus of the stomach.

Signs and Symptoms

1. Epigastric pain coming on soon after a meal in the case of gastric ulcers and perhaps two hours after in the case of duodenal ulcers.
2. Local tenderness.
3. Vomiting, more commonly in gastric ulcers, less so with duodenal ulcers.
4. 'Waterbrash'.
5. Loss of weight in the case of gastric ulcers, rarely with duodenal ulcers.
6. Presence of occult blood in the stools.
7. Pain relieved by food.

In duodenal ulceration the patient is often found to be of a worrying disposition and engaged in work that entails irregular hours and irregular meals.

Complications

1. Haemorrhage, i.e. haematemesis or melaena.
2. Perforation.
3. Pyloric stenosis.
4. Hour-glass stomach.
5. Malignant changes have been included in the past, as complicating, particularly gastric ulcers; it is now felt that any malignant lesion has probably been malignant all the time.

Haemorrhage

Haematemesis means that the ulcer has eroded a blood vessel; it causes the vomiting of coffee-ground acid vomitus, unless haemorrhage is very profuse, when bright red blood may be vomited, mixed with food. Treatment is usually conservative though operation may be needed in elderly patients with arteriosclerosis, or when there is so much local fibrosis that 'nature' cannot close the bleeding vessel down.

Melaena is similar except that partially digested blood, resembling a black tarry mass, is passed per rectum.

Perforation

Perforation means that the ulcer has eaten right through the stomach wall into the peritoneal cavity, so that the gastric or duodenal contents escape into the peritoneum and set up peritonitis.

These are usually slowly eroding ulcers, surrounded by a good deal of fibrosis; this latter has usually 'strangled' neighbouring blood vessels so haemorrhage is minimal.

Signs and symptoms of perforation:

1. Acute abdominal pain and tenderness, possibly but not invariably preceded by a history suggestive of peptic ulceration.
2. Rigid 'board-like' abdominal wall.
3. Vomiting may occur on account of the pain.
4. Pallor.
5. Subnormal temperature due to shock.
6. The pulse is at first little affected (70–90), but if shock remains untreated may increase in rate and decrease in volume.

After a few hours the effects of general peritonitis appear, the abdomen becomes distended, there is acute abdominal pain and tenderness and continuous vomiting, which becomes effortless; the rigidity lessens, the pulse becomes quick and weak and the temperature raised.

Treatment. Perforation may be treated by continuous aspiration of the gastric contents with the administration of morphine or by operation.

Operative treatment consists of either partial gastrectomy, if the patient's general condition is sufficiently good, or simple suture with cleansing of the peritoneal cavity. Operation will be carried out under cover of antibiotics to prevent and treat general peritonitis. If the patient is very ill on admission because a long period of time has elapsed since perforation occurred, resuscitation by means of blood transfusion or saline or dextran infusions, with gastric aspiration and the giving of antibiotics, may be necessary before operation is possible. When the condition has improved, simple suture will be necessary.

Pyloric stenosis

Narrowing of the pylorus due to scar contraction as the ulcer heals is a later complication and causes the vomiting of large amounts at long intervals; food which was taken some time earlier may be recognized in the vomit, the stomach being grossly dilated.

Hour-glass stomach

This is due to scar contraction in the centre of the stomach, dividing it into two cavities with a narrow opening between them. It is relatively rarely seen today, probably because in the increased incidence of peptic ulceration, the increase has been relatively great in duodenal ulceration.

Treatment

There is much controversy as regards the relative merits of medical and surgical treatment. Unless or until complications arise an attempt is usually made with medical treatment first and surgery resorted to either if exacerbations are so frequent and so severe as to cause prolonged and frequent absences from work, or if complications arise.

Medical treatment includes:

1. Physical rest, preferably in bed.
2. Removal of worry.
3. Sedation, e.g. phenobarbitone 30 mg twice or thrice daily.
4. Stopping smoking.
5. Small, frequent and bland meals. ⎫ to buffer
6. Milk drinks between meals. ⎬ the acid
7. Antacids, e.g. magnesium trisilicate mixture. ⎭ gastric juice
8. Biogastrone, to promote healing of gastric ulcers.

It has seemed that the very elaborate restrictions and modifications of normal meals have been of psychological rather than dietetic value!

Surgical treatment. Various operations have been devised, but almost all have aimed at removing the ulcer bearing area and/or cutting down the acid secretion powers of the stomach. This latter is achieved either by removing the area of the stomach normally concerned with secreting acid or cutting the nerve supply on which acid secretion depends. Operations therefore include:

1. Partial gastrectomy of one type or another.
2. Selective vagotomy (division of the branch supplying the stomach); a pyloroplasty is not required.
3. Vagotomy and pyloroplasty.

for oesophageal gastric and duodenal ulcers.

4. Local excision.

Operations used in the treatment of peptic ulceration and its complications

Partial gastrectomy. This is an extensive operation in which the lower two-thirds of the stomach is removed and the remainder joined to the jejunum or duodenum. Since the acid-forming gastric glands are found mainly at the pyloric end of the stomach and hyperacidity is often associated with the ulceration, this operation will hasten the healing of an ulcer even if it does not remove the actual ulcer. Shock may be considerable, but with advances in blood transfusion and saline or dextran infusions it can be treated successfully. Occasionally a fresh ulcer forms at the site of anastomosis, but as hyperacidity is reduced it is less likely to occur.

Gastroenterostomy. This is making a permanent opening from the stomach into the beginning of the jejunum. In a small proportion of cases fresh ulcers form at the site of this opening. This operation is generally carried out only in patients on whom gastrectomy cannot be performed.

Vagotomy. This is division of the branches of the vagus nerve, which stimulate gastric secretion and muscular activity. It may be performed to diminish acidity of the stomach. It is used with gastroenterostomy or pyloroplasty since without one of these the

GASTRIC AND DUODENAL SURGERY

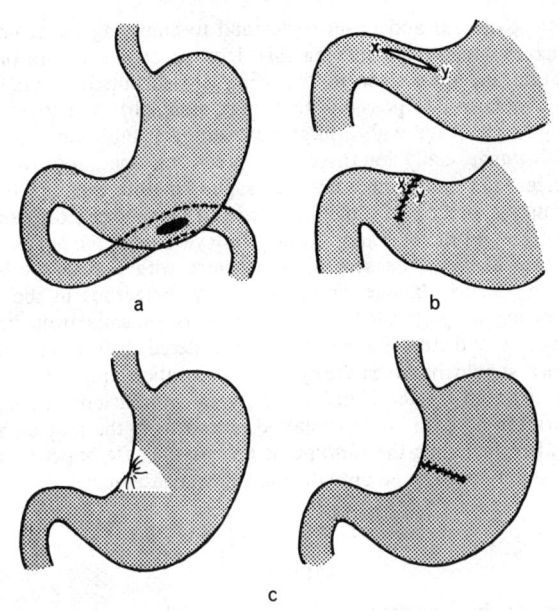

Fig. 27. Some stomach operations. (*a*) Gastroenterostomy. (*b*) Pyloroplasty. (*c*) Excision of a gastric ulcer.

diminished motility would make for problems in the stomach emptying.

Pyloroplasty. This is a plastic operation frequently carried out in association with vagotomy; the pylorus is incised longitudinally and so manipulated as to allow for suturing of the incision horizontally. By this means the passageway through the pylorus is enlarged.

Simple excision and repair is sometimes performed for emergency cases of perforation, but is liable to be followed by recurrence and therefore is not used except when the condition is urgent and does not permit the more extensive operations.

Preparation for Operation

In addition to the routine preparation, which must always include careful explanation and reassurance, special care should be paid to treatment of oral and nasal sepsis and to emptying the stomach. The exact means of achieving this depends on the nature of the operation and the reason for its being carried out. In the case of pyloric stenosis (or possibly hour-glass stomach) the patient may have gastric lavage with a large bore stomach tube, e.g. 22 to 24 English gauge, daily for three days preceding operation. In other instances the stomach may be aspirated the evening before (continuous suction is sometimes ordered by the surgeon) and on the morning of the operation through a Ryle's tube; the patient is in any case likely to be sent to the theatre with a Ryle's tube in position. Gastric lavage would be highly dangerous in the case of bleeding or perforated ulcer. If there is anaemia from haemorrhage, blood transfusion may be ordered before operation. Glucose should be given freely before operation and dehydration prevented, and treated if necessary by saline infusions. Such skin preparation as is to be done should extend from the nipple-line to the pubes, including the suprapubic hair; in the case of perforation, shaving may be delayed until the patient is anaesthetized.

After-care

Shock may be considerable so all nursing skills must be practised to reduce its severity. Blood transfusion may be continued after operation if there has been loss of blood before and during the operation to prevent anaemia. The blood pressure will indicate the need and also the blood count. If blood transfusion is not continued the patient is almost certain to be given other intravenous fluids and this will be continued until sufficient fluid is being taken (and absorbed by mouth). The actual volume and type of fluid depends on the patient's level of hydration and his serum electrolyte levels; usually between 2 and 3 litres are given per day.

When the patient's blood pressure has reached a 'safe' settled level he will be nursed in a sitting position.

Continuous suction may be used on the Ryle's tube, but usually it is aspirated at hourly intervals. This is continued until the volume of fluid aspirated is minimal, e.g. less than 100 ml in 12 hours, and until there are consistently good bowel sounds and flatus has been passed. Great care must be taken when aspirating the Ryle's tube to make sure that the tube is patent; neglect of this can result in a surgical emergency due to the stomach becoming distended with blood (should bleeding occur) or fluid.

GASTRIC AND DUODENAL SURGERY

Most surgeons allow the patient to take 15–30 ml of clear water as soon as the aspirate is becoming clear of blood. This fluid is given immediately following aspiration, so allowing time for it to be absorbed before the next aspiration. The volume is gradually increased to 60 ml hourly, when the Ryle's tube will be removed providing all other changes indicate improvement. Oral fluids are then gradually increased, and semi-solid food is introduced as soon as the patient is able to tolerate it and feels hungry. During this time a very strict fluid balance chart must be maintained. Most agree, particularly after partial gastrectomy, that meals should tend to be small and frequent rather than large and infrequent.

The mouth will require frequent attention and mouth-washes must be given hourly, with special care till the patient is eating a light diet. During this period the patient may be given small quantities of ice to suck to keep the mouth and throat moist. The use of boiled sweets to suck helps to keep the mouth moist by stimulating a flow of saliva. Chewing gum is also of great value in keeping the teeth and mouth clean. These may be given from the first day.

A chart of fluid intake and output is kept and the electrolyte balance is estimated while gastric suction and intravenous therapy continue.

An aperient is not given until the fourth or fifth day after operation. Senna or cascara preparations may be given twice daily, or liquid paraffin only after an initial dose with senna or cascara. Some surgeons do not like liquid paraffin as it may cause leakage at the suture line. Nowadays it is more likely that the patient will be given a suppository, bisacodyl or glycerin, on the second or third day after operation. If the patient is worried about the lack of bowel action, it is necessary to remind him that this is to be expected as he has not eaten solid food.

Chest complications are very liable to occur, as the patient may not use the diaphragm freely. The chest must be well protected, fresh air being provided without either draught or chill, a point which needs more thought than is often given to it. Deep breathing exercises are taught by the physiotherapist and the nurse should encourage the patient to carry them out frequently. Most surgeons get these patients up early to lessen the risk of chest complications—on the first day following the operation. If the patient's condition permits he will also be assisted out of bed during the afternoon of the first day and will be allowed to have a walk round his bed. This will be increased each day. If the patient just sits in a chair it will increase the risk of a deep venous thrombosis forming, so walking is essential.

No smoking is allowed at first and no alcohol. When the patient is up and walking about he may be allowed one cigarette a day after a main meal if he must smoke at all. He should smoke, if possible, only after meals and moderately and should take alcohol only moderately and with meals. He is advised to eat at frequent and regular intervals and to take sufficient time over his meals, chewing his food well. If his work makes meal times erratic, he should carry biscuits and chocolate to eat between meals so that his stomach does not remain empty for long periods. The manner of eating is more important than the content of the meal.

There is a psychosomatic factor in this illness, i.e. one in which the state of the mind can have a causative effect, mental stress helping to produce excessive gastric secretion and activity: if this is explained to the patient and he is encouraged to seek relief from emotional distress associated with either his work or domestic life, recurrence is less liable to occur. He should not, if possible, return to work for two months.

Complications are possible and include leakage from the duodenal stump, giving rise to generalized peritonitis or subphrenic abscess, obstruction due to oedema at the site of the anastomosis between the stomach and the small intestine, stagnation of the contents in the blind end of the duodenum, causing distension, pain and vomiting. If oedema does cause obstruction hypertonic saline or concentrated plasma may be administered. Hypertonic saline (1·8%) is passed down the Ryle's tube and then aspirated back after a period of two to four hours. This overcomes the oedema. Leakage and stagnation due to kinking will require a second operation. Post-gastrectomy dumping syndrome may occur, a feeling of weakness soon after a meal, and anaemia.

GASTRIC CARCINOMA

This occurs in older patients, generally over 50 years, and especially in men. There is a history of indigestion and loss of appetite over a relatively short period of time—weeks rather than years as with peptic ulceration; if the growth is in the body of the stomach there may be no other symptoms until the patient begins to show symptoms of cachexia, i.e. loss of weight, weakness and anaemia. The condition is therefore frequently undiagnosed until it is inoperable, as the patient does not come for advice. There may be haematemesis. A lump can be felt in the abdomen. If the growth is at the pylorus, obstruction occurs early.

Treatment

If seen in time, partial or total gastrectomy is performed. If the lymphatic glands and liver are already affected, gastroenterostomy is performed to relieve obstruction and prevent starvation, but it is merely palliative. Modern surgeons, because of the improved methods of anaesthesia, with the use of muscle relaxants and the introduction of antibiotics to overcome infection, may carry out more extensive operations. With the stomach, parts of the pancreas and the spleen and lymphatics may be removed, and even parts of the liver, the cut surface being quickly covered with alginate gauze to arrest bleeding from its surface. If operation is not undertaken to remove the growth, death will probably result from hepatic insufficiency, when a large part of the liver is involved. Secondary growths in the liver may still follow the more radical operations. Even when the growth appears to be in its very early stages at the time of operation, prognosis is very poor; however an operation like partial gastrectomy is well worth while, even when carried out at a late stage as the patient's end is made a little less distressing, both to him and to his relatives.

It has been estimated that 15% of patients with carcinoma of stomach have a five-year survival rate following surgery.

CONGENITAL HYPERTROPHIC PYLORIC STENOSIS

Pyloric stenosis in infants is due to congenital hypertrophy of the sphincter. It gives rise to vomiting, which comes on in the third to fourth week and becomes increasingly projectile, shooting out 30–60 cm from the child in advanced cases. There is a visible peristalsis from left to right in the left hypochondriac and epigastric regions. A tumour can be felt over the pylorus. The child rapidly becomes dehydrated, the skin becoming loose and wrinkled. There is loss of weight and constipation unless the condition is diagnosed and treated early.

The condition is generally seen in male infants and usually affects the first child.

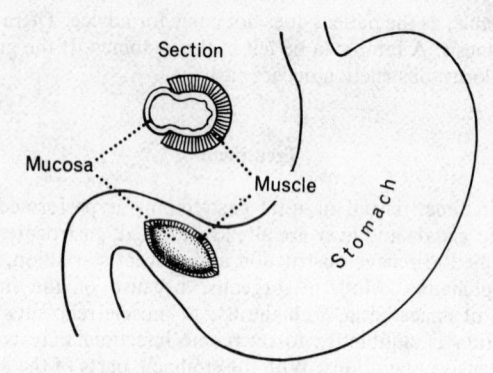

Fig. 28. Ramstedt's operation for congenital pyloric stenosis, showing the muscle fibres divided and the mucous membrane bulging through the incision.

Treatment

Medical treatment by special feeding and/or antispasmodic drugs such as methonitrate (Eumydrin) and stomach washouts was used in the past, but mortality was high, partly because of the prolonged hospitalization which was inevitable. Surgical treatment has given good results since Ramstedt's operation was introduced, provided it is done early, before there is much dehydration and wasting. This consists of dividing the muscle fibres at the pylorus, allowing the mucous membrane to bulge through.

Preparation for Operation

The stomach is washed out the evening before and the morning of the operation, using saline or water; it is usually repeated during the four hours prior to operation. Subcutaneous saline is given, and repeated four- to six-hourly if there is dehydration, giving the right proportions of normal saline and other fluids to keep the electrolyte balance correct, or an intravenous infusion is commenced, perhaps the preceding day. Care must be taken to prevent heat loss from the infant.

GASTRIC AND DUODENAL SURGERY

After-care

Infusions. Subcutaneous saline may be given on return to the ward, and repeated as required according to the condition and pulse. In severe cases intravenous saline and glucose infusions or blood transfusion may be given.

Diet. Postoperative feeding will be ordered by the specialist and the regimen varies considerably. The following is a specimen diet:

First day. Commence feeds four hours after operation, giving 5 ml of 5% glucose in water hourly for four feeds.

Increase to 7–8 ml of 5% glucose in water hourly for four feeds.

Increase to 10 ml of breast milk if procurable from the infant's own mother or from a breast milk 'bank', otherwise milk and water mixture, or half-cream dried milk, every one and a half hours for four feeds. Wherever possible, when a baby is admitted to hospital it is given the same milk preparation it had been having at home, unless this was *highly* unsuitable.

Increase to 20 ml every one and a half hours for four feeds.

Second day. Give 30 ml every two hours for six feeds.

Third day. Then give 90 ml three-hourly, at 6 a.m., 9 a.m., 12 noon, 3 p.m., 9 p.m., and 12 midnight daily.

If the child is breast fed, milk must be drawn off with a breast pump and given by bottle till the infant is well enough to be put to the breast on the second or third day. This procedure is considerably easier now that the practice of admitting mothers with their babies is increasing.

Prevention of infection. Great care is necessary to prevent cross-infection giving rise to gastroenteritis in these infants. Feeds should be prepared and given by nurses who do not also 'change' babies. They should be prepared in a special milk kitchen and both prepared and given with strict precautions to prevent infection. The infant should be sent home as early as possible—often towards the end of the first week—returning for removal of sutures at seventh to tenth day for the same reason, i.e. to shorten his contacts with possible sources of infection, as gastroenteritis following operation may prove fatal.

General care. The infant must be kept warm, but overheating carefully avoided. Any vomiting or diarrhoea after operation should be reported, and a record of the weight kept as an important indication of the child's progress.

FOREIGN BODIES IN THE STOMACH

Gastrotomy, or opening of the stomach for removal of foreign bodies, is sometimes necessary; most foreign bodies that have been swallowed will, however, pass through the tract, and meals of thick porridge are given to assist this. All stools should be carefully inspected till the foreign body is recovered.

Gastrostomy should not be confused with gastrotomy. In gastrotomy the opening into the stomach is closed straightaway; in gastrostomy a relatively permanent opening, or stoma is left, usually as a means of feeding the patient.

OTHER GASTRIC OPERATIONS

These consist mainly of anastomoses between the stomach and other neighbouring organs, e.g. the gall-bladder (see Chapter 18).

17

Conditions Affecting the Intestines

Conditions affecting the intestines and requiring surgical treatment include forms of inflammation, for example appendicitis, one of the most common; also ileitis, diverticulitis and ulcerative colitis when these conditions do not respond to medical treatment; new growths; intestinal obstruction due to a number of different causes; and trauma.

APPENDICITIS

Appendicitis is very common in affluent races and is frequently associated with a history of constipation. Concretions may be present in the appendix, which is inflamed.

The typical signs and symptoms are:

1. *Generalized abdominal pain* of sudden onset, with generalized tenderness and aggravated by movement.
2. *Nausea and vomiting* following the onset of pain.
3. *Rise of temperature*, usually to between 37·2 and 37·7°C.
4. *Rise of pulse rate* correspondingly.
5. The pain and tenderness later becoming *localized* in the right iliac fossa, together with muscle rigidity in the same area.
6. Usually a history of *constipation*, but diarrhoea may occur when the appendix lies behind the caecum.
7. The *tongue is furred* and appetite is lost.
8. The patient prefers to lie still with flexed knees.
9. The patient may give a history of previous 'milder' attacks.

In mild cases the symptoms are not so typical and the condition may be mistaken for gastric trouble or bilious attacks; unfortunately the patient is sometimes given a drastic aperient by well-meaning relatives and this may precipitate perforation. Pain is comparatively mild; there is vomiting, constipation and indigestion. The omentum may become adherent to the appendix and drag on the stomach; also the lymphatic glands draining the appendix run up towards the stomach and may become involved. These factors make diagnosis difficult, as the symptoms suggest gastric and duodenal conditions.

Causes

The appendix is invariably obstructed by a faecolith within its lumen, but the obstruction may be due to enlargement of lymphoid tissue or a 'kink' caused by adhesions. This obstruction causes bacteria to multiply within the obstructed appendix and these invade its walls causing obstruction to its blood supply. These blood vessels are end arteries from the ileocolic artery and so

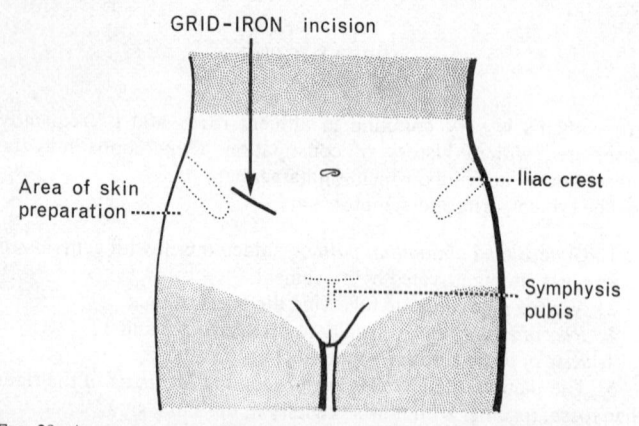

FIG. 29. A common appendicectomy incision. A grid-iron incision is about 7 cm long, starting just above the level of the anterior superior iliac spine and running a little nearer to the horizontal than does the groin crease. The area of skin usually prepared (unshaded) extends from the level of the umbilicus down to the top of the thighs. It extends to each side as far as can be reached without turning the patient. As much pubic hair as possible should be removed without separating the legs.

obstruction due to formation of thrombi results in gangrene of the appendix and the risk of perforation.

An attack of acute appendicitis may resolve, but on the other hand it may lead to gangrene, perforation and general peritonitis, with fatal results; even if it subsides it is liable to recur and adhesions (bands of fibrous tissue, due to the inflammatory reaction) are likely to form, binding the appendix to the neighbouring coils of intestine, the omentum and the abdominal wall.

In such cases a further attack may lead to a perforation into a small cavity shut off by adhesions, resulting in a localized abscess; if this is not opened and drained, it may rupture internally and give rise to a generalized peritonitis.

Pain may be colicky, due to obstruction by adhesions or concretions, and, especially in young subjects, may lead to the injudicious administration of castor oil, with serious results; this must always be borne in mind when treating children with colic. Even mild aperients should *never* be given in the presence of undiagnosed abdominal pain.

Treatment

Operative treatment, appendicectomy, is now advocated as a general rule, on account of the serious risks of perforation, gangrene and abscess formation. If the attack is not severe, the appendix is removed and the wound closed without drainage. In acute cases with peritonitis drainage is essential; in cases of appendix abscess, the abscess is opened and drained without removal of the appendix, and the appendix is removed later, when the inflammation has died down. In all cases where there is risk of peritonitis the use of systemic chemotherapy with the appropriate antibiotics has greatly improved the outlook.

Preparation

In acute cases the operation is an emergency one, and the only preparation is shaving of the site, if time and condition permit. In other cases the routine preparation for abdominal operations is required. The surgeon's wishes with regard to the giving of aperients and an enema preoperatively must be carefully followed; in the acute case nothing is done.

Preoperative urine testing is important, particularly for albumen. The presence of albumen, especially with a temperature over 37·7°C, suggests a right-sided kidney infection as a possible alternative diagnosis.

ULCERATIVE COLITIS

This is a common disease of the large intestine. It is most commonly diagnosed in females between the ages of 20 and 40 years and is suspected of being an autoimmune disease. It can affect any part of the large intestine, but is most commonly seen in the sigmoid colon and rectum.

Many patients are given conservative treatment by the physicians for many years before surgery is performed, but in some cases the decision to operate is made very early in the illness as it may present in an acute, rapidly progressive form, the patient suffering from severe blood loss and disturbance of his nutritional and electrolyte levels. A retention enema of prednisolone, 20 mg in 100 ml of fluid, may be given in the medical treatment.

When a patient has this condition he experiences varying levels of diarrhoea which, during acute phases, contains blood, mucus and pus. Abdominal pain will be present and this may be severe and colicky in nature. The patient will appear to be anaemic, weak and eventually emaciated.

The state of the patient's colon is assessed by means of a barium enema and sigmoidoscopy and the type of surgery will be decided. If the lesion is small and localized it may be possible to resect the affected area (colectomy), otherwise an ileostomy will be necessary. This may also involve a perineal excision of rectum in which case the ileostomy will be permanent.

Preoperatively the surgeon will prescribe oral medication, and the patient should be visited by a member of the Ileostomy Association, so that he may discuss his future with a person who can give positive advice and support from her or his own experience. Rectal wash-outs are *not* performed before an ileostomy when a patient has ulcerative colitis as this could be very dangerous.

Many patients with this condition are given corticosteroids and if this is so an increased dosage is prescribed to 'cover' the operative period. This is reduced gradually during the postoperative time.

CONDITIONS AFFECTING THE INTESTINES 253

After-care

When an ileostomy has been performed the patient will require a great deal of emotional support, as this is an aesthetically offensive operation, and the nurse must help the patient to overcome his initial repugnance by her attitude and explanations.

The ileostomy apparatus that is most suited to the patient will be chosen and great care will be taken to teach the patient about the care of his stoma and the surrounding skin. It is very important that the equipment fits perfectly round the stoma, but it must not constrict it. This is necessary as excoriation will occur if the faecal fluid comes in contact with the skin. In some cases, such as when the Chiron apparatus is used, a karaya gum washer is eased in between the stoma and the apparatus and this creates a protective seal. However, many types of apparatus entail sticking adhesive on the skin, and the patient may be allergic to it, but in other cases the adhesive is incorporated into a karaya gum disc which is very soothing and protects the skin. It is advisable that, before the operation, pieces of adhesive from the different types of apparatus are fixed to the patient's forearm. This will act like a patch test and will indicate which types of adhesive the patient is sensitive to, and so this type of adhesive will not be used. Sometimes it may be found necessary to use a combination of the different types of equipment as the most important thing is to ensure that the patient is equipped in the most suitable manner.

The patient will be encouraged to eat all types of food and observe the effect it has on his ileostomy action, and then to avoid the foods that 'upset him'.

Following discharge he will obtain supplies of equipment by prescription from his own doctor and should be capable of living a normal, active life.

INTESTINAL OBSTRUCTION

Intestinal obstruction may be considered in two main groups:

1. *Mechanical.*
    a. Conditions within the lumen, such as faecal impaction or gall-stone ileus.
    b. Conditions within the wall, such as tumours or Crohn's disease.

254 SURGICAL NURSING

   c. Conditions outside the wall, such as strangulated hernia, volvulus, intussusception or adhesions.
2. *Paralytic*, when the ileum is paralysed.

Obstruction may be acute or chronic. Acute conditions generally affect the small intestine; chronic obstruction particularly affects the large intestine.

Acute Obstruction

Causes of acute obstruction include:

1. Strangulated hernia.
2. Adhesions following surgery or deep X-ray therapy for carcinoma of the cervix.
3. Volvulus.
4. Intussusception.
5. The chronic case becoming acute.
6. Faecal impaction especially where growths are present.

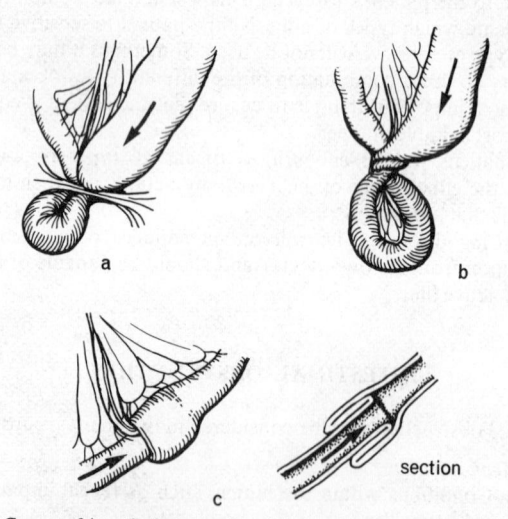

FIG. 30. Causes of intestinal obstruction. (*a*) An adhesion constricting a loop of bowel. (*b*) Volvulus, i.e. a loop of bowel which has twisted on itself. (*c*) Intussusception, i.e. the telescoping (or invagination) of one piece of bowel into another.

7. Rarely a large gall-stone may ulcerate from the gall-bladder into the bowel and produce obstruction.

8. Paralytic ileus also results in acute obstruction as nothing can pass along the gut owing to the paralysis of the inflamed intestinal muscles; this is a physiological rather than mechanical obstruction.

Signs and symptoms of acute obstruction

1. Acute pain, colicky in type, is usually the first symptom.

2. Vomiting; first the stomach contents, then bile-stained, and finally 'faecal' or stercoraceous vomit which has a definite faecal odour; the higher the obstruction, the earlier vomiting is likely to occur.

3. Absolute constipation; no passage of faeces or flatus.

4. Increasing abdominal distension, especially in chronic large bowel obstruction.

These may be associated with:

1. Shock: subnormal temperature, quick weak pulse, cold clammy skin, cold sweat and pallor.

2. Dehydration due to persistent vomiting, and causing collapse: low blood pressure, dry skin, hollow cheeks, sunken eyes.

3. Septic absorption. These effects will follow later; the higher the obstruction the more quickly they arise; temperature and pulse rate are raised; the skin is hot and the cheeks flushed; in severe cases there will be delirium and possibly a fatal result, as peritonitis will occur unless the condition is treated early by surgical interference.

If a patient presents with these signs and symptoms, then an X-ray of the abdomen will be carried out. This will show the distended bowel and fluid levels which will help to localize the site of the obstruction.

Strangulated hernia

In cases of strangulated hernia the bowel is nipped by the neck of the hernia sac and the return of blood by the veins is obstructed because of their thin walls; the blood pressure in the veins rises, becoming as high as in the arteries, resulting in rupture with haemorrhage into the bowel wall and obstruction to the flow of blood in the arteries. As a result gangrene of the bowel wall sets in and infection from the contents of the bowel causes acute inflammation which spreads to the peritoneal cavity, resulting in general peritonitis, unless early operation relieves the condition.

Adhesions

Adhesions are bands of fibrous tissue developed in the abdomen as a result of previous inflammation. These may nip the wall of a piece of the bowel in the same way and produce the same results (Fig. 30).

Volvulus

Volvulus is a twisting of the bowel on itself. This nips the mesentery supplying the twisted portion of the bowel, obstructing the blood vessels, and producing gangrene and peritonitis unless relieved. In the adult it occurs most frequently in the sigmoid flexure when there is constipation and a strong aperient is taken. This is due to the short attachments of the mesentery here. Vomiting occurs early in these cases, although the obstruction is low. In adults, operation and chemotherapy will save life, if early diagnosis and surgical intervention are practicable. In infants the whole small intestine may twist on itself and become gangrenous; this condition is always fatal.

Intussusception

Intussusception is the telescoping of one piece of bowel into another. It is often associated with over-vigorous peristalsis, which may be due to swelling of lymphatic tissue in the gut. When this condition develops in adults it is usually due to a benign tumour, but can be caused by a malignant form.

The signs and symptoms include the following:

1. The child becomes pale, draws up its legs and screams at intervals on account of colicky pain.
2. It passes one normal stool after the first attack, and then only blood and mucus, called the redcurrant jelly stool.
3. Between the attacks he will go to sleep and be quite comfortable.
4. Vomiting.
5. A sausage-shaped tumour may be felt in the abdomen (usually in the right hypochondrium); this hardens during an attack of colic.

If treated early by surgical operation, the piece of gut can be reduced by squeezing it out, with very successful results, but, if left, the mesentery supplying it will become severely nipped and gangrene and peritonitis will follow. Operation for removal of the gangrenous gut and anastomosis is carried out with intensive chemotherapy, using penicillin and other antibiotics, with or without sulphonamides. The condition is very serious and the earlier the operation is carried out the greater the chance of recovery. In infants resection of a strangulated bowel carries a high mortality.

Chronic obstruction due to a growth may become *acute* owing to a solid mass of faecal matter completely blocking the narrowed lumen of the bowel. In this case and in that of gall-stone there is not the same danger of gangrene of the bowel and peritonitis, but there will be septic absorption from the decomposing contents of the bowel above the obstruction, which cannot be evacuated.

Paralytic ileus

Paralytic ileus is always present for the first few hours following major abdominal surgery and so the alimentary tract is rested. In some cases gastric suction is used with the administration of a limited amount of fluid such as 30 ml per hour immediately after aspirating the stomach contents. The gastric suction helps to decompress the bowel. This is given to keep the patient's mouth and pharynx moist. Many cases which would previously have been hopeless make a satisfactory recovery with modern treatment, but the earlier diagnosis and treatment are carried out the less severe will be the patient's condition.

Treatment of acute obstruction

Immediate operation is the only means of saving life and must be undertaken within a few hours where there is a risk of gangrene and peritonitis. In doubtful cases the nurse may be asked to give a small gentle enema to see whether constipation is present. A second enema may be ordered as the first may empty the bowel below the obstruction; if the second enema results in the passage of flatus, it suggests the obstruction is not complete. Morphine may be ordered to relieve the pain and so improve the patient's general condition. The sulphonamides which are not readily absorbed may be given by mouth, together with the antibiotics that are effective by this route, e.g. neomycin, streptomycin or chlortetracycline; they serve as disinfectants to the intestinal contents and lessen the toxaemia which occurs from absorption from the obstructed bowel. A stomach wash-out is also sometimes ordered, so that the patient may not vomit foul material under the anaesthetic, to lessen the risk of pneumonia from the sucking of such matter into the lungs. A Ryle's tube may be used with aspiration and continuous suction after operation.

The operation will consist of relieving the obstruction and examining the gut; if it seems liable to become gangrenous, resection and anastomosis will be necessary, i.e. the affected part is cut away and the ends are joined. This is generally done by stitching up the two ends, placing them side by side and making an opening between them; this is called lateral anastomosis. End-to-end anastomosis, i.e. the joining of two ends after removal of the affected gut, is liable to result in narrowing of the lumen from scar contraction. Drainage of the abdominal cavity may be necessary.

The postoperative nursing will be similar to that needed after any abdominal operations. Shock is severe and the patient is often dangerously ill for a few days; vomiting may be troublesome on account of peritonitis, but this responds to treatment by resting of the alimentary tract, with intermittent or continuous gastric or duodenal suction postoperatively; anti-gas-gangrene serum may be given to lessen the risk of infection of the intestinal wall and intensive chemotherapy will be used. Dehydration will be treated or prevented by the giving of intravenous saline, with glucose, or other fluids such as dextran, during the postoperative period, when no fluids may be given by mouth. The usual safeguards of keeping a fluid intake and output chart, checking the electrolyte balance in the blood stream and the care of the mouth will be of great importance. The diet will be ordered by the surgeon and will vary with the severity of the conditions found at operation. The surgeon's instruction should be obtained with regard to the aperient, but usually aperients are better avoided. The passing of a flatus tube or the giving of enemata may be ordered for flatulence.

Chronic Obstruction

Chronic obstruction is usually due to malignant growths. These commonly occur in the sigmoid flexure and rectum, less commonly in the caecum and transverse colon. They are never found in the small intestine.

Signs and symptoms of chronic obstruction

1. A history of alteration in the bowel habit, with either constipation, or alternating constipation and diarrhoea. This latter is due to the solid faeces being held up by the obstruction, decomposing and so liquefying, and then being easily passed.
2. Attacks of colicky abdominal pain over a period of time.
3. Abdominal distension.
4. Visible peristalsis according to the site of obstruction.
5. Distended coils of gut may be obvious and produce the 'ladder abdomen'.
6. Blood may be passed per rectum, though this may only be due to haemorrhoids.
7. Wasting, weakness and anaemia will be obvious in late cases; these tend to result from the malignancy rather than the obstruction.

Treatment of chronic obstruction

Operation is essential. If the patient is seen early, removal and anastomosis is performed (Fig. 31); in rectal cases colostomy and excision of the rectum (see Chapter 20) may be carried out. If the condition has become acute, colostomy is performed for drainage, with the administration of a course of succinylsulphathiazole, sulphaguanidine or streptomycin by mouth: later an-

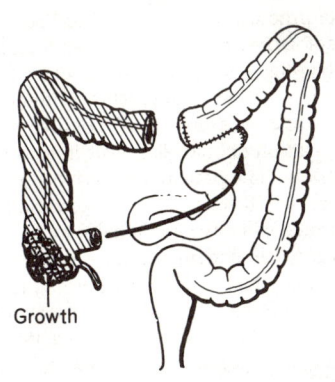

FIG. 31. Excision of the first part of the large intestine with lateral anastomosis of the ileum to the transverse colon. Shading indicates the area removed.

SURGICAL NURSING

astomosis is carried out when the general condition has improved. If the growth has already spread to glands or liver, removal may be impossible and permanent colostomy is necessary to prevent death from obstruction.

Colostomy

This name is derived from two Greek words, *kolon* meaning colon and *stoma* meaning mouth. There are two different types of colostomy.

1. *Temporary*, where a loop of bowel is brought out on to the abdominal wall and this consists of proximal (into colon on small intestine side of stoma) and distal (into colon on rectal side of stoma) parts of the loop.

2. *Permanent*, where the stoma is brought out and sutured to the abdominal wall, the rectal side of the colon having been excised.

With present-day availability of antibiotic and chemotherapeutic drugs, there is not the same need as formerly to bring an unopened loop of gut out and to wait for the peritoneal cavity to be sealed off prior to releasing intestinal contents; it is consequently practicable for the surgeons to form a proper stoma into the colon.

When colostomy is a planned operation, the patient *should* be told the nature of the operation and made to understand that, though very distressing at first, with care and training the working of the colostomy can be conveniently controlled, so that he can live a normal life.

It is a sensible practice for the patient to become accustomed to the 'feel' of the colostomy bag against his abdominal wall before the operation, so a bag has a small volume of warm fluid poured into it and is then fixed in position. The patient continues with his normal day's activities while wearing it. If possible a member of the Colostomy Association should also visit him to discuss his future life with a colostomy. The patient will derive a great deal of benefit from this visit as the discussion with a person who has had a colostomy performed will have much more meaning.

Following surgery the patient will have two wounds. One will be the colostomy stoma which will be discharging faecal fluid and the other will be an abdominal incision. This later wound must *not* be contaminated with the faecal fluid and *must* be dressed using the full aseptic technique. If possible it must be sealed off in such a way that it requires the minimum of attention.

There are many types of disposable colostomy equipment

CONDITIONS AFFECTING THE INTESTINES

available and their use makes the nursing care of the patients much easier and renders the operation much more acceptable to the patient. The Hollister loop ostomy method is very effective following surgery as it consists of a bag that can be emptied and re-used, a gasket and belt to hold it in position and an adhesive karaya gum seal that fixes it to and protects the skin. The adhesive karaya gum seal does not require changing each time the bag is changed and is left in position until it becomes loose and there is a risk of faecal substance coming in contact with the skin. If this does occur the karaya will protect the skin, but the seal should be changed as quickly as possible to prevent the skin being irritated by the faecal material.

The Translet colostomy equipment is also very effective but does not include a karaya gum seal. It is, however, fixed to the skin and has a detachable bag which is replaced with a fresh one as it is required.

During the first few days the discharge from the colostomy is fluid and drains from the colon at frequent intervals; however, once diet is commenced the patient may be given Isogel or Celvac granules and this will result in the discharge of a more normally formed stool. A light diet is given, avoiding excess of fruit, especially oranges, green vegetables and fluids at first, but the patient must learn from experience how much he can tolerate without inconvenience. Fruit with pips must be avoided. As new foods are being added to the diet they should be introduced singly, so that if there is any upset, the patient knows to which food it is attributed; that food should then be avoided for another week, when another attempt can be made to introduce it.

If this is a permanent colostomy the patient will be taught how to care for himself and so regain his independence. At first he will require a great deal of reassurance but usually by the time he is ready for discharge he will have overcome his initial repugnance and will be ready to resume normal life. Prior to discharge, if this has not already been arranged, the patient must be put in contact with the nearest branch of the Colostomy Association who will be able to give him a tremendous amount of support and encouragement as he will mix with and be able to discuss his problems with the other members.

ENTEROSTOMY, JEJUNOSTOMY AND ILEOSTOMY

Enterostomy may also be performed; this is the making of an opening into the small intestine.

Jejunostomy (opening the jejunum) may be carried out for patients too ill to tolerate operations on the stomach, in cases of carcinoma or ulcer, for feeding purposes. In ulcer cases, after feeding by this route, the patient may improve so that operation becomes possible. In cases of carcinoma it is generally merely palliative and prevents the patient dying of starvation.

The ileum may be opened (ileostomy) in a case of obstruction in the caecum when the patient's condition is such that the obstruction must be relieved, but the cause cannot be dealt with either because the patient is suffering severely from the effects of toxic absorption or because the condition is inoperable. The higher the obstruction in the gut is, the more serious are the toxic effects, as the contents of the gut contain many more living bacteria and are more fluid.

Postoperative care following an ileostomy is similar to that given when a patient has had a colostomy. However, due to the character of the faecal fluid great care must be taken by the doctors to ensure that an electrolyte imbalance does not occur. The main difficulty encountered following this operation is that of protecting the patient's skin to prevent excoriation occurring. This will develop if the faecal fluid is allowed to gain contact with the skin and so this must be prevented. Disposable ileostomy bags are used which incorporate a karaya gum seal. This protects the skin and prevents the faecal fluid gaining contact with it. When it is necessary to change the adhesive part of the equipment the skin must be very carefully washed, dried and be protected with cream, e.g. Chiron. The new adhesive may then be placed in position. If excoriation does occur then Chiron barrier cream or karaya gum powder is very effective. However, all nursing is aimed at preventing excoriation, not treating it.

18

Conditions Affecting the Gall-Bladder, Liver, Pancreas and Spleen

AFFECTIONS OF THE GALL-BLADDER AND BILE DUCTS

Inflammation of the gall-bladder (cholecystitis) and gall-stones (cholelithiasis) are the commonest affections of these organs. Gall-stones are always associated with inflammation, and are thought to be the result of infection, the stone resulting from the deposit of mineral salts round a nucleus of septic material. On the other hand, inflammation may be present without stone formation. The stones may be single or multiple, the latter being most common. They consist essentially of cholesterol and bile pigments and the multiple stones show many facets. They are found in approximately 10% of people over the age of 40 years, especially in females who are fat and middle aged.

Symptoms

Inflammation and gall-stones give rise only to vague symptoms of indigestion and flatulence as a general rule, until a stone enters the cystic duct, obstructs it and prevents the escape of bile from the gall-bladder, or passes down the cystic duct and obstructs the common bile duct, preventing bile passing into the duodenum. This gives rise to biliary or gall-stone colic, which may or may not be associated with jaundice, according to the site of obstruction.

Biliary Colic

Biliary colic generally causes agonizing pain, which comes on suddenly, possibly after a severe jolt. The pain is in the right hypochondriac region and shoots through to the back, often between the shoulders. Reflex vomiting accompanies the pain, with a varying degree of collapse, according to the severity and duration of the

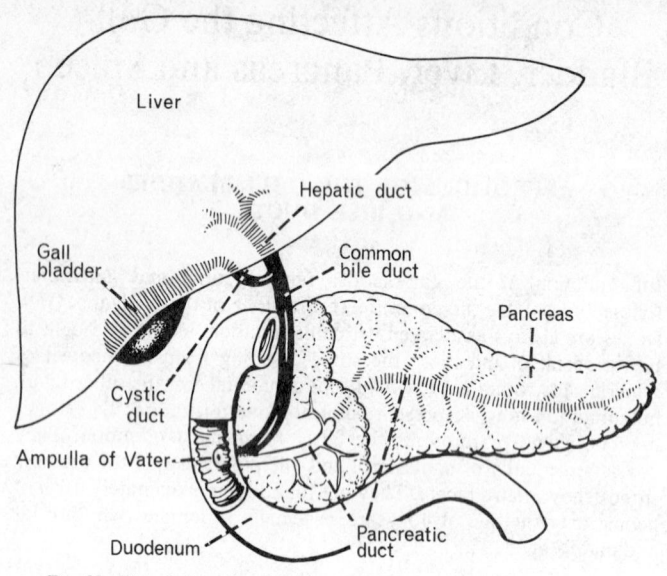

Fig. 32. The relationship of the biliary tract to its neighbouring structures.

attack. The pain continues till the stone falls back into the gall-bladder or passes into the intestine, when it ceases as suddenly as it began. Tenderness and slight jaundice may follow if the stone is in the cystic duct, the jaundice being due to inflammation of the bile duct following injury by the stone. Great care is taken to confirm the diagnosis as the condition can be confused with ureteric colic.

If the stone is in the common bile duct, jaundice will be marked, the skin and whites of the eyes being yellow, the urine dark greenish-brown or black and the stools clay-coloured, as no bile can now pass into the duodenum and it therefore gets into the blood stream. The skin irritates, the pulse is slow, and the patient is likely to be depressed. The stone may become impacted, especially at the entrance to the duodenum, in which case the colic and jaundice will continue, but will vary in intensity. If infection supervenes, fever and rigors develop owing to a severe state of toxaemia.

Investigations will include:

1. Straight abdominal X-ray.
2. Intravenous or oral cholangiogram.
3. Liver function tests.

Treatment of jaundice due to gall-stones

Medical treatment may relieve symptoms, but will never cure a case with gall-stones and operation is generally advocated unless there is some definite contraindication. However, many people have gall-stones but suffer no symptoms and require no treatment.

Gall-stone colic is generally so painful that pethidine 75–100 mg (depending upon the age and weight of the patient) is required to relieve it; this also helps to reduce muscle spasm.

If the condition is acute it is very unusual for surgery to be carried out at once. Usually the patient is given conservative treatment in hospital until his signs and symptoms subside. During this time a full course of antibiotics will be given. The patient will then be discharged home with an appointment to return to the out-patients' clinic. While at home he will be cared for by his general practitioner and will be given a fat-free diet. Instructions will also be given that the patient must not smoke; this is very important as obesity is usually present and these two factors suggest the likelihood of a postoperative chest complication developing. When the patient returns to the clinic the surgeon will evaluate his condition then arrange for readmission in two to three months so that a cholecystectomy may be performed.

The conservative hospital treatment consists of continuous or intermittent aspiration of the stomach, pethidine to relieve the pain and careful observation of the patient's signs and symptoms.

Pancreatitis is often present, in which case continuous aspiration of the stomach will be performed and intravenous normal saline or 5% glucose will be administered. The serum electrolytes will be carefully checked as it may be necessary to administer potassium (lost in the aspirate) and the serum amylase levels will be measured daily. Treatment will continue as long as the amylase levels are elevated.

Operations on the Gall-bladder and Bile Duct

Cholecystectomy

Removal of the gall-bladder is generally advocated as further stone may form if it is retained. The cystic duct is tied and the wound closed with drainage. The common bile duct is usually explored to ensure that it is patent and a T-tube inserted in case reactionary oedema causes obstruction as a result of local inflammation, or if gravel is present postoperatively in the common bile duct.

Cholecystostomy

Opening the gall-bladder, removing the stones and draining the gall-bladder, is carried out where it is found, for technical reasons, impossible to dissect out and remove the gall-bladder.

Choledochotomy

For impaction of stone in the common bile duct, the duct is opened, the stone removed and the duct drained (choledochotomy).

Cholecystgastrostomy or cholecystenterostomy

Where there is obstruction of the common bile duct due to outside pressure, e.g. in carcinoma of the head of the pancreas, the gall-bladder is anastomosed to the stomach or to the small intestine (cholecystgastrostomy or cholecystenterostomy). This relieves the jaundice, but is merely palliative. In a few cases the pancreas has been successfully removed or the head of the pancreas has been removed and the tip has been anastomosed to the small intestine.

Drainage of the gall-bladder

It may be necessary to perform this operation as an emergency as the patient will be hyperpyrexial and toxic with a very high white blood cell count. The surgeon will prescribe intramuscular penicillin 1 million units six-hourly for 24 hours and then will take the patient to the operating theatre where a drainage tube will be inserted into the gall-bladder and the pus will drain into a bag. This treatment will continue until the patient's condition improves sufficiently for

CONDITIONS AFFECTING THE GALL-BLADDER

either discharge home to the care of the patient's general practitioner (followed by readmission), or by a cholecystectomy.

Preparation for Biliary Tract Operation

In addition to the routine preparation there is special risk of haemorrhage since, in the presence of jaundice, fat-soluble vitamin K may not be absorbed from the intestine and, without it, the liver will not manufacture prothrombin adequately. This difficulty is overcome by the administration of some form of vitamin K which according to the preparation used will be given as a hypodermic, intramuscular or intravenous injection. Since there is failure in absorption, oral administration is obviously useless.

The blood should always be grouped and in severe cases arrangements are made for blood transfusion before, during or after the operation, as ordered. Glucose should be given freely to help to protect the liver from damage, usually in the form of intravenous Dextrose. During this time a fat-free diet is given to the patient.

After-care

The patient is nursed in the upright position as soon as the effect of the anaesthetic passes off. Deep breathing must be encouraged. The physiotherapist will teach the patient suitable exercises before operation and the nurse must encourage the patient to carry them out frequently. Since these patients are frequently very obese it is particularly important to encourage them to move freely in bed and to give them the necessary help.

Special watch must be kept for postoperative haemorrhage.

Flatulence and postoperative vomiting are rarely seen, but may occur.

The dressing must be changed daily; if cholecystectomy has been performed the tube or corrugated rubber drain from the gall-bladder bed is generally removed on the fourth or fifth day, having been previously shortened by withdrawing slightly and cutting off about 2·5 cm each day as ordered. When the common bile duct is drained, a T-tube is generally inserted, with one branch of the tube in the part of the duct leading from the liver and the other part leading into the duodenum. This tube drains into a sterile plastic 'Bardic Bile Bag', and is fixed to the skin by one suture. After seven to eight days a T-tube cholangiogram is performed in the X-ray department to see if there is a free flow of bile through the common bile duct into the duodenum. If the radiologist states that the appearance of the X-ray is satisfactory then the surgeon will ask the nursing staff to clamp off the T-tube with an artery forceps for a period of six hours and to watch the patient carefully for any sign of pain. The clamp will then be removed and the nurse will watch to see if there is a spurt of bile from the tube (indicating that there is some degree of obstruction). The clamp is left off for about one hour, then reapplied for a further six hours. This is continued for about 48 hours, and if everything appears to be satisfactory the tube is removed by an experienced member of the nursing staff. It is usual for the patient to be given an analgesic such as pentazocine 60 mg by intramuscular injection, before this procedure. If the patient is very nervous the surgeon may prescribe diazepam to be given at the same time. The tube is released by removing the skin suture, and the area round the tube is steadied with one hand while gentle traction is exerted on the tube with the other. The tube can be felt to leave the common bile duct but comes out easily. There may be an area of inflammation around the pucture hole so a wound swab must be taken. Culture and sensitivity testing will be carried out, then if necessary the appropriate oral antibiotic will be prescribed. The area is covered by a dry dressing which is changed as required.

In some cases it is the practise to transfer the patient home to the care of the community health care team 48 hours after the T-tube has been removed. The district nurse will remove the skin sutures on about the tenth day and the tension sutures on the fourteenth. The patient will be instructed to avoid excess fatty foods for the first month, and then to eat anything he likes, but to avoid foods that he finds are liable to cause him discomfort.

AFFECTIONS OF THE LIVER

The liver may be affected by:

1. Growths.
2. Trauma, i.e. rupture with internal haemorrhage.
3. Obstruction of the portal vein causing portal hypertension, associated with failure of the liver.
4. Portal pyaemia.
5. Hydatid cysts.

Growths

Growths in the liver are very rarely primary, but if this is so and the tumour involves only one lobe then it may be removed (hepatic lobectomy), with the use of alginates to arrest bleeding from the cut surface, but recurrence may follow and it is not often attempted. Most liver tumours, however, are secondary and resection is rarely of value. The common cause of death is liver insufficiency, but this does not occur until seven-tenths of the organ has been destroyed by the growth.

Trauma

Trauma may arise in a variety of ways, such as when a car driver is thrown against the steering wheel in a car accident, or when a patient receives a stab wound which involves the liver. Emergency surgery plus massive blood transfusions are required, otherwise the patient may die. Many surgeons perform a hemihepatectomy when they remove the area of damaged liver. Within a very short period of time the liver grows to its normal size again, as demonstrated by liver scans. When a liver scan is performed the physicist administers an intravenous injection of specific radioactive material. A Geiger counter is then used to build up a 'picture' of the liver by measuring the amount of radioactive material that the liver has taken up. (Other substances are used to perform scans on other organs.)

Portal Hypertension

Portal hypertension can be relieved by operation: the portal vein may be anastomosed to the inferior vena cava or splenectomy (a portacaval shunt) may be performed and the splenic vein anastomosed to the inferior vena cava. These operations allow the portal vein to drain into the general circulation and, provided the operation is undertaken before the liver cells are too seriously affected, may give marked relief. The patient is seriously ill and the operation a grave one, especially when there is haematemesis due to rupture of the distended veins at the lower end of the oesophagus and the cardiac end of the stomach. Bleeding at this site where the portal and general circulations anastomose may be severe. It may

270   SURGICAL NURSING

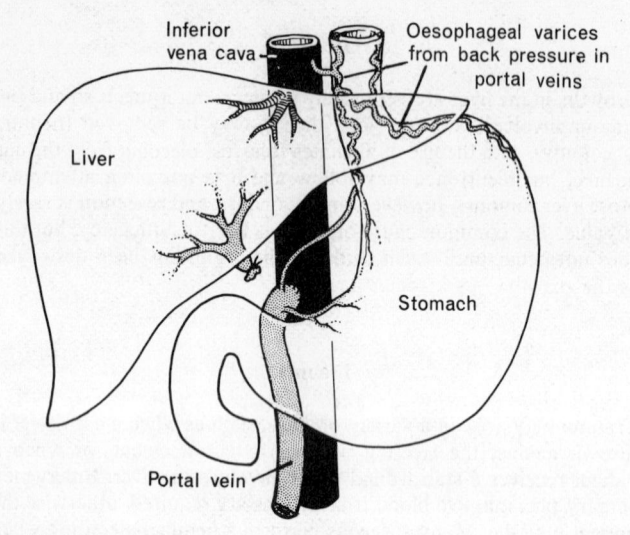

Fig. 33. Anastomosis of the portal vein with the inferior vena cava, performed for the relief of portal hypertension.

be necessary to control it before operation by the use of a special gastric tube fitted with inflatable cuffs to press on vessels in both the oesophagus and cardia.

Portal Pyaemia

This infection may reach the liver via the bile ducts, when it may be due to *Escherichia coli*, or via the hepatic artery or portal vein. If the infection has been transmitted through the artery then other abscesses will be found in other parts of the body; if it has been transmitted via the vein then it may be due to amoebic dysentery. Chemotherapy is given and it may be necessary to drain a single large abscess.

Hydatid Cyst

This disease is due to a tapeworm called *Echinococcus granulosus* which infests the gut of dogs that have contracted the infestation from sheep. It is most common in sheep-rearing areas of the world (sometimes seen in South Wales). The treatment is for the cyst to be surgically exposed, then for 2% formalin to be injected into it so that the daughter cysts within the main cyst are killed. If possible the main cyst is then removed intact.

AFFECTIONS OF THE PANCREAS

The pancreas may be affected by:

1. Cysts and tumours.
2. Inflammation.
3. Trauma.

Cysts and Tumours

Cysts of the pancreas may occur and are treated by opening and draining.

Tumours. Carcinoma of the pancreas is twice as common in male patients, especially among the middle-aged and elderly. Some 60% of lesions are found in the head of the pancreas, 25% in the body and 15% in the tail. This condition is suspected if the patient has a progressive jaundice.

Removal of the pancreas (*pancreatectomy*) is a very severe operation, but may be carried out. The pylorus and duodenum are generally also removed, the bile duct is anastomosed to the jejunum, as is also the stomach. Total pancreatectomy creates a diabetic state which must then be treated with insulin. A Whipple's operation may be performed, when the involved area of pancreas is excised and the bile ducts are reconstructed.

Inflammation

Inflammation may be acute or chronic. Acute suppurative cases are the ones which come for surgical treatment; these are frequently associated with gall-stones and cholecystitis, and fat necrosis is often present. It may not be possible to distinguish pancreatitis from peritonitis until laparotomy has been performed.

Symptoms include acute abdominal pain, with vomiting, distension, rapid pulse and collapse.

Treatment varies depending upon the surgeon's decision. In some cases an immediate laparotomy is performed and the peritoneal cavity is drained. In other cases conservative treatment is used; the patient is fed intravenously, continuous aspiration of the stomach is performed and antibiotics are administered together with propantheline 15 mg three times a day to reduce the output of pancreatic enzymes.

Some cases are due to a small tumour that may be blocking the pancreatic duct. In this case the tumour is removed surgically and this cures the pancreatitis.

Trauma

Rupture may occur in 'run-over' accidents and stab wounds, and gives rise to internal haemorrhage and pain due to the escape of pancreatic juice into the abdominal cavity.

Treatment consists of a partial pancreatectomy at the earliest opportunity; the after-care is similar to that for any acute abdominal case.

AFFECTIONS OF THE SPLEEN

Removal is the only surgery carried out on this organ.

Rupture

Rupture of the spleen occurs in 'run-over' accidents, and in penetrating wounds, and is especially liable to occur when the spleen is enlarged, as in malaria. It results in serious internal haemorrhage, except when the damage if very slight. Immediate operation is essential to save life, the spleen being excised (*splenectomy*). Massive blood transfusion is likely to be necessary.

When a patient is suspected of having damage to the spleen he must be admitted for observation for a period of five to seven days. This is essential as the signs and symptoms of haemorrhage may not at first be apparent, as the splenic capsule retains the blood. The abdomen is tender, especially on the left side, but bruising is only slight. The patient will develop tachycardia and left shoulder tip pain: emergency surgery is then necessary.

CONDITIONS AFFECTING THE GALL-BLADDER

Splenectomy may also be performed in some cases of disease associated with enlargement and abnormalities in the blood, such as haemolytic anaemia. Blood transfusions will always be required in such cases to overcome the associated anaemia.

This operation may also be performed if a patient has Hodgkin's disease.

19

Hernia

A hernia is present when part of the contents of a cavity, e.g. the peritoneal cavity, protrudes through its coverings into an abnormal situation. Hernias develop where there is a weakness in the abdominal wall, this weakness being either:

1. *Congenital*, due to failure of closure of the umbilicus.
2. *Acquired*. This form may be due to the presence of structures that penetrate the abdominal wall, such as the femoral canal, or may occur when a surgical incision weakens the layers of the abdominal wall. The actual formation of the hernia may be precipitated by anything that causes an increase in the intra-abdominal pressure, such as a chronic cough or conditions that weaken the abdominal muscles such as gross obesity.

Abdominal hernias are the most frequent and consist of a sac of peritoneum containing, most commonly, a loop of small intestine or omentum, more rarely the caecum, appendix, ovary or tube. The sac leads from the peritoneal cavity at its neck, which may be broad, so that organs will readily slip in and out of the sac, but may be narrow and surrounded by a dense ring of fibrous tissue due to irritation from the wearing of a truss, especially if this fits badly.

ABDOMINAL HERNIAS

Types of Abdominal Hernia

The following varieties of hernia may be found: (*a*) inguinal; (*b*) femoral; (*c*) umbilical; (*d*) incisional; (*e*) diaphragmatic; (*f*) hiatus.

HERNIA 275

Inguinal hernia. Protrusion of an organ through the inguinal canal, which runs through the abdominal wall just above the inguinal (Poupart's) ligament in the groin, is more common in the male sex, because the testes descend from the abdomen, where they first develop, into the scrotum through this canal before birth, and bring down a pouch of peritoneum. The pouch should be obliterated except around the testes themselves, but may persist and form a hernial sac, hence inguinal herniae are more common in males than females.

Femoral hernia. Protrusion of an organ through the femoral canal, i.e. between the inguinal ligament and the pelvic bone in the groin alongside the femoral artery and vein, is more common in the female than in the male, owing to the canal being wider because of the broader, rounder female pelvis.

Umbilical hernia. The congenital type is seen in babies and the acquired type in fat middle-aged women, especially after multiple pregnancy.

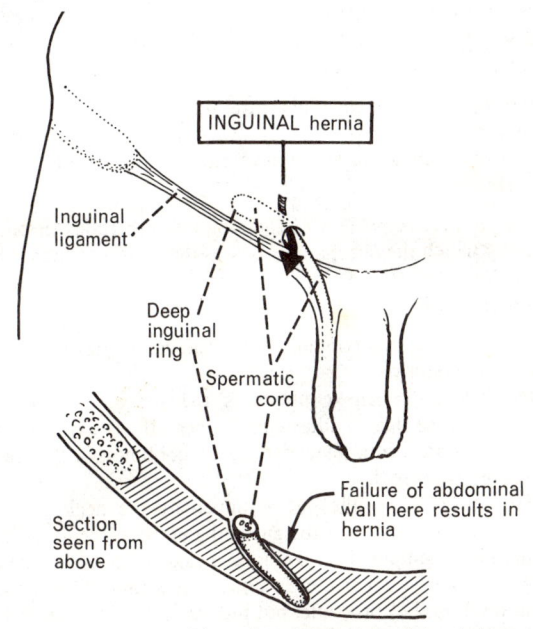

FIG. 34. The structures of the groin and their relation in inguinal hernia.

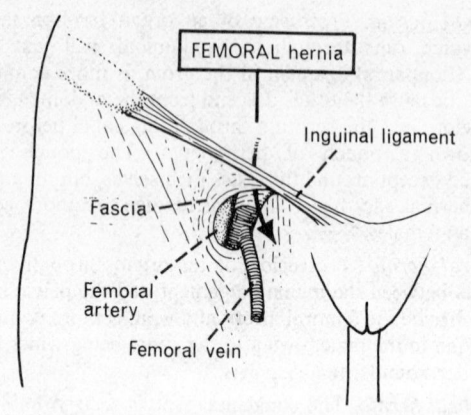

FIG. 35. The structures in the groin and their relation in femoral hernia.

Incisional hernia. This form occurs at the site of an operation wound when the muscle has failed to unite properly on account of sepsis or poor general condition.

Diaphragmatic hernia. This rare form may be a congenital deformity or may follow a 'run-over' accident, the diaphragm rupturing under pressure and allowing abdominal organs to escape into the thorax.

Hiatus hernia. A portion of the stomach protrudes through the opening by which the oesophagus passes through the diaphragm.

A hernia may be:

1. *Reducible,* i.e. the contents of the sac can be pushed back into the abdominal cavity.
2. *Irreducible,* i.e. the contents of the sac cannot be pushed back; this may be due to adhesions between the organ and the sac or to the intestine being distended by its contents: in this case the blood supply is normal.
3. *Strangulated,* i.e. the gut is nipped by the neck of the sac, which causes obstruction of the gut and gangrene due to the cutting off of the blood supply. This is due to a ring of fibrous tissue at the neck of the sac, which stretches under the strain of heavy lifting, allowing the bowel to protrude, but recoils directly the strain is over and contracts on the intestine at the neck of the sac. This obstructs

the thin-walled veins, so that blood cannot return; the pressure therefore rises in the veins, becoming as high as in the arteries and obstructing the flow from them; the veins finally rupture and bleed into the walls of the bowel, gangrene sets in and the dead tissue is readily infected by micro-organisms present in the intestine, such as *Cl. perfringens* (*welchii*), and general peritonitis follows. Strangulation therefore necessitates immediate operation or the result will be fatal, owing to acute obstruction and peritonitis. Strangulated hernia does not occur in infants, but an infant's hernia may become irreducible and cause the child to scream with pain, which increases the intra-abdominal pressure. This is not due to adhesions and can generally be rendered reducible by fixing the child up so that the hernia sac drains by gravity into the abdominal cavity. The loop of intestine empties and can generally be easily pushed back. The child's legs may be tied up to a cradle by soft flannel bandage. In the home the child can be fixed up in an armchair, with a thick book under the buttocks and the legs secured so that they rest against the back of the chair and the head towards the edge of the seat. Use something soft round the ankles to hold the legs up. The child will soon stop crying, as a general rule, and drop off to sleep.

The signs of hernia are a swelling at the site, which can be reduced unless the hernia is irreducible or strangulated; there is an impulse in the swelling on coughing. Often a hernia will reduce itself when the patient is lying flat, hence the doctor will invariably want the patient to stand up for part of his examination.

Treatment of Abdominal Hernia

Hernia may be treated by (*a*) surgical operation, resulting in cure, or (*b*) the wearing of a truss, a palliative measure in cases where operation is impracticable or must be delayed. The treatment varies in different cases.

Medical treatment

Umbilical hernia. In the umbilical hernia of children operation is not necessary as a rule as it is usually corrected spontaneously as growth proceeds; but a pad may be applied at the site and can be improvised from a penny or 'tiddlywink' covered with lint and fixed in position by means of a piece of strapping. Alternatively,

278 SURGICAL NURSING

strapping alone may be used. These treatments though not necessary may relieve the mother's worries. However, the hernia may be extensive, with the bowel contained only in a translucent sac. In this case immediate surgical repair is essential because if it ruptures, death will result from peritonitis. The umbilical hernia of fat middle-aged women is not easily cured by operation, because of the obesity and because it is often not seen till the gut is adherent to the sac. Operation is mainly undertaken if strangulation occurs and in cases where the sac is small; trusses are advised in other cases.

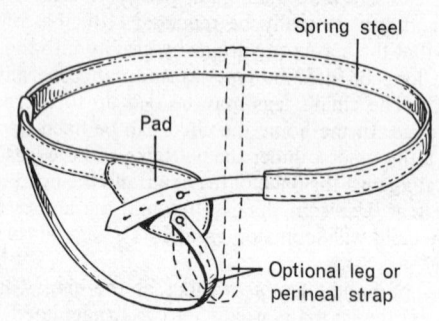

FIG. 36. A truss of the type sometimes used for inguinal hernia.

Inguinal hernia. In cases of inguinal hernia a truss may be used (Fig. 36), but it is merely palliative and is not recommended for adults unless an operation is undesirable or impracticable, the surgeon preferring to repair the hernia to prevent the risk of strangulation developing. The truss is worn for nine to twelve months, and if cure has not then taken place, operation is advised.

In children occasionally obliteration of the sac occurs spontaneously in the early months of life, so although operation is nearly always needed ultimately, it is usually postponed till the child is one and a half to two years old to allow for this possibility of spontaneous closure.

Femoral hernia. In cases of femoral hernia the use of a truss is not desirable, because the neck of the femoral canal is narrow and so an irreducible or strangulated hernia is liable to occur. Operative treatment is always the treatment of choice unless the patient's condition makes it impracticable.

Operative treatment

Herniotomy gives good results in suitable cases. The sac is opened, its contents returned to the abdomen, the sac removed and the abdominal wall strengthened, with great care in inguinal hernia to avoid injury to or pressure on the spermatic cord. To strengthen the abdominal wall strips of fascia removed from the thigh may be stitched round the hernial orifice or artificial materials such as Teflon may be used.

Preoperative Care

Preparation is as for any abdominal operation. It is particularly undesirable that the patient should put strain on the repair from coughing or constipation in the early postoperative days; hence if the patient has a respiratory infection at the time of admission, even though it is slight, operation should be delayed till it has been effectively treated. Elderly patients are especially prone to develop constipation so a mild aperient such as Milpar is given preoperatively and continued following the operation. Ideally patients suffering from chronic bronchitis should be operated on in summer

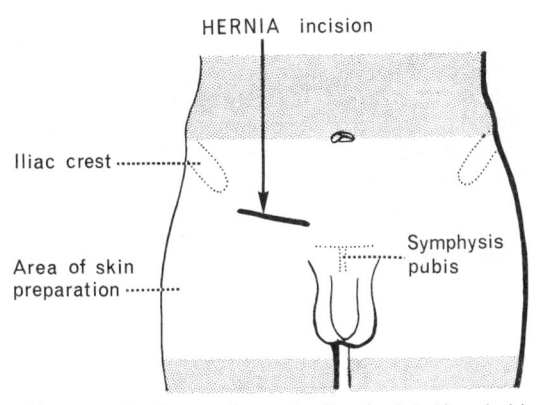

FIG. 37. Skin preparation for operative repair of hernia. A 7–10 cm incision along the groin crease is often used for both femoral and inguinal hernia. The skin to be prepared (unshaded) usually extends from the level of the umbilicus to an imaginary line 7 cm down the thighs. It extends from side to side as far as can be reached without turning the patient.

280 SURGICAL NURSING

when the disease is more quiescent; in practice, with such long waiting lists as many surgeons have, this is a counsel of perfection.

Special Nursing Points

In infants no dressing is applied, as it is liable to be contaminated by urine. Whitehead's varnish or Nobecutane may be applied.

It may be better for a child to lie on several folds of napkin, rather than to have a napkin applied in the traditional manner so that urine is not held in contact with the wound. To keep the child's hands from the wound, a cradle may be placed under the nightdress and the skirt pinned to the cradle like a tent.

The old rule, that the patient must lie flat for an appreciable period, rarely applies today and the patient is almost always allowed to assume the position he finds most comfortable, even sitting up if he has any 'chest trouble'. He is particularly encouraged to practise breathing exercises and to move his legs freely. Analgesia will be administered as required. He usually sits out of bed on the day after operation and becomes gradually more and more active. This earlier and freer movement has lessened the difficulties with micturition which used to be so common. Strain on the wound should be avoided for six weeks, and heavy strain for three months in young persons and longer in the older patients. Careful watch should be kept for (a) constipation, (b) retention of urine, (c) haematoma of scrotum and (d) sepsis, which are possible complications in all cases. In cases of strangulated hernia, the patient's condition will depend on the time interval before operation is undertaken and the extent to which the peritoneum is affected. Particularly in the case of strangulated hernia, generalized peritonitis may occur and endanger the patient's life, though early operation with the use of penicillin, streptomycin and other antibiotics, with or without a sulphonamide, usually gives satisfactory results.

HIATUS HERNIA

Hiatus hernia is the protrusion of part of the stomach through the opening in the diaphragm by which the oesophagus passes to join the cardiac sphincter of the stomach. It gives rise to regurgitation of acid into the oesophagus because the muscle of the diaphragm no longer helps to grip the tube when abdominal pressure is increased, e.g. on coughing or passing a stool or flatus. This may result in ulceration in the lower end of the oesophagus which causes the symptoms of peptic ulcer. It may be treated by operation to repair the diaphragm either from the thorax or from the abdomen after a barium meal has been given to confirm the diagnosis and guide the surgeon in the treatment required, though medical treatment, with special emphasis on posture after meals, is almost always tried first.

(See also Chapter 10.)

20

Surgery of the Rectum

Surgical conditions affecting the rectum include:

1. Imperforate anus.
2. Fissure-in-ano.
3. Fistula-in-ano.
4. Prolapse of the rectum.
5. Haemorrhoids.
6. Polyps.
7. Malignant disease, usually carcinoma.
8. Pruritus ani is normally considered 'medical' but very occasionally, where the condition is particularly resistant, a surgeon's help may be required.

Methods of Examination

A full rectal examination consists of:

Digital examination. The examiner's finger is protected either with a caped finger-stall, or a finger-cot, or he wears a disposable glove. A lubricant is needed and the patient lies in the left lateral position, with his buttocks near the edge of the bed and his knees drawn well up. Clothing should have been adjusted so that the doctor can palpate the abdomen at the same time if necessary.

Examination by rectal speculum. The speculum or proctoscope is passed with the patient in the knee–chest or lithotomy position. It should be *warmed* and lubricated. The surgeon may wear a head mirror; this makes it possible to see the lower part of the rectum; alternatively an Anglepoise lamp can be used to direct a beam of light down the speculum. Some instruments have a bulb incorporated receiving current from, for example, a battery in the handle.

Examination by sigmoidoscope. This is a graduated tube fitted with electric light and hand pump by which air can be introduced to distend the rectum. This makes it possible to examine the upper part of the rectum and the pelvic colon.

For these examinations the rectum must be empty and an enema must be used to ensure this if necessary. It is also important that the bladder is empty.

A barium enema is requested if the doctor suspects some conditions other than haemorrhoids.

IMPERFORATE ANUS

Imperforate anus is a congenital condition in which there is no opening from the rectum to the external skin. Failure to pass meconium during the first 24 hours draws attention to this and prompt treatment, of at least a palliative kind, is needed. There may be only a thin piece of tissue between rectum and skin, the anal canal being partially formed and marked by a depression in the skin. In such cases an opening can be made with relative ease. In other cases the colon may end many centimetres from the anus and it is then possible only to perform a permanent colostomy or to carry out a major repair operation.

FISSURE-IN-ANO

Fissure-in-ano is a crack in the anus and is often associated with a single pile lying over it, called the sentinel pile. The crack is opened up every time the bowels are opened, causing acute pain during and after the act of defaecation, which is very distressing to the patient. It is often associated with constipation and may tend to cause it, as the patient dreads the pain associated with an action. It may be relieved by careful regulation of the bowels and the application of cinchocaine ointment. The use of an aperient that lubricates is also advocated. In persistent cases the anal sphincter may be stretched under a general anaesthetic and proctocaine may be infiltrated into the fissure. If the condition is chronic then excision is necessary.

284   SURGICAL NURSING

FISTULA-IN-ANO

Fistula-in-ano is a tract leading from the rectum to the external skin. It is generally due to an abscess which had formed in one of the anal glands and had not been drained efficiently, and will not heal because it is constantly reinfected from the rectum.

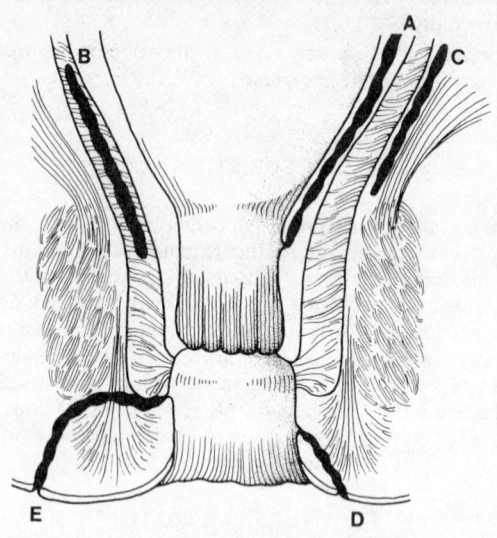

Fig. 38. Various forms of sinus and fistula-in-ano. (A) Submucous. (B) Intermuscular. (C) Anorectal. (D) Subcutaneous. (E) Subsphincteric or anal.

An open saucer wound is made which heals by granulation. It is constructed so that the final portion to heal lies outside the anocutaneous margin. This ensures complete and permanent healing.

The bowels are confined for three to four days. The dressing is not changed for 24–48 hours, as ordered. The wound should be dressed with a flat piece of gauze, the corner being pressed into the apex of the triangle. When the bowels act the dressing must be changed; otherwise the wound is dressed morning and evening. Baths may be used after the bowels have acted, before dressing.

SURGERY OF THE HEART 187

treatment, and her observations will help her greatly in her postoperative care of the patient.

Diagnosis

Diagnostic procedures which may be carried out include the following.

X-ray of chest will indicate the condition of the lungs, the size of the heart and the presence or absence of calcification in the valves.

Screening. When posterior, anterior, lateral and penetrating X-rays are taken, they will show the presence and position of a calcified valve. When this condition is diagnosed the affected valve is replaced by a prosthesis. If the valve is not calcified it may be possible for it to be 'stretched'.

Barium swallow. This procedure is not often carried out, but it demonstrates the indentation made by the left atrium on the oesophagus and thus shows up any enlargement of the chamber.

Cardiac catheterization often yields valuable information, especially when a valve replacement is being considered. A radiopaque catheter, rather similar in appearance to a ureteric catheter, is introduced into the antecubital vein, in front of the elbow. The patient usually has a sedative and a local anaesthetic. A general anaesthetic may be used for the nervous and the very young. In a darkened room, by using fluoroscopy, the tip of the catheter can be seen entering the right atrium, ventricle and pulmonary artery and any abnormal communications can be demonstrated. Heparinized saline, 1 ml heparin (1000 units in 1 ml) to 500 ml normal saline, is dripped in to prevent clotting and pressure readings can be taken in the various chambers and vessels by connecting the catheter with an electric manometer. Blood samples are also obtained, the oxygen content is analysed and intracardiac pressures are measured.

Angiocardiography is usually carried out at the same time as the cardiac catheterization. It may be performed under a general anaesthetic or following sedation with omnopon 10 mg or promethazine 25 mg by intramuscular injection. An opaque medium such as 70% diodone (10 ml for an infant and 60 ml for an adult) is injected into an arm vein and reaches the heart in 0·5 seconds. Serial radiographs with exposure frequencies of up to one-sixth of a second are taken in two planes at right angles to each other on a continuously moving X-ray film. In this way serial pictures are obtained of all the chambers of the heart and their outflow tracts. In many hospitals a video tape recording is also made so that it can be replayed.

Electrocardiogram. This measures the electric impulses generated by the heart muscle and gives information about cardiac rhythm and function.

Oxygen saturation of the arterial blood. This, before and after exercise, is estimated in cyanotic heart disease to assist the surgeon to determine the degree of shunt of blood from right to left in the heart and if any respiratory disease is present.

Exercise tolerance tests. These are usually supervised by the doctor, but the nurse's help may be enlisted. The test can be arranged to suit the individual patient and may be walking on the level or walking up and down a set number of stairs a set number of times at a given pace. It is necessary to have the patient's full cooperation. Pulse and respiration must be recorded immediately before and after the test. The time taken for pulse and respiration to return to pre-exercise level must be noted. The normal time is two minutes. The length of time taken to perform the test must be stated. The condition of the patient at the end of the test and the reason for stopping must be recorded. Some patients are distressed by mild dyspnoea, others will tolerate a severe degree with equanimity. The time of day in relation to meals, and the weather, can make a considerable difference to the result of the test. The results are less good immediately after a meal or in foggy weather.

Clinical estimate of respiratory efficiency. This is always made. Vital capacity and respiratory excursion may be measured and bronchospirometry readings may be taken. Vital capacity includes tidal air, that is the normal quantity of air a patient breathes in, plus a deep intake of breath and plus the additional air above the normal that a patient can breathe out. For respiratory excursion the expansion of the chest is measured at various levels. A bronchospirometer is an instrument for measuring respiration. It has a special type of catheter for intrabronchial use so that the function of a single lung can be determined.

Routine blood tests are carried out, including electrolytes, urea, haemoglobin, erythrocyte sedimentation rate, grouping and cross-matching, coagulation studies and blood count.

PROLAPSE OF THE RECTUM

Prolapse of the rectum may occur in children and in adults, when it is generally associated with haemorrhoids. In infants the protruding mass should be washed, smeared with petroleum jelly and gently pushed up. The buttocks are then strapped together or a pad and bandage are applied. The bowels should be carefully regulated and the child made to defaecate lying on his side on some form of disposable protection if necessary. His general condition should be improved by a holiday in the country and good simple food. It can, however, occur in well-nourished children where there is congenital laxity or malformation of the tissues around the rectum. Rectal polyps constitute a predisposing cause, as does constipation.

In the adult, prolapse may be complicated by prolapsed haemorrhoids or incompetence of the anal sphincter and operation may be necessary. Cutting away the prolapse is unsatisfactory and liable to cause stricture. An opening is made behind the anus and plugging is introduced to cause adhesions to form between rectum and sacrum, so that the condition cannot recur. This is called rectopexy.

HAEMORRHOIDS

The very common condition of haemorrhoids or piles is a varicose state of the veins surrounding the anus. Haemorrhoids are very prone to occur because the veins run longitudinally and are linked up by anastomosing branches at the anus, which become affected, this being the lowest point of the portal circulation; also this is a link between the portal and general circulations, and thus very liable to congestion. Haemorrhoids are associated with pregnancy, chronic constipation and cardiac failure. They may be (*a*) external, covered with skin, or (*b*) internal, covered with mucous membrane; the latter may prolapse and therefore be visible externally.

Symptoms

The chief symptom is the passage of bright blood in the stool in the later stages associated with a good deal of discomfort and pain. If this is allowed to continue anaemia may result. Haemorrhoids may

286 SURGICAL NURSING

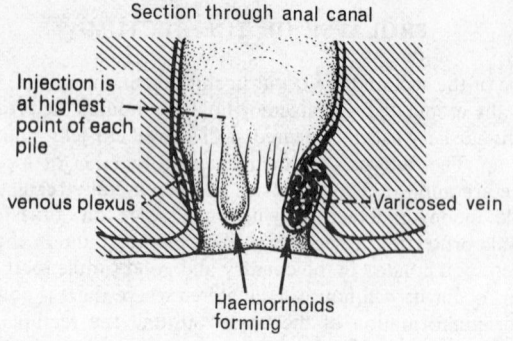

FIG. 39. Internal haemorrhoids prolapsing towards the anal opening. If a sclerosing agent is given, it must be injected into the tissues and not into the vein itself.

be associated with prolapse or thrombosis; the latter is really due to rupture and clotting of blood outside the vein; it is very painful. When prolapse occurs and the piles are not pushed up, the sphincter contracts, interfering with venous return, and inflammation and acute discomfort follow, with infection and ulceration if the condition is neglected.

Treatment

Haemorrhoids may be treated by:

1. Injection.
2. Digital dilatation.
3. Operation.
4. Conservative treatment.

Injection is satisfactory in the mild stages and does not necessitate anaesthetic or confinement to bed. Phenol (5–20%) in almond oil is generally used, sometimes urethane solution (5%). A 10 ml syringe should be prepared, fitted with special needles that cannot be accidentally disconnected. A straight and an angled needle should be prepared. The injection is given into the tissues around the veins and not into the veins themselves in this condition. Treatments are given once a week; usually one pile is treated at a time and three injections are necessary for each as a general rule. One regimen is known as 'the rule of three': 3 ml are injected into the base of each site (usually three), three times, at three-weekly intervals. The patient should keep the bowels from becoming constipated during treatment, with liquid paraffin, senna, etc., but must avoid purging. He should rest for a short period after injection and avoid long standing, if possible.

Digital dilatation. Dilatation of the anal sphincter under a general anaesthetic often results in a definite improvement of the condition.

Operation. Haemorrhoids may be treated by (*a*) ligature and excision or (*b*) clamp and cautery. Whitehead's operation, removal of the whole pile-bearing area, has been advocated, but is liable to be followed by stricture and is therefore not recommended.

Conservative treatment. If the haemorrhoids are strangulated and thrombosed, the foot of the patient's bed is elevated, warm or cold compresses are applied to the painful area and morphine may be prescribed for the pain. At this stage operation is contra-indicated because of the risk of portal pyaemia.

Treatment for prolapsed and inflamed piles. The patient should push up prolapsed piles and anaesthetic ointment, e.g. ointment of gall and opium or witch-hazel (hamamelis) may be applied. If the piles have become inflamed the patient should be kept in bed; fomentations are applied and the foot of the bed is raised on blocks. When inflammation has subsided treatment by operation or injection should be advised.

After-care

This varies greatly but due to the advances in surgery the following routine is generally observed.

If the patient has had a haemorrhoidectomy performed in the morning and the postoperative observations are satisfactory he will be encouraged to have a bath on the evening of operation. This is very soothing and relieves the rectal discomfort. Following this a saline bath (one cup full of salt per bath) will be given to the patient each day. Initially when the patient returns from theatre a gauze pack will be in the rectum, and this is used to create local pressure which reduces the risk of bleeding. This pack is not removed by the nurse but is allowed to fall out when the patient has a bath, or when he first has a bowel action.

To ensure that the bowel action is easy a combination of aperients will be prescribed by the doctor such as Milpar 5 ml, Isogel 15 ml and liquid paraffin 15 ml. This will be given prior to surgery and then twice a day. It is very unusual for the nurse to have to administer an olive oil enema if this form of medication is administered and it is much more comfortable for the patient.

Occasionally anal dilators are used, but if possible this is avoided as it causes anal stretch which may result in incontinence of faeces at a later date.

If possible this patient should be discharged home to the care of the community members of the health care team. The actual timing varies in different hospitals but usually the patient is discharged after he has had a satisfactory bowel action and this once again varies in different patients. If the patient does not have a bath at home early discharge is not possible, as this is a very important part of the required after-care.

Haemorrhage, urinary retention, stricture and sepsis are common complications.

GROWTHS IN THE RECTUM

Polyp

A polyp is an innocent growth and is a common cause of the passing of blood per rectum in children. It may be removed by operation, or may be passed as a result of rupture of its pedicle during defaecation.

Carcinoma of the Rectum

Malignant growth of the rectum is generally a carcinoma. It tends in this site to spread particularly by direct extension into the neighbouring tissues, usually by the circulation, and may spread forward into the bladder, peritoneum, vagina or prostate, or backwards into the sacrum, possibly causing sciatica.

Symptoms

1. The passage of fresh blood and 'slime' or mucus.
2. A sense of fullness of the rectum when the bowels have been emptied.

SURGERY OF THE RECTUM

3. Constipation or diarrhoea according to the site of the growth, or these may alternate with each other.

4. Obstruction does not occur till late, as the growth spreads longitudinally because of the circulation: the blood vessels here tend to run lengthways and not circularly round the rectum. This develops when the lumen of the bowel is occluded.

Treatment

If seen before the appearance of secondary growths and before it has spread into the neighbouring tissues fixing the growth, a radical cure is attempted by excision of the rectum and permanent colostomy. Before operation a course of treatment with one of the sulphonamide or antibiotic preparations which are not absorbed, and therefore disinfect the bowel contents, may be used, e.g. nystatin, phthalylsulphathiazole, neomycin, streptomycin or chlortetracycline may be given. Sometimes local wash-outs may be ordered preoperatively, in addition to treatment by mouth, to lessen local ulceration, either by the anus or by the lower opening of a previously performed colostomy. After rectal wash-out, an infusion of succinylsulphathiazole emulsion may be run into the rectum, e.g. 7·5 g/100 ml, to be retained for four hours; blocks at the foot of the bed are used to help the patient to retain the enema. Anaemia must be corrected, often by means of blood transfusion. The operation may be performed from the perineum only after a preliminary colostomy performed two to three weeks earlier. Other surgeons perform the operation by the abdominoperineal method, first opening the abdomen and dividing the gut above the growth, then removing it by a perineal incision. This is usually carried out by two surgeons, one undertaking the abdominal and the other the perineal operation, at the same time. In either case there is a colostomy and a large cavity in the perineum, which is either sewn up with drainage or more often packed with gauze. Oiled silk may be inserted between the wound and the gauze to prevent sticking. A Foley's catheter is introduced and kept in position for three days. Chemotherapy will be used before and immediately after the operation. Ryle's tube may be used with gastric aspiration or suction. Dehydration will be prevented by the use of intravenous infusion of saline after operation, till the patient can take fluids by mouth. The packing will be changed daily, using the antiseptic ordered by the surgeon, e.g. Milton 5% solution, to cleanse the wound, and repacking. The pack is gradually decreased in size as the granulations grow up from the base of the wound.

These patients are generally elderly and will require special protection from chest complications and bedsores. They should be nursed on sorbo mattresses or even ripple beds, lying on the side, on account of the perineal wound, with the shoulders raised as far as is comfortable. They should be turned regularly from side to side at least four-hourly in order to lessen the risk of collapse of the lung or bedsores. Breathing and other exercises are of special importance in the prevention of chest complications and deep vein thrombosis. Everything should be done to keep the mouth clean and improve the patient's general condition. Shock and heart failure may cause a fatal result.

A large percentage of cases seen in hospital practice are inoperable (95%), owing to the fact that the patient, and even his doctor, may think the bleeding is due to haemorrhoids and no examination is made. Of the operable cases, those will be cured in which the growth has only invaded the mucous membrane. If it has reached the muscle coat, there will probably be a recurrence within five years; if the glands are already affected, the patient will probably be dead within three years; nevertheless most people feel it is justifiable to subject such a patient to a major operation since removal of what will become (if it is not so already) a foul, ulcerating mass, makes his last years or months rather more tolerable. If the condition is completely inoperable then palliative treatment for temporary relief may be given by deep X-ray, diathermy of the tumour or cytotoxic drugs.

PRURITUS ANI

Pruritus ani is intense irritation of the skin around the anus. This may be due to local or general causes such as lack of cleanliness, leakage of mucus from haemorrhoids, rectal neoplasms, threadworms, scabies, fungal infections and obstructive jaundice. It may also accompany pruritus vulvae in severe untreated diabetes mellitus. If the cause is known this is treated, but if it is idiopathic then hydrocortisone ointment and care with personal hygiene gives great relief.

21

Surgery of the Sympathetic Nervous System

Surgery of the sympathetic nervous system is undertaken for the relief of symptoms in a number of conditions. The *sympathetic nervous system* consists of a chain of ganglia running down on either side of the spinal column and derived from nerve cells in the thoracic and upper lumbar segments of the cord; it is antagonistic to the *parasympathetic system*, which is derived from the cranial nerves and the sacral ganglia. These two sets of nerves form together the autonomic nervous system and supply among others the heart and blood vessels, the muscular wall of the alimentary canal and the glands associated with it. They have opposite or antagonistic effects. The sympathetic nerves contract the blood vessels and stimulate the sweat glands; the parasympathetic nerves dilate the vessels and check sweating. The sympathetic nerves check the digestive processes, both the muscular action of the canal wall and the secretion of the digestive juices; the parasympathetic nerves stimulate digestion. On the other hand, both respiration and circulation are stimulated by the sympathetic nerves and depressed by the parasympathetic nerves.

The autonomic system is mainly an outward pathway for stimuli to muscle in the walls of organs and blood vessels, and to glands. There are, however, a small number of sensory fibres, so that pain may be felt through these nerves, for example, the acute pain of coronary thrombosis, renal colic and intestinal colic. Spinal nerves, leaving the spine in the thoracic region from the first and second lumbar vertebrae, give off white branches (or rami) to the chain of ganglia which lie outside the spinal canal, against the bodies of the vertebrae. The upper thoracic nerves are linked with cervical

292 SURGICAL NURSING

ganglia, as well as the thoracic ganglia, there being no links from the cervical nerves to these ganglia. The ganglia give off (*a*) branches to the internal organs—the heart, the lungs, stomach,

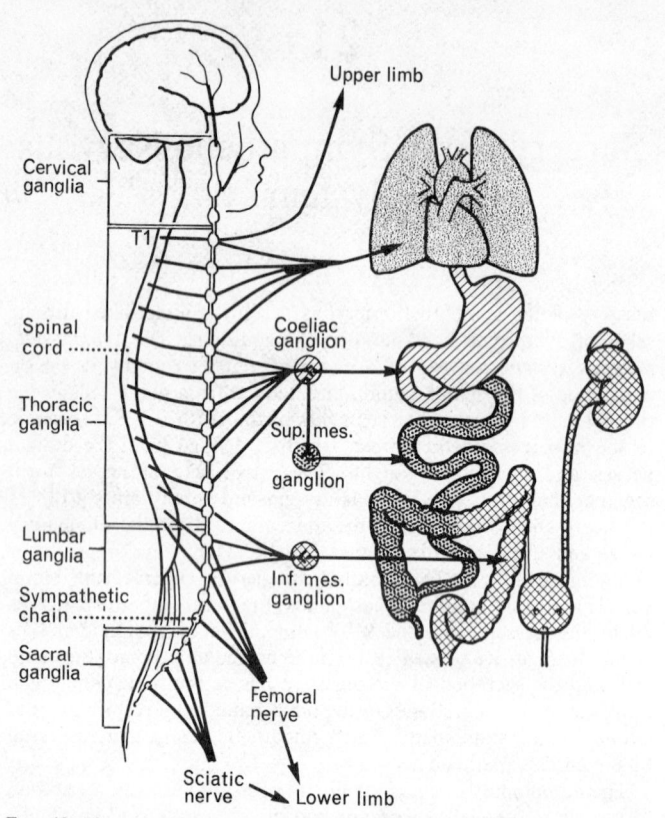

FIG. 40. The sympathetic nervous system and the main structures it supplies (simplified).

intestine, liver and pancreas; (*b*) branches (grey rami) to join the spinal nerves again for distribution to the blood vessels in the muscles of the limbs and trunk, and the skin covering them. These accompany the spinal nerves and the branch nerves which they form (the peripheral nerves). The operations undertaken on the sympathetic chain stop the functioning of the sympathetic nerve fibres without affecting the functioning of the peripheral nerves in any other way.

SYMPATHECTOMY

Sympathectomy consists of removal of parts of the sympathetic chain; it may be used for relieving the restricted circulation in the limbs in cases of Raynaud's disease, thrombo-angiitis obliterans

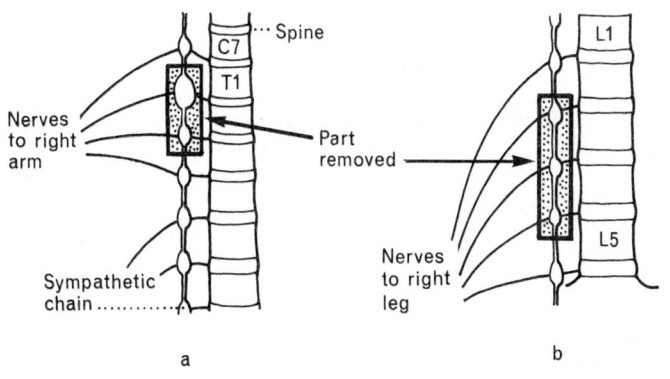

FIG. 41. Sympathectomy, showing the area of the sympathetic chain removed to affect the upper (*a*) and the lower (*b*) limb.

(Buerger's disease) and the intermittent claudication that is an early sign of this condition. In both these cases the operation is undertaken if there is an indication that spasm of the blood vessels is present. Raynaud's disease particularly affects the upper limbs, and this is treated by cervicothoracic sympathectomy with a dramatic improvement; unfortunately the result may not be permanent. This lessens the pain felt in the extremities and the cyanosis, and sores resulting from the impoverished circulation may heal. Before operation the limb is tested for the effect of relief of spasm, by a hot-air bath, by an injection of a local or regional anaesthetic or by inducing fever and noting the effect on the skin temperature of the limb. If there is improvement when these tests are carried out, operation will relieve the symptoms. If the lower limbs are also affected, a lumbar sympathectomy will also be carried out. After operation the limb becomes warm and dry, because the blood vessels become dilated and sweating is checked.

The operation is not a serious one, but complications may occur, viz: (*a*) postoperative pain of a burning nature over the back of the shoulder (this passes off after four to eight weeks as a general rule); (*b*) chest complications if the pleural cavity is opened (air or fluid may collect in it and require aspiration—an X-ray after operation will show the need for this measure); (*c*) local swelling from haematoma, or injury to the thoracic duct on the left side. More recently, the use of reserpine has made medical treatment of Raynaud's disease more effective and lessened the need for surgery.

Indications for Sympathectomy

Thrombo-angiitis obliterans is a condition which attacks men, particularly men between 40 and 50 years of age. There is superficial phlebitis associated with thrombosis in the arteries; it affects the lower limbs. One of the early symptoms is an attack of cramp-like pain in the calves of the legs, which is relieved by rest but recurs with exercise; this is termed intermittent claudication. Lumbar sympathectomy may relieve this pain and again tests are carried out to determine whether the condition is associated with spasm of the blood vessel walls before operation, e.g. spinal anaesthesia is administered and the skin temperature of the limbs tested before and after. If there is a marked rise in temperature, improvement is likely to follow sympathectomy, which can be carried out under spinal anaesthetic. The operation is generally carried out on both sides, as both limbs are finally affected. Patients should be encouraged to give up smoking as smoking reduces the ability of haemoglobin to carry oxygen.

Angina pectoris. Sympathectomy has been used for the relief of pain in cases of angina pectoris. A cervicothoracic ganglionectomy is performed. This relieves the very acute pain felt by these patients. Some feel that the pain is valuable in determining the limit of the patient's capacity for exertion. The operation only relieves the symptoms and does not, like cardio-omentopexy, improve the circulation of the heart wall.

High blood pressure. Sympathectomy has also been used for severe cases of high blood pressure, but is today reserved for those cases of *malignant hypertension* which do not respond to other forms of treatment, as the improvement after the operation is not maintained in many cases. In these patients both sides are operated on (Smethwick's operation), usually in two operations, carried out with an interval of about three weeks between them. When the operation of lumbar sympathectomy is carried out for high blood pressure, the incision involves removal of the twelfth rib and may be associated with damage to the pleura and pneumothorax. The lumbar chain on both sides and the splanchnic nerves supplying the abdominal organs are removed: this will embarrass respiration and the action of the heart. After operation the blood pressure may become very low and the patient is nursed flat to ensure a sufficient blood supply to the brain. It may be necessary to lower the head, bandage the limbs and give stimulants, e.g. adrenaline. After operation the patients cannot stand sudden change of position and cannot rise quickly after stooping. When they first get up, the legs are bandaged and an abdominal support provided to ensure a sufficient blood supply to the brain. As the peritoneum is not involved, the operation is not associated with any risk of peritoneal infection and the wound should heal in the normal time and require the routine postoperative care.

Other indications. Incipent *gangrene* may also be treated in this way. The sympathectomy improves the circulation to the skin and abolishes rest pain caused by the impaired circulation. This may then allow reconstructive arterial surgery to be carried out instead of an amputation of a limb. Sympathectomy may also be carried out to relieve *excessive sweating* of face, hands and feet, especially where these interfere with the patient's work and medical treatment is not effective. The excessive sweating may be general or localized and the treatment will depend on the case. It may be used also for *cardiospasm*, causing obstruction on swallowing, and sometimes for the relief of *Méniere's disease* and *migraine*.

22

Diseases of the Genitourinary System

Methods of Examination

The urinary system may be examined in various ways.

Examination of the urine. The following tests should be done:

1. Observation of colour, clots, debris, quantity, specific gravity, reaction and smell.
2. Chemical tests for abnormal contents, e.g. albumen, sugar, acetone.
3. Microscopical tests for the presence of casts, crystals, bacteria and blood or pus cells.
4. Bacteriological examination. This must be carried out at once.

Examination of blood. Blood is examined for:

1. Urea, normal levels being 2·5–7·5 mmol/litre.
2. Acid phosphatase which is found in excessive quantities (normal is 0–12 IU/litre) if there is a carcinoma of prostate which has already produced metastases.
3. Electrolyte and serum calcium levels.

Palpation. The patient is examined in the dorsal position for enlargement and tenderness in the kidney area and to detect lesions of the bladder, scrotum and penis. For enlarged prostate rectal examination is also used, often in the genupectoral position.

Examinations in theatre. Bimanual examination under anaesthetic ensures that the patient is relaxed and so allows the surgeon to feel the prostate and the bladder.

Urethroscopy involves internal examination of the urethra.

DISEASES OF THE GENITOURINARY SYSTEM

Cytoscopy is looking into the bladder by means of a cytoscope, a hollow metal tube fitted with lenses and electric light. This is passed into the bladder after catheterizing and washing out the bladder, leaving about 250 ml of lotion in it to distend the walls so that they do not come into contact with the instrument. This enables the surgeon to see the condition of the bladder walls, the orifices of the ureters and the presence of stones. Further, it is possible by means of a special cytoscope to pass catheters directly into the ureters and collect specimens of urine from each kidney separately for testing the function of each kidney in secreting urea, or for examination for bacteria.

Ureteric catheterization is performed so that a specimen of urine may be collected from the pelvis of either kidney, and prior to a retrograde pyelogram.

The steroid addis count. An injection of a test dose of steroids is given before a specimen of urine is obtained; the steroids stimulate the excretion of pus and blood cells from a kidney in which there is latent infection.

X-ray of the urinary tract. For details see Chapter 25. A straight X-ray may be performed. In addition a retrograde pyelogram or an intravenous pyelogram is available for special examination of the genitourinary tract.

Aortography. This detects abnormalities in the renal vessels and assists the surgeon to distinguish between a cyst and a new growth.

Renogram. This assesses kidney function by the injection into a vein of a radioactive substance such as Hippuran ^{131}I. A 'counter' can be put over the kidneys and the amount of radioactivity assessed, since approximately 1 litre per minute of blood is passing through the kidneys, the amount should be quite considerable.

Renal function tests. These would include creatinine clearance, which measures the glomerular filtration rate, or the urea concentration test.

CONGENITAL ABNORMALITIES

The presence of congenital abnormalities in the urinary tract is very likely to result in impeded drainage of urine; localized stagnation is then very liable to lead to infection.

Affecting the Kidney and Ureters

Double ureter. There are two or even three ureters on one side.

Congenital cystic kidney. Some of the collecting tubules of the kidney may fail to empty into the pelvis, with the result that urine collects in such tubules, forming cysts. These gradually increase in size and press upon the normal substance of the kidney, ultimately destroying it. In this condition the patient may have either a polycystic or a solitary cystic disease. The polycystic disease is bilateral and the solitary type may be bilateral or unilateral. It produces marked enlargement of the kidneys with increasing loss of function, so that the patient dies between 30 and 40 years of age from uraemia, due to the retention of waste products which the kidneys should excrete. Operation to drain the cysts may be undertaken and this consists of draining and de-roofing them. This is necessary to prevent the cysts filling up again.

Errors of position. These may take a variety of forms. Rotated kidneys face forward not sideways. Horse-shoe kidneys have the lower poles fused in front of the aorta. Pelvic kidney is in the pelvis or on the iliac fossa.

Absence of one kidney. Rarely one kidney is absent; less rarely one is atrophied. These last two conditions are important in that, since there is, in effect, only one kidney, its removal in case of disease is impossible.

Aberrant renal vessels.

Congenital hydronephrosis. This is probably secondary to some other congenital condition which causes obstruction to the bladder outlet such as a congenital urethral stricture or the presence of abnormal urethral valves.

Affecting the Bladder and Urethra

Ectopia vesicae or extroversion of the bladder. The anterior wall of the bladder and the abdomen fail to develop, but the posterior wall and trigone at the base of the bladder are present and urine gushes from the orifices of the ureters. In this case a rectal prolapse may be present so it is not possible to transplant the ureters into the colon, as this would only result in incontinence of urine and faeces

DISEASES OF THE GENITOURINARY SYSTEM

because of the malfunctioning anal sphincter. So the abdominal wall is repaired and the ureters are transplanted into a portion of defunctioned colon (a colcystoplasty or an ileocystoplasty). Before surgery sulphafurazole may be ordered by the surgeon to disinfect the bowel and a broad-spectrum antibiotic may be used to 'cover the operation'.

Diverticula may be present in the bladder and do not empty satisfactorily, so that residual urine remains and gives rise to cystitis, and possibly stone formation. Excision is necessary.

Hypospadias. The urethra opens in the perineum or undersurface of the penis. The operation is usually done in two stages: (*a*) to correct the deformity of the penis and (*b*) to repair the urethra.

Epispadias. The urethra opens on the upper surface of the penis and plastic operation is required.

LESIONS OF THE KIDNEYS

The kidneys may be affected by:

1. Trauma.
2. Pyelonephritis.
3. Hydronephrosis.
4. Renal calculi.
5. Neoplasia.
6. Chronic infections.

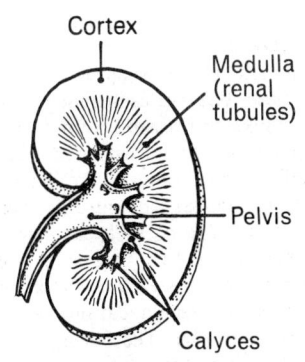

FIG. 42. Longitudinal section of the normal kidney.

Trauma to the Kidney

Rupture causes internal haemorrhage, with the passage of blood in the urine associated with pain and shock. If the tear is slight, the bleeding will quickly cease and the specimens of urine gradually show less blood. It is advisable to save all urine, labelled with the time of passing. A careful watch must be kept on the pulse rate. Rest in bed, with the giving of fluids by mouth and urinary antiseptics, is all that is necessary in these mild cases. Renal colic may occur from the passage of blood clots down the ureter.

In severe cases operation to repair the rent or, more frequently, for excision of the kidney is necessary. These cases are likely to require blood (or plasma) transfusions, if there has been severe internal haemorrhage.

Pyelonephritis

In this condition inflammation is present in both the kidney substance and the kidney pelvis. Treatment is given to the underlying cause which is usually an infected obstruction.

Hydronephrosis

Hydronephrosis is usually a pelvicalyceal distension; it is due to intermittent or partial obstruction of the outflow of urine. Complete sudden obstruction results in suppression of urine, so that distension does not arise. The causes include blockage of the ureters by stones, stricture, kinks or pressure from a tumour, or muscular spasm. First the pelvis becomes distended and later the kidney substance is gradually thinned out and the kidney becomes a thin-walled bag of fluid, the cortex and medulla being gradually destroyed by back-pressure. The partially stagnant urine is prone to infection, causing the fluid to turn to pus, a condition known as *pyonephrosis*; as the pus cannot escape, the kidney may give way and surrounding tissues are infected, causing perinephric abscess.

Diagnosis is by pyelography. The normal pelvis holds about 7 ml; if it holds more there is hydronephrosis.

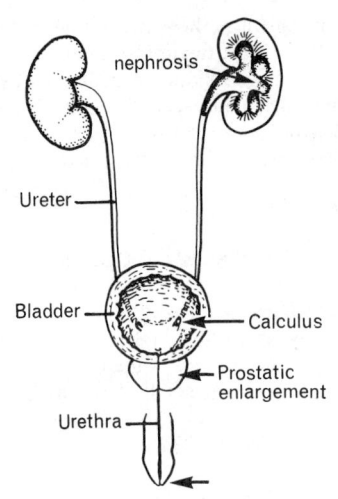

Fig. 43. The male urinary tract, showing some of the common causes of obstruction to the flow of urine.

Signs and symptoms

1. This condition is asymptomatic until infection occurs when manifestations of pyelonephritis are seen: pain, fever, haematuria and pyuria.
2. Enlargement of the kidney gradually becomes apparent.
3. If both kidneys are affected uraemic symptoms will follow, as the kidneys are destroyed.

Treatment

The cause should be removed, if early diagnosis is made. Sometimes plastic operation may be carried out to reduce the size of the pelvis of the kidney, after relief of pressure which may be due to kinks in a post-caval ureter which is compressed by the inferior vena cava.

If the blockage cannot be removed or the kidney is functionally useless, nephrectomy is performed because of the risk of infection. Nephrectomy may also be performed in cases of hydronephrosis with high blood pressure, as, in some cases, removal of such an abnormal kidney may result in a fall in blood pressure.

An alternative treatment in these cases is tying the renal artery to cause atrophy of the kidney: the improvement is thought to be due to the fact that the damaged kidney produces an excess of renin, a pressor substance which causes contraction of the blood vessels and therefore raises the blood pressure.

If pyonephrosis occurs, nephrectomy is necessary.

Renal Stones or Calculi

Renal stones or calculi are deposits of mineral salts that form in the tubules of the kidney and often make their way into the pelvis, ureter and bladder, where they may increase in size very considerably. Though generally small, they may fill the whole of the pelvis of the kidney.

Types of calculi

1. *Phosphates* are smooth but may be large, filling the whole pelvis of the kidney. These are commonly called 'staghorn' calculi.
2. *Carbonates* are grey/white in colour and often very large. Especially seen following infection.
3. *Urates*. Ammonium urate stones are often found in young children.
4. *Oxalate* stones are small, hard, dark in colour and have an irregular spiky surface. These are liable to injure the tissues and cause bleeding.
5. *Uric acid* stones are generally found in adults and are hard, smooth and brownish in colour. They are not radiopaque.
6. *Cystine* stones are also not radiopaque.

Signs and symptoms

Symptoms and signs vary considerably. Large stones filling the kidney pelvis may give rise to little in the way of symptoms and their presence may be unsuspected until some complication arises. There may be slight pain and traces of blood in the urine occasionally, especially on jolting. Small stones, on the other hand, are likely to enter the ureter and give rise to renal colic, until the stone either slips back into the pelvis or is passed into the bladder.

Treatment of renal calculi

This depends upon the size and site of the calculi. Surgery is generally advocated unless there is some contraindication. Several operations are available:

1. *Nephrolithotomy*, removal of a stone from the kidney. There is a risk of secondary haemorrhage due to incision into kidney substance.
2. *Pyelolithotomy*, removal of a stone from the pelvis of a kidney.
3. *Ureterolithotomy* may be necessary if a stone has passed down from the kidney and is held in the ureter.
4. *Partial nephrectomy* may be performed if a stone is confined to one pole of a kidney.
5. *Nephrectomy* may be necessary if the stone is large and fills the pelvis of the kidney (such as a staghorn calculus); however, the other kidney must have an adequate degree of function.

Renal Colic

Renal colic is characterized by:

1. Acute agonizing pain of sudden onset, starting in the loin and shooting down to the groin, scrotum or thigh as far as the knee. The patient writhes with pain in typical cases and vomits.
2. Signs of shock and collapse, e.g. rapid, weak pulse, subnormal temperature, pallor and sweating.
3. Blood may be passed in the urine; there may be frequency of micturition with the constant passage of small quantities of blood-stained urine (strangury).

The type of drug and its dose depends upon the patient's age and general condition, but morphine, pethidine, pentazocine and DF 118 are commonly prescribed to relieve the patient's pain. Atropine may be ordered to paralyse the parasympathetic nerves and relax the spasm. Other treatments will not relieve the patient for long, but while waiting for the doctor some benefit will follow the application of heat.

The patient must be encouraged to drink large volumes of fluids, but not if the calculi has caused an obstruction, or if the patient is vomiting. Urine must be carefully observed and all specimens must be filtered so that any calculi passed can be saved for inspection (sometimes the calculus can be heard as it falls into the glass or metal urinal or bed pan). The doctor may prescribe exercise for the patient, especially in the form of skipping; this is very useful as it helps to dislodge the calculus if it is in the ureter. This form of treatment is only ordered if the patient is fit enough and not experiencing severe pain.

Growths in the Kidney

Growths may occur in infants and in adults and are commonly malignant. *Sarcoma* occurs in children under five years of age; it is bilateral and always fatal. There is bilateral swelling in the kidney region. *Teratoma* may occur attached to one kidney and may become a carcinoma or a sarcoma. This is called Wilms's tumour.

In adults both hypernephroma and carcinoma of kidney pelvis are commonly seen. In many cases the patient first complains of feeling generally unwell and has some gastrointestinal symptoms and this may be the first indication of serious illness. Irregular haematuria may be present and in some cases a blood clot colic may develop. In other cases the first symptoms noted are due to metastases in other organs as these occur very early, especially in bone.

Early cases can be cured by nephroureterectomy with, in some cases, the removal of a cuff of bladder, but there is a great risk of spread by the tumour cells 'seeding' down the ureter from the kidney to the bladder. The patient is followed-up with cystoscopies so that the condition can be diagnosed early should a neoplasia of bladder develop.

If a secondary growth has occurred in the lungs then satisfactory treatment is impossible.

Chronic Infection

Renal tuberculosis is an important example of this type of infection which unfortunately is increasing in incidence in the United Kingdom at the present time. It is always secondary to a primary lesion which has occurred elsewhere in the body, most commonly in the lungs. The commonest symptom is painless haematuria. Frequency of micturition only develops when the bladder is involved and this is very distressing as the patient is disturbed very frequently day and night.

Typical tuberculous changes occur, the kidney substance being destroyed; natural cure by fibrosis and calcification may occur, but if both kidneys are affected uraemia is likely to follow and prove fatal.

The disease also affects the epididymis, and in either case the infection may spread by direct extension via the ureter and vas deferens from one of these organs to the other. The uterine tubes are liable to infection in the female and will give rise to sterility.

The pathologist will require a series of three early morning specimens (the first urine voided after a night's sleep); these are examined microscopically and guinea-pig inoculations are carried out. The result is not known for six weeks. If difficulty is experienced in culturing the tubercle bacillus then the patient may have to provide 24-hour specimens of urine.

Antitubercular drugs will be prescribed when the diagnosis has been confirmed; when the course of drugs is complete a nephroureterectomy will be performed (removal of the affected kidney together with the whole of its ureter, plus in some cases a cuff of bladder).

If both kidneys are affected sanatorium treatment is advocated, together with the antituberculous drugs.

If the bladder was involved in the infection then treatment may leave a healed, scarred, contracted bladder. In this case surgery may be performed when the bladder is enlarged with piece of colon. This operation is generally very successful but the patient is 'followed-up' for many years. The passage of mucus may worry the patient but this is of little significance as it is secreted by the piece of colon used to enlarge the bladder.

Renal Transplant

This operation may be carried out in the treatment of terminal renal failure. Usually the patient has been receiving chronic renal dialysis for some time, and has been carefully selected for transplant surgery.

The donor kidneys may be obtained from a living person or a cadaver; in either case tissue typing is carried out on the white blood corpuscles of both recipient and donor. The highest incidence of success occurs when the kidney is transplanted from a near relative.

The donor kidney is transplanted into the iliac fossa of the

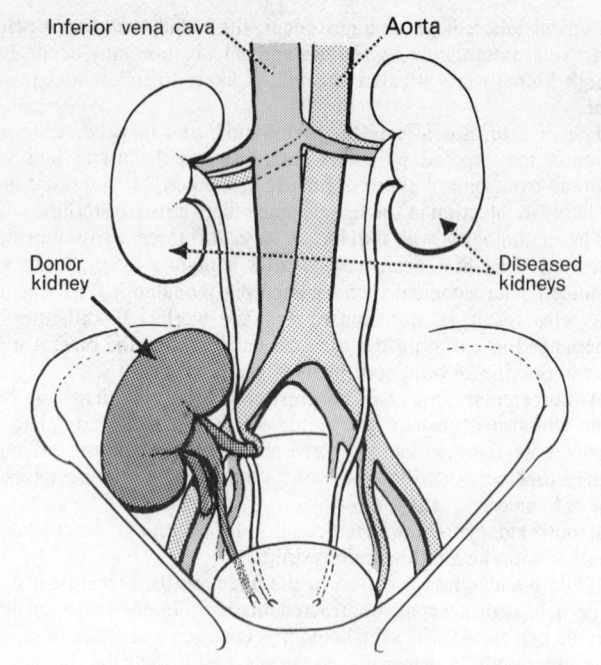

FIG. 44. A renal transplant.

recipient, and the blood vessels and ureter are united as in Fig. 44. A ureteric catheter is inserted to act as a splint and to drain urine from the transplanted kidney. A self-retaining urethral catheter also drains the bladder. Intravenous dextrose or dextrose/saline (saline is not used if the patient is hypertensive) is administered according to the amount of urine passed by the patient.

The wound area is drained by Redivac drains and the amount is carefully recorded. Fluids are administered and a low-protein diet is started the next day. Sometimes the patients are nursed in isolation, and in other cases small doses of radiotherapy are administered to the transplant area. Drugs (Imuran and prednisone) are also given to reduce the risk of rejection. As there is a risk of urinary tract infection, chemotherapy (gentamicin and ampicillin) is also given.

Rejection can be recognized by the development of a spiking temperature, tachycardia, decreased urinary output and elevation of blood urea and creatinine. The treatment consists of the

DISEASES OF THE GENITOURINARY SYSTEM 307

administration of methylprednisolone and the kidney is investigated by a renal scan and biopsy. It may be necessary to perform a second transplant.

Patients who receive this form of treatment are usually very well informed about their illness, so the nurse must be aware of the unique needs of the patient in this specialized type of unit.

Preparation of the Patient for Kidney Operation

A good nurse will *reassure the patient* at all times and make sure that he has a basic understanding of everything that is happening or is going to happen.

In all cases an *intravenous pyelogram* is carried out and the patient's blood urea is estimated. These investigations are very important as the surgeon must be sure that the patient has adequate renal function which is compatible with life.

Skin preparation consists of rendering the required area clinically clean. A lumbar incision is commonly used, and for this the back must be prepared from the scapula to the pelvic crest, and

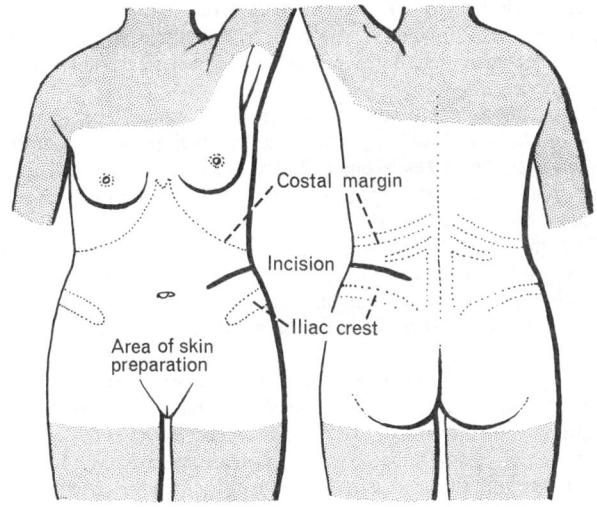

FIG. 45. A common incision for operations on the kidney. The skin area to be prepared is unshaded.

the abdominal wall on the affected side to the midline. Sometimes an abdominal incision is employed when there is great enlargement and then the whole abdomen is prepared in the usual way, including the skin round to the back on the affected side.

The nurse must make sure that the patient's *bowels* are empty and that he has a good night's *sleep* before surgery.

The patient is usually encouraged *to drink freely*, being supplied with a jug of lemon barley water or lemonade at the bedside, up to within six hours of surgery. After this time fluids are restricted and the patient is also fasted.

If necessary a *broad-spectrum antibiotic* is ordered and administered.

A complete *measurement of urine* is kept and the urine passed must be watched carefully for any abnormalities such as the passage of stones or blood.

Postoperative Care

The bed must be prepared while the patient is in the theatre/recovery room so that his care and observations may be continuous on return to the ward. If he has been in the recovery room all vital signs will be stable and the patient conscious, in which case he is placed in the most comfortable position. Drains are connected up and intravenous fluids suspended after checking on the flow.

Observations are made and recorded at once. These are continued half-hourly at first then the interval increased as postoperative recovery takes place. There is a risk of a pneumothorax developing so it is important that the movement of both sides of the chest is carefully observed.

The intravenous fluids will be continued until the patient is able to take sufficient fluids orally, usually for a period of about three days. Initially only small amounts are allowed orally because of the risk of paralytic ileus developing, the return of bowel sounds being a good sign.

Analgesics are given to keep the patient pain-free; this is important as the incision is extensive and pain is caused by deep breathing and movement. Analgesia should be given 30 minutes before the physiotherapist gives deep breathing exercises; the nurse must make sure that the patient continues them in the absence of the physiotherapist. Urine drainage must be carefully observed, particularly the volume and colour.

DISEASES OF THE GENITOURINARY SYSTEM

The wound may have both a round and a suction drain in situ; the round drain is shortened and removed when drainage has ceased for a period of 48 hours. The suction drain may be taken out as soon as drainage has stopped.

Mobilization is commenced gently and is increased daily; by the third day the patient may be able to have a shower (after carefully protecting the wound). If possible the wound is not disturbed unless the patient is pyrexial or complains of undue wound discomfort.

LESIONS OF THE URINARY BLADDER

The bladder may be affected by:

1. Inflammation.
2. Retention of urine.
3. Vesical calculus.
4. Neoplasia.
5. Trauma.

Inflammation of the Bladder

Inflammation of the bladder is termed cystitis. It is due to infection and is treated medically. Surgery will be called for only if there is some other associated condition, e.g. calculus.

Retention of Urine

Retention of urine means that the bladder is full of urine but the patient is unable to pass it, as opposed to suppression, when the kidney fails to secrete urine.

It may be due to:

1. Obstruction to the outflow from the bladder due to:
    a. Bladder neck obstruction.
    b. Enlargement of the prostate gland.
    c. Stricture of the urethra.
    d. Retroverted gravid uterus.
    e. Bladder calculus.
2. Inability to carry out the act on account of:
    a. Fear or nervous shock, as after operation.

SURGICAL NURSING

    b. Abnormal position for micturition.
    c. Paralysis of the sphincter guarding the urethra, as in fracture or disease involving the spinal cord.

Treatment for obstruction to the outflow is, in most cases, surgical but may have to be preceded by catheterization. Treatment for inability to carry out the act may also, ultimately, have to be catheterization. It is very important that this procedure be carried out with full aseptic precautions.

Bladder Neck Obstruction

In this condition the patient will have retention of urine but the prostate gland is normal. Hypertrophy of muscle and fibrosis of the posterior lip of the internal meatus are present. It is thought to be congenital in origin. This form of obstruction may also be due to calculus formation in the prostate.

The patient is usually from a younger age group and will have a long history of difficulty in micturition. The condition is diagnosed by means of a cystoscopy and the treatment consists of resection of the posterior part of the internal meatus, by the transurethral route.

Enlargement of the Prostate

Enlargement of the prostate is seen in patients over 50 years of age and is generally simple, though it may be due to malignant disease. As the prostate gland encircles the urethra at the base of the bladder, enlargement interferes with the act of micturition and may endanger life by the destructive effect of back-pressure on the substance of the kidney, causing uraemia, or by infective processes following the introduction of infection by catheterization and encouraged by stagnation of urine in the bladder.

Symptoms include:

1. Difficulty in micturition, especially in starting the act, there is a poor 'stream'.
2. Frequency, especially troublesome to the patient at night, as little urine is passed at one time. Often there is superimposed infection.
3. Haematuria.
4. Signs of uraemia, i.e. drowsiness, headache, dry dirty tongue, followed in the later stages by twitching, convulsions and coma.

DISEASES OF THE GENITOURINARY SYSTEM

The patient's first visit to the general practitioner may be because of the early signs and symptoms of uraemia. Symptoms of an enlarged prostate may have been present for some time but the patient has 'ignored' them.

5. Acute retention of urine.

Diagnosis is confirmed by rectal examination, and an intravenous pyelogram is carried out to investigate the condition of the upper renal tract.

Simple enlargement may be treated by prostatectomy. Malignant conditions respond satisfactorily to drugs such as tetrasodium fosfestrol, ethinyloestrol and occasionally stilboestrol. These drugs are used if the patient has neoplasia of the prostate.

Prostatectomy

Prostatectomy may be carried out retropubically, transvesically or transurethrally, each surgeon having his favourite route. If the surgeon favours the retropubic route he makes a suprapubic incision but he dissects down to reach the prostate through the gap between the symphysis pubis and the bladder wall instead of approaching it from within the bladder, the earliest method. On reaching the prostate gland he incises the capsule, shelling out the gland tissue and leaving the capsule which he sews up to surround the urinary passage. He leaves a catheter in the urethra for drainage and bladder wash-outs. The suprapubic incision is closed except for a small drainage tube to prevent the formation of a haematoma or the leakage and collection of urine in the retropubic space.

If there is a catheter in the urethra, it is controlled by a spigot or drains into a receptacle at the bedside; it is very important that this should be a closed receptacle which is either a 'disposable', to be replaced completely when full, or which can be sterilized each time it is emptied. Some surgeons tie off the vas deferens on each side to lessen the risks of epididymitis and orchitis in this and all other operations on the prostate.

The operation is associated with some risk owing to the possible age of the patient and the possibility of severe haemorrhage and shock. The outlook also depends on the previous condition of the patient's kidneys and bladder, uraemia and toxaemia both being possible causes of a fatal ending. There is danger of pneumonia and heart failure and this increases with age, especially where there is any previous weakness of the chest.

PREPARATION FOR OPERATION

The routine preparation for abdominal operation is required and in addition an attempt is made to reduce the patient's blood urea level but this is not essential if the anaesthetist is willing to anaesthetize the patient. He may decide to administer a spinal anaesthetic especially if the patient is elderly and has some form of chronic lung or heart condition which is a contraindication to general anaesthesia.

The patient is encouraged to drink freely by giving plenty of bland fluids such as barley water. A fluid intake and output chart should be kept.

It may be necessary to operate under the 'cover' of an antibiotic especially if the patient has a chest infection. Established infection of the urine will be treated by the administration of the appropriate antibiotic.

It is important to make the patient believe that the operation will cure him, although it is well to prepare him for a little discomfort during the two or three weeks while the wound is healing. He may need reassurance concerning his sexual capacity, i.e. though through the tying of the vas deferens he will be sterile, he will not be impotent.

POSTOPERATIVE CARE

Patients requiring a prostatectomy are often elderly, so very careful basic nursing is necessary to prevent the many complications that could arise. He will be nursed in a sitting position as soon as his condition allows, but it may be better to leave him in his most comfortable position for the first few hours with the head of the bed raised. In some cases spinal anaesthesia is used and these patients must be nursed flat for 24 hours postoperatively and sensation in the lower limbs must be checked carefully. However, if he has a chronic chest condition such as bronchitis the anaesthetist may request that he be nursed in the sitting position as soon as possible. Intravenous therapy is always employed as it may be necessary to give the patient a blood transfusion and he will only receive limited amounts of fluid until his bowel sounds return. After this time the patient is encouraged to drink large volumes of fluid frequently and a very careful fluid balance chart is maintained. The patient's bladder will be drained continuously and a 'milking' tube will be incorporated to allow this to be carried out. Skilful 'milking' will prevent clot retention but if this does occur bladder irrigation may be necessary; normal saline at body temperature is used by an experienced nurse or a doctor. A pre-sterilized plastic bladder syringe with a capacity of 50–100 ml is used, taking care to aspirate the fluid back and not just to rely on it draining out. The wash-out is continued until the returned fluid is completely clear. If the amount of urine excreted is abnormal or if haematuria is excessive and not decreasing the medical staff must be informed.

The urethral catheter is removed when the urine is clear and in a satisfactory case this may be in four to five days, but it must remain in position if the urine is still blood-stained. This must also apply if the patient is very confused and unable to cooperate in bladder training. If the patient is unable to understand instructions, and so unable to train his own bladder, he will dribble urine or not pass any at all and this would result in leakage of urine from the wound. Bladder training demands the cooperation of the patient and consists of holding urine in his bladder first for thirty minutes, then one hour, then for three hours. Some patients train their bladders very quickly and others may take days. A very important aspect of this training is that the nurse must remove the urinal when the patient has used it and *not* return it until the patient is due to void again. Mobilization is commenced gradually and this is controlled by the patient's possible limitations, e.g. those due to age.

A transurethral prostatectomy does not require an abdominal incision but there is an increased risk of bleeding as haemostasis is very difficult to secure. As a result even though the risk of paralytic ileus is minimal an intravenous infusion is still used, partially to allow the rapid administration of blood if necessary but also to maintain the fluid intake and output so reducing the risk of clot retention developing.

Some surgeons request that a catheter specimen of urine is obtained and that a bladder washout with Hibitane 1 in 5000 is performed leaving 50 ml in the bladder before the catheter is removed. This ensures that the first fluid passed from the bladder down the urethra is not acid in reaction and soothes the traumatized urethra.

Vesical Calculus or Stone in the Bladder

Stone in the bladder causes the following symptoms:

1. Pain, especially at the end of micturition and referred to the tip of the penis.

2. Haematuria; this is slight and occurs at the end of micturition.
3. Frequency, which is diminished at night unless there is also cystitis.
4. The flow of urine sometimes stops suddenly during the act of micturition, due to a small stone falling over the outlet to the urethra.
5. Occasionally a small stone is passed, often accompanied by severe pain.

There may be a history of previous attacks of renal colic. The diagnosis is confirmed by X-ray and cystoscopy.

Treatment consists of either crushing the stone and washing out the fragments (litholapaxy) or suprapubic cystotomy for removal of the stone (lithotomy).

Before carrying out either of these treatments the condition of the bladder should be improved by the giving of urinary antiseptics and plenty of fluids by mouth, if cystitis is present.

Suprapubic lithotomy is carried out by opening the bladder by suprapubic incision, but it may be subsequently sewn up unless the bladder is septic and drainage is considered advisable. A small tube will always be present in the wound in case any leakage of urine through the bladder incision occurs.

After-care will be similar to that for prostatectomy.

New Growths in the Bladder

Transitional cell tumours of the bladder are very common. They are usually primary, but sometimes a bladder tumour may have spread from the rectum or uterus. The majority of tumours are either carcinomas or papillomas. Sarcoma is rarely seen at this site. The tumours give rise to painless haematuria and in the later stages frequency of micturition and pain develop. Diagnosis is confirmed by cystoscopy and an intravenous pyelogram will be performed to assess renal function.

Treatment may be surgical, by radiotherapy or by the administration of cytotoxic substances in the bladder lumen, but psychological care must also be given to the patient and the relatives throughout the whole of the preparation, treatment and after-care.

In early cases papilloma may be treated by diathermy through the cystoscope, with successful results. In cases where the growth is larger, suprapubic cystostomy may be necessary and excision of the growth. If malignant changes have taken place, or if the original growth is malignant partial cystectomy may be practical, but only if the tumour is in a part of the bladder that can be resected. This is not possible if the trigone is involved. Complete cystectomy may be carried out with urinary diversion. There are many operations that can be performed and the site used depends on the age and general condition of the patient. A ureterocolic anastomosis is usually limited to advanced cases, when it is only a palliative measure. If the patient is expected to live for a long period of time this operation could result in a variety of problems, such as electrolyte imbalance. One of the operations of choice is a rectal baldder where a colostomy is performed and the patient's rectum is defunctioned. The ureters are then implanted into the rectum and this acts as a reservoir for the urine. The patient then passes urine from the rectum and faeces from the colostomy.

It is possible for the ureters or kidneys to be drained permanently on to the external skin in the loin, but apparatus is difficult to adjust and the patient is liable to become very depressed. Transplantation into the rectum is therefore generally advocated, though there is some risk of infection spreading from the bowel to the pelvis of the kidney. Intestinal disinfectants, either antibiotics or sulphonamides, are ordered before operation and the operation is carried out under cover of these drugs systemically. Patients can eventually gain control over the fluid in the bowel quite satisfactorily.

The stoma therapist should be involved in this patient's rehabilitation from an early preoperative stage.

Radiotherapy tends to be used when the surgeon considers the patient's condition to be operable and it is performed prior to surgery. Radon seeds may be implanted at the time of operation by the radiotherapist and their use does not entail any special nursing techniques as radon has a very short half-life. The seeds are left in position and remain visible on future X-rays. The only precaution that should be taken is that any necessary bladder irrigation should be done gently to avoid dislodging the seeds. The urethral catheter is left in a little longer as wounds tend not to heal as quickly when a patient has had radiotherapy treatment.

The nursing of these patients is similar to that for suprapubic cystotomy if operation is undertaken for excision. Special emphasis is given to prevention of chest complications and bedsores; observation of the quantity of urine passed and its nature; chemotherapy and the giving of urinary antiseptics; and general observation for any symptoms of uraemia and toxaemia, especially where cystitis is already present.

Rupture of the Bladder

Trauma may result in rupture of the bladder, e.g. a blow or crushing, especially when the bladder is full. This allows the urine to escape, and generally the peritoneal cavity is involved, resulting in peritonitis; in other cases pelvic cellulitis may occur.

Operation is performed at the earliest moment to repair the rent and drain the abdominal cavity.

LESIONS OF THE URETHRA AND PENIS

The urethra may be affected by:

1. Stricture.
2. Phimosis.
3. Trauma.

Stricture of the Urethra

Stricture causes difficulty in passing urine and may be treated by either:

1. Dilatation in early cases.
2. Urethrotomy, internal or external.

It may follow injury to the urethra if preventive treatment by dilatation is not taken during healing. Following inflammation it is now less common on account of the curative effects of penicillin in gonorrhoeal infection.

For dilatation, graduated bougies may be employed or bougies of elastic gum in suitable cases.

For urethrotomy, the internal operation is generally employed, Wheelhouse's staff being passed; this is grooved for the passage of a special knife called the urethrotome, which divides the stricture.

After these operations either a catheter is sutured to the penis (if the bladder has not been opened) or a self-retaining catheter is used to prevent extravasation of urine during healing of the wound, and bougies are introduced to prevent contraction recurring, as fibrous scar tissue forms. The patient should be encouraged to drink freely, and daily bladder wash-outs are ordered as long as the catheter is left in the urethra. Antibiotics and sulphonamides are used to cover the operation period, as necessary.

Phimosis

Phimosis is a tight foreskin, i.e. a foreskin or prepuce which has a very small opening, so that it may interfere with the passage of urine and cannot be drawn back over the glans penis for cleansing In severe cases this will prevent the escape of urine, so that the foreskin is distended during micturition, the stream is reduced to a dribble and the infant screams with pain and strains during the act. In less severe cases there may not be this disability, but there is a risk of (*a*) *balanitis*, i.e. inflammation, due to lack of cleanliness; and (*b*) *paraphimosis*, a condition due to a tight foreskin being

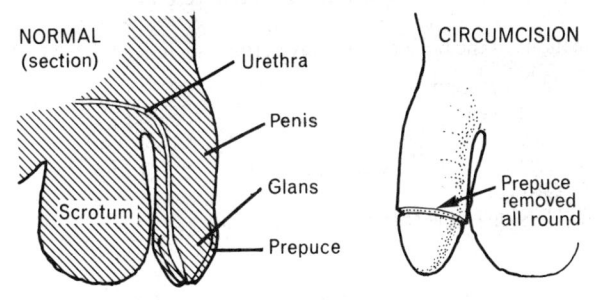

FIG. 46. The operation of circumcision, showing the removal of the prepuce.

pushed up and constricting the circulation, causing swelling of the parts below so that the foreskin cannot be pushed down again, and requiring operative treatment. Ice packs to reduce the oedema and manual reduction may avoid the need for surgery, but this will eventually be necessary.

If chronic balanitis is present the surgeon may decide only to make a dorsal slit in the prepuce, but if possible a circumcision, i.e. cutting away the prepuce, is preferable. After this operation the wound must be kept clean, antiseptic dressings applied and the parts cleansed after the passing of urine. In out-patient cases a strip of gauze soaked in tincture of benzoin in oil, 1 part to 7 parts, wrapped round the penis at the site of the wound is useful. Mild cases of phimosis can be relieved by gradually stretching the foreskin by pulling it back over the glans penis when bathing and attending to the child, so that operation is obviated.

Trauma

Trauma may result from such accidents as falling on to a spiked railing. It should be treated by catheterization, the catheter being tied in, so that there is no extravasation of urine into the tissues, since this is liable to lead to pelvic cellulitis, with serious and possibly fatal results, owing to the irritating effect of the acid urine.

As healing occurs there is danger of stricture from scar contraction, and bougies must be passed at regular intervals to prevent this, the patient being kept under observation.

LESIONS OF THE MALE REPRODUCTIVE ORGANS

Affections of the male reproductive organs include:

1. Inflammation.
2. Hydrocele.
3. Varicocele.
4. Undescended testicle.
5. Growths.
6. Torsion of the spermatic cord.

Inflammation of the Testis and Epididymis

Inflammation may be acute or chronic and may attack the testicle proper (orchitis) or the epididymis (epididymitis). Surgery plays little part in treatment.

Hydrocele

A hydrocele is an excessive collection of serum in the tunica vaginalis surrounding the testicles; it occurs as a result of inflammation in this membrane. In children it often subsides without surgical interference. It is treated in chronic cases by tapping with trocar and cannula and palpation to exclude any primary lesion of the testicle. If the condition tends to recur, satisfactory results can be obtained by operation for excision of the sac under local or general anaesthesia. In postoperative care retention of urine may be a troublesome complication, but can usually be overcome by the giving of a simple enema, if other measures fail.

Varicocele

Varicocele is a varicose condition of the veins draining the testicle. It may give rise to no symptoms beyond the distortion due to the enlargement of the veins, but pain of an aching character may be present. The patient is often subfertile as spermatogenesis may be defective.

In mild cases a suspensory bandage may relieve the condition. Treatment is necessary for entry into the Armed Forces and may be either by injection or excision, as in other cases of varicose veins. In operative cases the nursing points are similar to hydrocele.

Undescended Testicle

The testicles first develop high up at the back of the abdomen close to the kidneys and gradually descend through the abdomen and inguinal canal, reaching the scrotum shortly before birth. They may fail to reach the scrotum, so that it is empty on the affected side; this is normal in the premature baby. Descent may be completed after birth, but if the testicles fail to descend they fail to develop at puberty. There is also a suggestion that failure in descent may be followed by malignant changes.

Operation may be undertaken to stitch the testicle down in the scrotum. The operation is undertaken before puberty, but is liable to be followed by atrophy of the testicles, as the spermatic cord is short and the blood vessels are obstructed by the tension put on them. Hernia is often also present and may be treated at the same time. Treatment is generally given between six years and the onset of puberty.

Growths

Both carcinoma and sarcoma may affect the testes, scrotum and penis and will require excision with bilateral removal of the lymphatic glands draining the part, if seen early enough to be curable. Postoperatively pressure dressings must be used to avoid seepage of lymph which would delay healing. Redivac drainage is used for the same reason. If the testicle is affected, dissemination occurs early and secondary growths in the abdomen or bones may be present before the diagnosis is suspected. Radiotherapy may be used for metastases or for carcinoma of the penis.

Torsion of the Spermatic Cord

If not treated promptly an orchidectomy may be necessary; however, the torsion can be reduced in the early stages.

23

Surgery in Bone and Joint Diseases

INFECTIONS OF BONE

These are now uncommon in developed countries as a result of improved health care and the implementation of preventative measures. They include:

1. Osteomyelitis.
2. Chronic inflammation, either syphilitic or tuberculous.

Osteomyelitis

Osteomyelitis is an acute inflammation of the bone and bone marrow. It is due to staphylococcal infection, which may reach the bone through the blood stream, as a result of spread from some septic focus, or through a wound involving the bone, e.g. when micro-organisms track down from the skin and along a pin when skeletal traction is in use. The staff must have a high standard of asepsis to prevent this. It is seen in the chronic form except in adults who have a long history as earlier energetic treatment now cures the condition.

Systemic antibiotics given immediately the condition is suspected give very good results and a large proportion of patients will recover without local treatment. If penicillin and other antibiotics are only given at a later stage, the formation of pus and local necrosis of the bone will necessitate open operation; with this surgical interference, local treatment with antibiotics can also be used, penicillin being employed as a solution or a powder. In these cases, the bone must be freely opened with drill or gouge for the drainage of pus and infected blood and lymph; dead bone must also be removed in the later stages, when sequestra have formed (a sequestrum is a loose piece of dead bone).

General treatment to improve resistance to infection is of great importance. The diet should be light and nourishing, with plenty of fluids to promote free excretion. Fresh air and light treatment are very beneficial.

Chronic Inflammation

Chronic inflammation may be either syphilitic or tuberculous.

Syphilis

Syphilis particularly attacks the bone in the tertiary stages; gummas occur in the bone, causing local swelling, which if not treated will be followed by breaking down of the part with the typical gummy discharge. Treatment is with antisyphilitic remedies.

Tuberculosis of bone and joints

All these types of tuberculosis have become rare in Great Britain with the elimination of bovine tuberculosis and the pasteurization of milk, but it is seen among immigrant children and the population from underdeveloped countries.

Tuberculosis of the joint actually starts in the bone extremity and spreads from it into the joint cavity, causing a tuberculous ulcer in the bone with the typical undermined edge. The joint reacts and fluid is formed in the joint cavity; there is pain, so that the muscles are thrown into spasm to prevent movement and rest the part during the waking state.

Treatment is usually medical and includes extension of the limb to separate the inflamed joint surfaces. Recovery is slow but with constitutional treatment and the use of anti-tuberculous drugs, results, in the end, are usually good. If in spite of this treatment the condition does not improve, excision of the joint may be undertaken; the limb is usually then immobilized in plaster of paris until bony union has occurred. If the joint affected is the hip it may be fixed surgically by a bridge of bone from the ilium to the femur.

Tuberculosis of the spine

Tuberculosis of the spine (Pott's disease) can attack the bone in two places: (*a*) in the body of the vertebra, tuberculous osteitis or spinal caries, and (*b*) under the periosteum, tuberculous periostitis.

Where the tuberculous disease in the spine is not arrested by constitutional treatment and rest, transversectomy may be advocated for the adult. A piece of bone is removed from the adult patient's iliac crest (from the tibia if the patient is a child) and used as a bone graft applied to the spinous processes of the affected vertebrae and those adjacent to it as a splint. The patient is nursed in a plaster bed.

RICKETS

Rickets is essentially a medical condition, but may give rise to bony deformities which require surgical treatment. It is due to lack of vitamin D and can be cured in the early stages by giving animal fats rich in this vitamin, especially cod-liver or halibut oil, and exposing the body to sun or artificial light.

Osteomalacia gives the general appearance of rickets and may be seen in elderly people.

In the early stages splinting may be required to correct deformities and take the weight off the bone. Later, when the child is three to four years old, if the condition has been allowed to become severe, osteotomy may be necessary; the bone is cut through with an osteotome, placed in good position and put up in a plaster splint. The nursing care is similar to that required in the case of fractures. These operations are only necessary to improve appearance, as the bent bones become naturally strengthened by a special buttress of bone laid down to take the strain at the bend; this makes the bone ultimately very strong and gives additional surface for muscle attachment, so that the limbs are sturdy, though shorter than normal.

ARTHRITIS

Arthritis is inflammation of a joint and may be acute or chronic.

324 SURGICAL NURSING

Acute Septic Arthritis

Acute septic arthritis may be due to:

1. Infection from the blood stream.
2. Septic wounds involving the joint cavity.
3. Extension of infection from neighbouring tissues.

Local signs of inflammation will be present, the joint being swollen, red and extremely painful on the slightest movement. There will be also general symptoms of septic absorption, which may be very severe.

If the case is diagnosed early before the discharge is purulent, the joint cavity may be aspirated with hollow needle and syringe and injected with an antibiotic dissolved in as much sterile solution as has been removed; however, this is not often necessary if systemic antibiotics, such as amoxycillin, or cloxacillin, are administered. The appropriate antibiotic is prescribed after the causative organism has been identified. Rest is obtained by the application of splints or extension with the joint in the position of rest, e.g. 5° flexion of the knee.

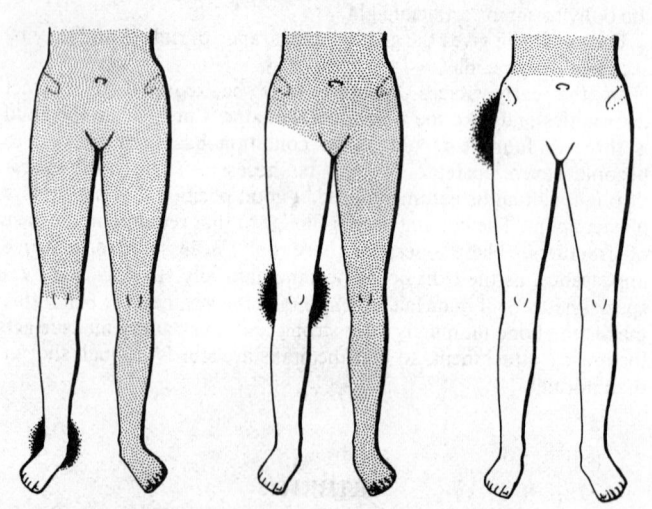

Fig. 47. The areas of skin preparation (unshaded) for operations on the ankle (*left*), knee (*centre*) and hip (*right*).

Chronic Rheumatoid Arthritis

Chronic rheumatoid arthritis is a very common and disabling condition where the synovial tissue in the joints proliferates and eventually the joint becomes ankylosed by fibrous tissue. Treatment is invariably medical but some patients require surgery when the disease has become quiescent in order to correct severe deformities which usually result from wasting of some muscles and contraction of others. These deformities tend to be the result of neglect, and immobilization in the optimum position earlier on during the acute phase should prevent most of them developing.

The small hand joints may be replaced with Silastic joints which give a pain-free useful hand; other joints can be given similar surgical treatment using materials such as titanium or carbon. Postoperatively active movement is encouraged to prevent the patient generally 'stiffening up' as a result of the rheumatoid condition.

Osteo-arthritis

This is an extremely common degenerative process of the articular cartilage which occurs spontaneously in the older age groups. It is also seen in younger people after lesions involving joints, such as a congenital dislocation. It usually affects the large weight-bearing joints. A variety of different operations may be performed including:

1. Arthroplasty.
2. Osteotomy.
3. Arthrodesis.

Of these arthroplasty is most commonly carried out, the head of the femur being replaced by a prostheses made of titanium, vitallium or stainless steel, etc. which is fixed in position by 'cement'.

Arthroplasty of the Hip

Preoperative care

It is very important that the skin is rendered socially clean, so the patient is requested to have a bath on the three days prior to surgery. The required area must also be carefully shaved. On the morning of operation the skin is also prepared with povidone iodine, for example. Suppositories are given 24 hours prior to the operation to make sure that the bowel is clear and to reduce the risk of bowel problems during the first postoperative days. It is also advisable for the patient to have experience in the use of bed pans and urinals. Breathing exercises will be taught by the physiotherapist and the leg on the affected side is measured so that a suitable shoe can be prepared to compensate for the shortening. This is very important as the patient's shoe must be 'broken in' and ready for use when he starts walking again. Slippers would hinder the patient's progress and could be dangerous. Patients who have arthritis of the hip are accustomed to a great deal of pain in the joint so the nurses must make sure that they know that the operation will allow them to walk without pain. This is important as many patients are amazed by the absence of joint pain on movement.

Postoperative care

When the patient returns to the ward he must be positioned with the affected leg in gentle abduction (to reduce the risk of hip dislocation occurring) and the dressing must be inspected for any signs of bleeding. A suction drain, e.g. Redivac, may be used and this is generally removed on the second day. On the second day the patient is usually lifted out of bed still with the leg in gentle abduction and is placed in a comfortable chair with his legs supported on a stool. The physiotherapist will then gradually start to mobilize the patient. Firstly she will teach the patient to use crutches, moving the legs as in normal walking but without weight-bearing, then with elbow crutches and sticks and finally to walk without support. The surgeon may give permission for the patient to start weight-bearing from about the seventh day. If possible the occupational therapist should check the patient's home to ascertain if any problems are present which could hinder the patient's freedom of action. If these are present efforts should be made to solve them prior to the patient's discharge. This will be about the sixteenth day, providing the patient has made an uneventful recovery.

When *arthrodesis* is carried out, movement of the hip will be lost and pain may be overcome, but the stiff hip may throw added strain on some other part of the skeleton, e.g. the lumbar spine, and again exercises, both breathing exercises and exercises for muscles of the back, knee and foot, must be carried out, even where they can consist only of a tensing of the muscle without actual movement of the joint.

These major operations on the hip are used in the later stages, when medical treatment is no longer sufficient to relieve the pain and make an active life possible.

SOFT TISSUE DISORDERS

Bursitis

Bursitis is inflammation of a bursa, e.g. prepatellar bursitis, or 'housemaid's knee'. It may be acute or chronic. Acute cases are treated by rest, followed, if necessary, by excision. Suppurative bursitis requires operative treatment to open and drain the sac. Chronic bursitis is commonly due to kneeling on the prepatellar bursa. Treatment is usually given in the out-patients department.

Tenosynovitis

Tenosynovitis is inflammation of the synovial lining of tendon sheaths. It may be simple, when rest, followed by massage, is the only treatment required, or suppurative, requiring treatment with a five-day course of antibiotics and, if necessary, incision and drainage. In the suppurative cases movement may be impaired.

A *ganglion* is a sac containing glairy fluid connected with the synovial tendon sheath. It may be punctured or ruptured, but the fluid may collect again unless the sac is excised.

Protrusion of the Intervertebral Disc

An injury other than fracture which may require surgical treatment is one which has become well recognized during the last ten to twenty years—namely, protrusion of one or more of the intervertebral discs, causing pressure on the roots of the spinal nerves. This results as a general rule either in an acute attack of sciatica or lumbar pain or in chronic pain in the back and leg, since prolapse of the disc is most common in the lower lumbar region; it can,

328 SURGICAL NURSING

however, occur in the neck and give rise to a brachial neuritis. Like fracture, it seems to occur most often where the more movable sections of the spine meet the more rigid, particularly where the lumbar spine meets the sacrum, or where the cervical spine meets the dorsal. Each disc consists of a central gelatinous part enclosed in a fibrous ring, and if the fibrous part is injured the gelatinous material can escape and bulge out, usually towards the back, as the fibrous ring is least strong here. If the bulge of gelatinous material is to one side of the middle line, it presses on the posterior sensory nerve root at the site and causes pain: most commonly the pressure is on the

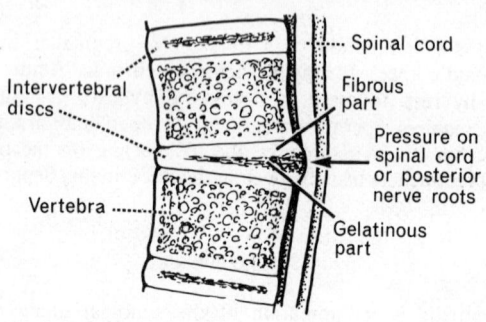

Fig. 48. Vertebral disc lesion. The prolapsed part of the disc protrudes posteriorly into the spinal canal.

fifth lumbar and first sacral nerve roots. It may result from strain due to bad lifting techniques; nurses should protect themselves by learning to lift patients and heavy equipment, keeping the spine straight and bending and straightening the hips and the knees.

The onset of pain may be sudden or gradual; it will be sudden if the prolapse is large, gradual if the bulge is small at first and later increases or becomes swollen. The patient may suddenly complain of agonizing pain in the back which spreads down the back of the thigh and leg to the foot. He cannot move on account of the pain, once acute sciatica develops. With the knee straight he cannot lift the leg on the affected side more than half-way to the horizontal position (to an angle of 45°) because of the stretching of the affected nerve roots. The pain increases with any attempt to stoop and with coughing or sneezing. There may be other sensory abnormalities, i.e. numbness or tingling. In the gradual onset, the patient suffers with chronic pain in the back, thigh or calf, according to the site of the prolapse, and cannot raise the leg fully when the knee is straight; he cannot bend or extend the spine well because of pain, though he can move the spine sideways without pain. Numbness or tingling may be present. There may be alterations in the reflexes, e.g. the knee jerk. The lumbar forward curve of the spine is generally lessened.

Treatment

The patient will be seen by a neurologist and then by a neurosurgeon, and as the symptom of backache can be due to other conditions it may be necessary for a female patient to be seen by a gynaecologist. X-rays are carried out as the patient may be suffering from arthritis of spine. If the examinations indicate that a prolapsed disc is in fact present the doctor will request that a myelogram be performed to pinpoint the actual site of protrusion. In some cases the neurosurgeon will suggest that a laminectomy be performed at once, but in others conservative treatment is used. An attempt may be made to treat the condition by supporting the affected part of the spine in a plaster jacket. This is applied in the out-patients department and the patient returns home with strict instructions about not lifting anything which is heavy. The symptoms gradually subside a few days after the application of the jacket, which is worn for two to three months. After this a steel-support corset may be worn for three to six months, especially if the patient returns to work which involves any strain on the back, particularly heavy lifting. If the patient still experiences frequent attacks of pain then hospital treatment will be suggested. This generally consists of skin traction with the foot of the bed elevated. This form of treatment can be very uncomfortable so the patient requires a great deal of encouragement. During this time muscular tone should be maintained by contracting the muscles of the back and abdominal wall and exercises of the limb muscles under a physiotherapist's supervision. Many nursing problems are present during this form of treatment and the nurse must face each one and handle it in an intelligent manner. A firm knowledge of anatomy and physiology will be of the greatest assistance.

If this treatment does not result in cure and the patient complains of repeated attacks of disabling pain, operative treatment is undertaken. The operation consists of removal of parts of the laminae to give access to the site, followed by removal of the prolapsed material. In the typical case the areas between the fifth lumbar vertebra and the sacrum and between the fourth and fifth lumbar vertebrae on the affected side are both examined, as it is not possible to say definitely from the symptoms at which site the prolapse has occurred and both may be affected. The skin is prepared over the back and buttocks, according to the surgeon's orders. Prior to surgery it may be necessary for the patient to discuss his future occupation with his surgeon and the disablement resettlement officer. This will allow him to be retrained for a career, or job, which will enable him to support himself and his family.

If the operation is straightforward the patient will be nursed in a semi-recumbent position and assisted out of bed on the first postoperative day, when weight-bearing is allowed according to the surgeon's instructions. The patient is usually discharged home on the tenth day. A suction drain may be inserted into the wound to prevent haematoma formation and this is removed on the second day. In a more complex situation ambulation is a little slower and the patient remains in hospital for a longer period of time. Intensive physiotherapy is given from the early postoperative days to strengthen the extensor muscles of the back, such as 'press-up' exercises in a prone position. Relief from pain may occur at once and no return of pain occur after operation: in other cases some backache may remain for several months, and patients engaged in work which involves heavy lifting may need to seek lighter work. Occupational therapy is valuable for those patients who have to spend long periods in bed in the flat position, and, where necessary, may not only be used to prevent boredom and distract the patient's attention from pain, but also to train the patient for more suitable work on his recovery, if this be necessary.

In very severe cases a spinal fusion may be carried out by an orthopaedic surgeon, in which case the patient will be nursed in a plaster bed. The plaster case may be raised on pieces of wood to allow giving of the bedpan without lifting the patient. The plaster may alternatively be slung from a metal framework erected on the bedstead, called a Nangle frame. If this is done, and the whole slung with suitable pulleys and weights, the patient's position can be changed, the head being raised for working during occupational therapy, for eating and to prevent chest complications. It can be lowered at night for sleeping, if this is more natural for the patient. Hospitalization is likely to be for a period of ten months if a spinal fusion has been necessary.

Injury to the Knee Joint

Injury to the *semilunar cartilage* or *meniscus* is an internal injury to the knee joint which may require surgical treatment, namely removal of the cartilage or *meniscectomy*. The condition generally results from sudden violence to the knee. It may follow slips with twisting of the joint, and may occur playing football or tennis. It causes sickening pain which may be followed by 'lock-up' of the joint, due to the displaced cartilage getting caught between the ligaments: or it may slip back into place to be displaced again when subjected to violence again. Operation is advised in cases which do not respond to treatment by pressure bandage, rest and active treatment to tone up the quadriceps muscle.

Preparation for operation

In addition to normal preparation, intensive quadriceps drill is ordered as the stability of the joint after operation depends on this muscle.

Postoperative treatment

The leg should be raised and protected with a large cradle. Effusion *into* the knee joint is prevented by a *pressure* bandage usually kept in position up to ten days after operation. A pressure bandage consists of three layers of gamgee and three layers of bandage which extends in a simple spiral from the thigh to the ankle, the aim being to prevent flexion at the knee. Generally a 15 cm crêpe bandage is used. Quadriceps drill or physiotherapy is started again, directly after operation. The patient is allowed up at varying periods after operation depending on the surgeon's orders and whether there is any effusion into the joint. It has been found that the amount of effusion is much less if the patient is kept in bed for a period of ten days postoperatively, when the sutures and pressure bandage are removed, but this causes many nursing problems with healthy patients who wish to be up and about. The patient must be re-educated in normal walking.

DEFORMITIES

Torticollis or wry neck is a deformity due to contraction of the sternomastoid muscle; it may be constant or spasmodic. The head is drawn down towards the shoulder and the face turned to the opposite side.

Manipulations to stretch the affected muscle are used in early cases. In severe cases the affected muscle is divided, with fixation in plaster of paris in a position of overcorrection. Exercises and manipulations will be required during after-treatment. Spasmodic cases are treated by dividing the nerves supplying the part. This condition can also be due to hysterical causes, in which case psychiatric treatment is necessary.

Cervical rib. This is a short extra rib which sometimes occurs on the seventh cervical vertebra. It is often bilateral and may give rise to no symptoms. It may, however, cause neuralgia and is then treated by excision.

Dupuytren's contracture is a contraction of the palmar fascia, occurring especially in men whose occupation involves pressure on the palm of the hand. It causes the ring and little fingers to be drawn down towards the palm of the hand, so that they cannot be extended. In late cases the affected fascia must be excised, called a palmar fasciectomy. A firm dressing is applied and the patient is instructed to keep the hand up. In this case the hand is immobilized for 48 hours following surgery, then finger exercises are commenced. Wax baths are given to the hand after the sutures have been removed.

Syndactylism is webbing of the fingers or toes. It is treated in the hand by plastic operations to provide a skin surface on the affected side of each finger to its base; otherwise the fingers will unite again.

Coxa vara is a decrease in the angle between the neck and shaft of the femur; it may be associated with rickets, disease of the joint, or injury to the neck of the bone. It results in shortening and outward rotation of the limb, with limitation of abduction.

Treatment consists of fixation in a position of abduction and internal rotation, rickets being treated also, if present. Osteotomy may be necessary, followed by fixation in good position and the use of a walking caliper for some time.

Genu varum (bow legs) and *genu valgum* (knock knees) are generally due to rickets and are treated by splinting or osteotomy. Sometimes young children, with no other abnormality, appear to have knock knees; usually the condition disappears and no treatment is needed.

SURGERY IN BONE AND JOINT DISEASES

Talipes equinovarus, or club foot, is a deformity in which the foot does not lie at the normal angle to the leg. There are various types: *talipes equinus*, when the heel is drawn up; *talipes calcaneus*, when the toes are drawn up; *talipes varus*, when the foot is inverted and the patient walks on the outer border; *talipes valgus*, when the foot is everted; and *pes cavus*, or hollow club foot, when the natural arch is exaggerated. These conditions may be combined.

The condition may be congenital or acquired; the acquired variety is generally a late result of anterior poliomyelitis, due to muscular contractions.

Treatment is by manipulation, with fixation by strapping, night shoes or splints, if required. In more severe cases the manipulations may be carried out under anaesthesia, using Thomas's wrench, and plaster of paris splints are then applied.

Sometimes operations such as lengthening the tendon of Achilles or division of tendons or ligaments may be necessary, and occasionally fixation of the joints, termed arthrodesis, and removal of portions of bone.

Hammer toe is a deformity produced by hyperextension of the first phalanx, acute flexion of the second, and extension or flexion of the third. It may be congenital, or acquired as a result of crowding of the toes from small or pointed shoes, or displacement to the big toe. Splinting or operation to excise the head of the first phalanx is necessary.

Hallux valgus is an outward displacement of the big toe from the middle line of the body, possibly due to wearing pointed shoes. (From the anatomical point of view, it may be described as an inward displacement towards the middle line of the foot.) This causes pressure on the joint between the metatarsal bone and the first phalanx, the structures becoming thickened. A bursitis may occur at the site and is known as a bunion.

Treatment consists in correcting the type of shoe worn, using strapping or a toe peg in the boot to keep the big toe in good position. Operation may be necessary in severe cases, especially where severe bunions are present.

24

Fractures: Dislocations: Sprains and Strains

FRACTURES

A fractured bone is a broken bone, whether the 'break' consists of an almost microscopic crack or whether the fragments of bone are widely separated. There are two main varieties of fracture:

1. *Simple or closed fracture* in which the bone is broken, but there is no external wound leading to the site of fracture and only slight damage to the surrounding soft parts.
2. *Compound or open fracture*, where there is a wound leading to the site of fracture, exposing it to infection.

Signs and Symptoms of Fracture

Local signs and symptoms

1. Signs of local injury, i.e. pain, swelling and bruising at the site, with possibly the formation of small blisters or blebs. These are important, as they may break and allow infection to enter. The bruising may appear superficially some distance from the site of fracture, the blood travelling by gravity to the lowest point, tracking down between the muscles.
2. Abnormal mobility in the part, except in an impacted fracture. Do not test for this, as a simple fracture may be made compound or complicated by so doing and pain and shock are increased.
3. Deformity produced partly by the violence causing the fracture, partly by the contraction of the surrounding muscles. It may be increased in injudicious handling and movement.
4. Loss of use in the part.

5. Crepitus or grating of the bone fragments on one another. Never test for this, as further damage to the soft parts may be produced and pain and therefore shock be caused.

6. Shortening, due to impaction or the muscle contraction, producing overriding of the fragments; this is especially marked in oblique fractures.

A history of hearing or feeling the bone snap may be procured. The broken bone may protrude through the flesh.

In all cases of fracture X-ray photographs of the limb in two different planes are required. They assist in diagnosis and in subsequent treatment.

General signs and symptoms

In all cases shock is liable to be present. In fractures of long bones, even if not compound, there may be severe haemorrhage into tissues. It is the shock and the haemorrhage which, in the main, produce the general signs and symptoms in fractures. Haemorrhage into the tissues around a fractured shaft of femur in the young contributes to the severe degree of shock which is often seen. Early blood transfusion has reduced the mortality in such cases. In the simple fracture, after the shock has passed off, beyond a slight rise of temperature for one or two days as a result of the trauma, there should be no general symptoms. In compound fractures sepsis is liable to occur, with the usual signs of septic absorption.

Healing of Bone

In the first place the bone ends will be embedded in blood clot. White blood corpuscles will be attracted to the site and phagocytes will digest the blood clot in the course of a few days, while the multiplication of the surrounding tissue cells will result in the formation of fibrous tissue in which mineral salts will be deposited to form a hard cement-like substance known as callus. This is due to the presence of bone-building cells or osteoblasts in the fibrous tissue. At first the callus is comparatively soft and forms a mass around and between the bone ends. Gradually the callus between the bone ends becomes harder and is converted into bone. This is known as permanent callus. Meanwhile the surrounding callus, called temporary callus, is absorbed and, the medullary canal is gradually established again if the fracture has been well set. Finally there may be little sign that the bone has been broken.

Complications of Fractures

The possible complications of a fracture must be considered, but with good nursing care they should not arise.

Local complications

1. Pressure sores, due to inefficiently padded splints.
2. Joint stiffness, which should be prevented by putting the part regularly through a full range of movement.
3. Malunion, i.e. union in a bad position, causing deformity and restricting function.
4. Shortening of the limb.
5. Gangrene, due to injury to the main artery supplying the part or to overtight splinting.
6. Postural deformities, especially drop foot caused by allowing the foot to remain in a bad position so that the muscles become useless.
7. Haemorrhage due to injury or sepsis.
8. Sepsis, in compound fractures, sometimes leading to osteomyelitis.
9. Paralysis, due to pressure injury to a nerve or muscle, resulting from over-tight splinting or severe haemorrhage within the muscle sheath interfering with the blood supply. This causes degeneration of the muscle fibres, which are replaced by fibrous tissue (myositis fibrosa). This is termed ischaemic paralysis and is most commonly seen in Volkmann's ischaemic contracture, which follows fracture of the forearm or near the elbow joint, particularly in children. It can be relieved by treatment to make the hand useful again, but progress is slow.
10. Non-union, especially in elderly patient.

General complications

1. Bedsores, due to immobilization in one position.
2. Hypostatic pneumonia, especially in old persons or those with a chronic heart lesion.
3. Renal calculi, which occur readily if the patient is immobilized too long in a supine position.
4. Embolism is rare, but fat embolism from the site of the fracture may cause a pulmonary obstruction, with fatal results.

5. Delirium tremens, from sudden cutting off of all alcohol when the patient is used to taking it regularly. This can be countered by giving alcohol in moderation to patients at risk.

6. Infection such as gas gangrene or tetanus.

Treatment of Fractures

The aim of the modern treatment of fractures is to get a useful limb or part with as full a range of movement in the joints and muscles as possible. If the bone ends are brought together and kept in place they will unite by the natural processes of repair.

Union is essential for restoring the use of the limb, but a perfect union is less important than full movement of muscles and joints. Until about forty years ago the limb or part was immobilized as completely as possible in an effort to obtain a perfect join, but this often resulted in stiff joints and muscles or tendons which were bound down by fibrous adhesions during the period of immobilization. Largely as a result of the teaching of a Viennese surgeon, Böhler, early movement came into common use with better final results for the patient.

Treatment may be considered under two headings:

1. Reduction and fixation.
2. Restoration of function.

Reduction and fixation

Reduction means getting the bone fragments into good apposition and alignment. It is usually carried out under anaesthetic, as this relaxes the muscles which are pulling the bone fragments out of position.

The surgeon first tries to manipulate the fragments into the correct position. This may be comparatively easy, especially where the muscles attached to the bone are not powerful. In such cases suitable splints or support are employed to keep the fragments in position until there is union. In other cases it is impossible to get a good result without either open operation or extension. Extension is particularly used for fracture of the femur, where the muscles attached to the broken bone are numerous and powerful, and for the compound fracture of tibia and fibula and radius and ulna, as it facilitates dressing of the wound and the tension lessens the risk of pocketing of pus in the limb.

Restoration of function

The patient's cooperation in restoration of function is essential if the maximum benefit is to be gained. A great deal of encouragement may be necessary to ensure that the prescribed exercises are carried out, because the motivation and morale of both the patient and his relatives may be very low, especially when progress is slow.

To ensure the fullest use of the part, the surgeon calls in the physiotherapists early in the treatment and, as pain subsides, these workers, together with the nursing staff, encourage the patient to exercise the part. Care must be taken not to displace the bone fragments, but within the limits of safety the more the patient moves the surrounding joints, and uses the muscles which move them, the less stiffness, fixation by adhesions and wasting of muscle there will be. Active movements are those made by the patient himself (and are considered the safer by many authorities since most patients will not carry them out if they are extremely painful); passive movements are those brought about by someone else, e.g. the physiotherapist, the patient lying quite relaxed.

Muscles not inserted into the broken bone, but crossing the site of fracture, can be used from the outset; for example, the fingers can be moved from the first day when there is a fracture of radius or ulna, e.g. a Colles's fracture, and the toes and ankle joint can be moved in cases of fracture of the femur and tibia, if the method of extension or splinting permits it. Muscles can be contracted slightly or 'tensed' without producing movement of actual parts while limbs are splinted or on extension where such movement is not possible. The broken bone must not be subjected to too great a strain and exercises have been devised which permit the physiotherapist to increase gradually the weight which the muscles are required to lift. Weight-bearing by the bones of the lower limb, when the patient begins to walk, throws a strain on the site of fracture and extension apparatus or plaster may be replaced by a walking caliper when the lower limb is first put to the ground. In the lower limb the importance of good setting to make the limb the correct length is important: a shorter leg will mean a permanent limp, even if there is no stiffness of joint or muscle. In the upper limb movement is more important than length. Some surgeons today employ open operation and plating of radius and ulna to hasten the time when hand and forearm can be freely used, as loss of use may mean that the individual can no longer carry out the work by which he or she earns a living. If deformity is likely to arise, the deformity is planned as far as possible to make a useful arm with the elbow bent at a suitable angle for the patient's work, e.g. slightly bent for the gardener and bent at a right angle for the writer, clerk or typist. The wrist is fixed in slight hyperextension with the fingers flexed to hold spoon and fork, pen and pencil, if possible. A collar and cuff sling is useful for fracture of the humerus and beyond this, frequently no other treatment is given. During convalescence various forms of occupational therapy and remedial therapy are used, not only to interest the patient and prevent boredom, but to re-educate the part in those movements which the injury has particularly affected. Where the patient cannot hope to return to his previous occupation, he is taught, where possible, occupations at which he can subsequently earn a living, as soon as it is practicable. This last part of rehabilitation is usually decided upon if not actually undertaken at a Department of Health Rehabilitation Centre which the patient usually attends on a daily basis for a period of weeks.

Splinting

Splinting may be external or internal.

EXTERNAL SPLINTS

These fall into two classes:

1. Those made to fit the patient—of plaster of paris, celluloid, plastic and poroplastic material. These give better support, but are unsuitable when there is, or is likely to be, great swelling, since they may become too loose or too tight.

2. Splints of wood and metal made in stock sizes and padded to fit the individual. These are useful in first aid and in the early stages when there is much swelling. They have been largely superseded by plaster of paris in modern surgery.

Plaster of paris is usually used for splints for patients who have fractures or to prevent deformity in patients suffering from illness which is producing unconsciousness or paralysis (e.g. the patient who has had a 'stroke'). Celluloid, plastic and poroplastic material are used for crippled children; they are lighter, but celluloid is more expensive, since it must be non-inflammable, and the splint takes longer to make. Plaster is strong when once dry, cheap, reasonably light and easy to apply. The plaster must be of good quality, fresh, and kept dry.

SURGICAL NURSING

To apply a plaster of paris splint. The limb is rendered socially clean, bony prominences are padded and either tubular stockinette or Orthoban is used beneath the plaster bandage. These are first placed vertically in a bucket of warm water and left till bubbles cease to rise. They are then lifted out with a hand over each end to keep in the plaster, gently squeezed and applied immediately to the limb. Frequently the plaster bandage is first made into a slab of eight to sixteen thicknesses, according to the strain to which it will be exposed. These slabs are applied direct to the skin where they are needed and moulded to the part. They are then secured, as necessary, by circular turns. In this way the splint is made thickest where need for support is greatest, and the remainder of the splint will be comparatively light. Ready prepared slabs are now available. Alternatively, the bandage may be applied to the limb firmly with circular turns, avoiding reverses and moulding it to the part. Pressure on bony prominences must be prevented.

When sufficiently strong, the plaster is polished by rubbing with the bare hand, and the edges trimmed with a plaster knife if necessary. If tubular stockinette has been applied to the limb first, it would have been left long enough so that 5–6 cm could be turned over the end of the plaster and incorporated in the last layer of bandage, which would not extend quite to the end of the plaster case (by about 1 cm). The part must be supported till the plaster is dry, or it may crack and be useless. Drying is best achieved in the open air.

The extremities should *always* be exposed so that they may be watched to ensure that the splint is not too tight.

If, for any reason it is desirable to remove the splint, it is split up both sides with plaster shears or an electric saw is used and then 'separators', the edges are bound with adhesive plaster and the splint secured by straps and buckles or firm bandages.

PATIENT CARE FOLLOWING THE APPLICATION OF A PLASTER OF PARIS SPLINT

The bed should be prepared to receive the patient with fracture boards and a firm pillow with a plastic cover.

If possible the limb should be exposed to the air outside the bedclothes (which are suitably protected with polythene sheeting) or, failing this, it should be covered with a cradle left completely open at the end. Artificial heat is undesirable as it tends to dry the surface of the plaster completely so that moisture cannot escape from the deeper layers of the plaster. It takes 48 hours to dry a thick plaster really thoroughly.

The nurse will prepare the patient's bed for his return from the plaster room, operating theatre or casualty department. Fracture boards are placed beneath the mattress and the bedding is made up into a pack so that the patient can be covered quickly and easily. All items of equipment that will be required for the care of the patient or his plaster are also assembled. If a leg plaster has been applied a protective pillow or pillows are placed beneath the wet plaster to support it and the doctor may request that the foot of the bed be raised in an effort to control any swelling. If the arm has been immobilized it may be necessary to elevate the fingers and hand to a vertical position. In some hospitals this is achieved by using a roller towel suspended from a drip stand.

One of the reasons why plaster has been applied is to make the patient comfortable, so that any undue complaint of discomfort must not be ignored and action must be taken. The nurse must also make certain routine, but very important, observations and her findings must be recorded. If she suspects that any problems have arisen, the relevant facts must be reported at once.

1. *Colour of the skin.* The skin should be a 'normal' colour and any change such as whiteness, congestion or blueness must be reported promptly. The skin will blanch when finger pressure is applied, but the colour will return to normal immediately upon removal if the circulation is adequate.

2. *Movement.* The surgeon will make sure that all digits are clearly visible and the nurse must ask the patient to move *all* of them. This is especially important when a patient has sustained a Colles's fracture, as such patients are reluctant to extend the fingers but will flex them quite happily.

3. *Sensation.* The sensation in all digits must be tested by asking the patient to look away and tell the nurse when she is touching the various digits. Any complaint of 'pins and needles' must also be reported, including the distribution of the sensation.

4. *Staining of the plaster* must also be observed and recorded. This will occur after open surgery or if the patient has a compound fracture. It is not advisable to write on the plaster as this can cause hair-line fractures which weaken the plaster splint.

5. *Cracks or rough edges on the plaster.* These will reduce the efficiency of the plaster and cause discomfort to the patient.

The patient's plaster must be handled very carefully with the flat of the hand until it is dry and the patient must be positioned so that all areas of the plaster have a chance to dry uniformly. If the patient's leg is enclosed in plaster care must be taken to avoid pressure on the toes when he is being nursed in a prone position.

6. *Odour.* Nurses must appreciate the significance of a 'sickly smell', which may suggest infection as this may be the first sign.

7. *Temperature* of the plaster is also very important as an area of local heat also indicates the possibility of infection.

INTERNAL SPLINTS

These splints involve open operation and are chiefly employed when good results cannot be obtained by other means, especially for fracture of the bones in the upper limb, where early movement is important for the restoration of function, and in, say, fractures of the neck of femur in the elderly, when early ambulation can be life-saving in preventing such complications as hypostatic pneumonia. The limb must be carefully cleansed as for any bone operation, though in many units this cleansing is delayed until the patient is anaesthetized to lessen the pain felt, both on grounds of humanity and to prevent increasing shock. The fragments are brought together and fixed by a metal plate screwed to the bone or by bone pegs or silver wire. These may be left in position, since they are chiefly employed in fractures where there is no sepsis and are introduced with the most strict aseptic precautions. Antibiotics may be used as a prophylactic measure. There is no direct handling of the wound, forceps being employed to handle all instruments, sutures, ligatures and swabs. These methods, however, produce some rarefaction of the bone at the site and by completely immobilizing the site of fracture prevent the natural friction of the bone surfaces on one another, which appears to stimulate the natural processes of repair. Delayed union or non-union may therefore result. Autogenous bone pegs are the most valuable of these measures, bone being generally taken from the subcutaneous portion of the tibia by Albee's saw, or from the ilium, and suitably shaped. Bone banks of sterile bone from another person may supply bone when autogenous bone pegs and grafts are not practicable.

Extension

Extensions provide a means of applying traction, i.e. a continuous pull on a fractured limb—commonly a leg. Traction may be fixed (usually to the end of a Thomas's splint) or sliding (when the cord through which the traction is exerted passes over a pulley wheel and has weights attached to it).

Traction may be:

1. *Skin traction*, usually fixed, when the pull is exerted first on the skin by means of Extension Elastoplast, zinc oxide strapping or Holland's strapping. Ventfoam is used if a patient is allergic to strapping, but this needs very careful attention.

2. *Skeletal traction*, often sliding, when the pull is exerted directly on bone by means of a Steinmann's pin, Kirschner wire or Denham's pin.

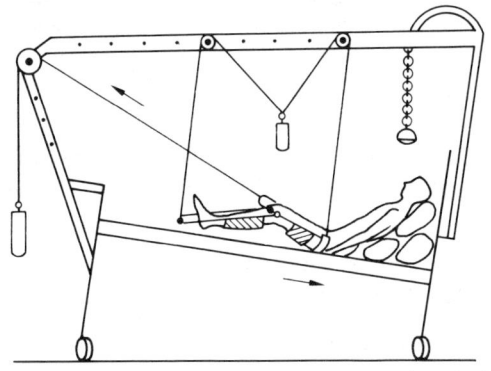

FIG. 49. The principles of counterextension using skeletal traction. The foot of the bed is raised so that the weight of the patient's body counteracts the pull of the extension apparatus on the fractured limb. This technique is used in particular for fractures of the femur.

3. *Pulp traction*, usually fixed, when, say, a suture is passed through the pulp of finger or toe and fastened to an extension piece incorporated in a plaster applied to hand or foot.

When an extension is applied to the leg, the latter is usually supported on a Thomas's splint or Braun's frame and particularly if sliding traction is to be used a frame of some sort is needed over the head of the bed, e.g. a Balkan beam.

SETTING FOR THE APPLICATION OF SKIN EXTENSION

Trolley containing:

Hot water, soap swabs, and towel on tray, if the leg is to be shaved—some authorities prefer this to be omitted.

Extension Elastoplast or Holland strapping (alternatively a complete skin traction kit may be used).

Spreader, cord (and weights if sliding traction is to be used).

344 SURGICAL NURSING

Pulleys and either a Balkan beam or other extention poles.
Thomas's splint, flannel bandages, safety-pins and foot support.
Calico or woven bandages.
Two wool pads covered in gauze.

Method of applying skin extension

The skin of the leg must be scrupulously clean and dry. Some surgeons like the skin to be shaved but others prefer not since they feel shaving sets up irritation, especially if Elastoplast is to be used and the new hairs growing out of the skin are more likely to penetrate and grow into and through it than if there were relatively long hairs already lying flat along the skin. Some surgeons also like the skin to be painted with tincture of benzoin to lessen the likelihood of irritation from the Elastoplast or strapping.

Bony prominences must be protected by the foam rubber which is included in the extension kits, by chiropodists' felt or by several turns of soft muslin bandage. If the extension kits are being used for simple traction they are cut to the correct length for the patient and are carefully applied to the skin, care being taken not to allow any folds to develop in the material. The Elastoplast is then cut to fit to the shape of the knee without causing any tension. Care must be taken to make sure that the spreader is exactly central otherwise unequal pulls will take place on the skin on either side of the leg. If the patient is having skin traction applied prior to the use of a Thomas's splint, it is advisable to apply two separate extensions so that they can be applied to the splint in such a way as to correct rotation. This cannot be done if a kit is used as the spreader interferes with the direction of pull.

The Elastoplast or Holland strapping is then applied smoothly and firmly to the leg so that the tibial tuberosities come exactly in the midline of the strapping. During this, a gentle pull should be exerted on the limb by a second person. Holland strapping, which is rather old fashioned but claimed to be much less of an irritant, needs to be warmed before application to make it slightly tacky. The free ends of the extension, distal to the foot, are attached round the spreader.

The whole leg is then bandaged, e.g. with a muslin bandage.

A previously prepared Thomas's splint, of the correct size, is then applied. (Its slings should be secured by large safety-pins, not clips, and they should be put in the slings as near to the metal sides of the splint as possible.)

If fixed traction is to be used (especially likely on old ladies with delicate skin), blind cord is fastened through the hole in the spreader and the Elastoplast or strapping and tied to the end of the Thomas's splint, or the ends of the Elastoplast or strapping, previously stitched to 1 cm lampwick, are tied directly to the end of the Thomas's splint.

A footpiece should be attached to the Thomas's splint in such a position that, with a sling attached to it, it will support the foot at right angles to the leg.

A thick pad of wool (three thicknesses), approximately 12 by 24 cm is placed behind the tibial tuberosities (to prevent hyperextension of the knee) and a similar pad is placed behind the foot.

Domette bandages 15 cm wide are then applied to enclose leg and splint, from toes (tips of which should be left just visible) to groin, taking care to leave the patella exposed.

As a means of applying some counter traction the foot of the bed can be elevated on about 20 cm blocks and, when the bed is made up, the weight of the top bedclothes is supported by a bed cradle.

To prevent footdrop the patient is encouraged to exercise his ankle, performing dorsi- and plantar flexion exercises.

Whereas an experienced nurse may have to apply skin extension, it is a doctor's responsibility to introduce a Steinmann's pin, the nurse preparing the equipment and helping him during the procedure.

When a patient's leg is fixed in a Thomas's splint great care must be taken to prevent soreness developing beneath the ring. This is particularly important if the patient is unconscious, elderly or incontinent. A cooperative patient must be taught to change the area of skin that is exposed to pressure from the ring and great care must be taken to prevent the leather of the splint becoming hard or cracked. The bandage must be checked daily and the skin extensions must be checked by an experienced nurse at frequent intervals to make sure that they are still attached firmly to the skin and are not causing soreness. Once again it is essential that the nurse should not ignore any complaint of discomfort by the patient and that the patient's limb and splint are sensibly observed at frequent intervals.

General Nursing Care of Patients with Fractures

The patient should have a liberal mixed diet with plenty of protein, also milk, eggs and green vegetables to supply calcium and animal fat to provide vitamin D. Vitamin C is also important, and it may have to be given medicinally, e.g. ascorbic acid tablets, 50 mg thrice daily. He should drink freely to help prevent the formation of kidney and bladder stones which is a possibility with prolonged immobilization.

The pressure areas need care, especially since movement is likely to be limited. Where the patient's position *can* be changed, this should be done—*at least* four-hourly and two-hourly in the aged.

The patient should be encouraged to exercise freely those parts of the body not immobilized, particularly perhaps the uninjured leg, and to this end he should be encouraged to do as much for himself as possible, e.g. in relation to his toilet needs. However care must be taken, especially with elderly patients, that this encouragement of self-help is not mistaken for neglect. Occupational therapy can be of great value.

Elderly patients especially, and younger ones who suffer from chronic bronchitis, should be encouraged to do deep breathing exercises. In relation to exercises, physiotherapists do very valuable work.

Drugs which these patients are likely to need include antibiotics or sulphonamides, especially if the fracture is compound or there is risk of hypostatic pneumonia, analgesics, e.g. morphine and then aspirin compounds, especially in the first forty-eight hours, and sedatives for the first few nights since immobilization and strange postures will make sleep elusive.

Fractures of the Skull

A fracture of the skull may be:

1. Fissured, involving the vault or base of the skull.
2. Depressed.

It may result from direct or indirect violence.

Fractures of the skull unite readily and, as fractures, cause little trouble, but are always serious because of the involvement of the brain. If a head injury has been sufficiently severe as to produce a fracture, concussion is almost certain to be present. Compound fractures also involve the risk of septic meningitis and septic inflammation of the brain itself, which may prove fatal.

Concussion

What consitutes concussion is not really understood. It appears to be a state following a severe jarring of the brain associated with unconsciousness lasting seconds, hours or days. It seems there is at least a momentary cessation of all brain activity. In the great majority of instances the injury is trivial and may pass unrecognized, but in a few cases the outcome can be very serious or fatal; hence the importance of very careful observation of those patients who have apparently sustained only a trivial injury.

The main dangers concern the development of oedema or the formation of blood clot consequent on haemorrhage. Serious harm can result from even small degrees of these because of the tension created in the enclosed cavity of the skull and resultant pressure on the brain.

Observations of patients who have sustained head injuries

The importance of these cannot be over emphasized as they may indicate a rising intracranial pressure due to clot formation. The earlier this can be recognized so that operative measures can be taken to evacuate the clot, the better the patient's chance of recovery. A slowing pulse rate and rising blood pressure constitute danger signs.

1. The pulse should be taken and recorded, preferably in the form of a graph, quarter-hourly at first, and then according to the surgeon's instructions, half-hourly, then hourly and later two-hourly, and then four-hourly.

2. The respirations should be observed at the same time as the pulse—depth, ease of breathing and regularity being noted as well as the rate.

3. The temperature should be taken, preferably rectally, usually hourly to begin with.

4. The blood pressure, both systolic and diastolic, is usually taken at the same time as the pulse.

5. The patient's colour, especially in relation to pallor of skin and mucous membranes, or cyanosis of the circumoral area, ear lobes or nail areas, should be noted.

6. His conscious level should be described, again usually at the times the pulse is taken. It is not enough to state, e.g. 'conscious',

348 SURGICAL NURSING

'semiconscious' or 'unconscious'. The nurse should write brief comments such as:

a. *Conscious:*
   i. Fully alert and orientated.
   ii. Alert but confused.
   iii. Drowsy but rousable.
b. *Unconscious:*
   i. Localizes to pain (physically resists it).
   ii. Flexes in response to pain.
   iii. Extends in response to pain.
   iv. Does not respond at all.

Pain can be caused by means of supraorbital pressure or by pressing on the sternum with the knuckles.

7. The state of the pupils should be noted, whether they are small or large and equal and whether they react to light. If there is abnormality in relation to size or equality it is important to check their normal condition with relatives, as occasionally a patient may normally have unusual pupils.

The above observations are usually recorded on a neurological chart, the exact design of which varies from hospital to hospital. In addition the nurse should note any deformities of limbs or reluctance on the patient's part either to move a part or to lie in a particular position; she should note any willingness or unwillingness to drink and the state of the appetite if conscious; she should note the patient's ability to pass urine, especially in relation to retention, urgency, frequency or incontinence: also bowel movements should be noted.

Nursing care

The bed should be in a corner position or a side ward, where lighting can be subdued, since a bright light disturbs the patient; cot sides should be available; there should be waterproof protection for the mattress in case of incontinence.

The patient is usually nursed flat, or at most with one pillow. Care is taken to keep the patient cool, even though actual hypothermia is not employed. He may well be covered with a sheet and quilt only and wear no pyjamas. His position should be *changed* frequently to prevent the development of both pressure sores and hypostatic pneumonia.

The patient should be encouraged to keep quiet; visitors should be close friends or members of the patient's immediate family only, and the *number* of people rather than *duration* of visiting hours should be restricted.

The bowels are opened by enemas if necessary.

Fluid diet is given, increasing to light diet as the patient improves. If the patient is unconscious, nutrition must be maintained by intragastric tube feeding.

Morphine is not allowed, as it may mask symptoms; codeine phosphate is sometimes ordered if it is thought that restlessness may be due to headache. (N.B. Restlessness in a semiconscious patient is often due to a full bladder and is relieved by putting the patient on a bedpan or putting a urinal in position.)

To relieve either retention of urine or incontinence it may be necessary for the patient to be nursed with a self-retaining, e.g. Foley, catheter in position.

In very severe head injuries hypothermia may be employed, the patient's temperature being drastically reduced to lower the oxygen needs of the body, including the brain, and to overcome the hyperpyrexia from which these patients may suffer.

Treatment

Treatment can frequently only be conservative, providing opportunity for natural 'cure' to come about, or symptomatic, e.g. tracheostomy, where unconsciousness is prolonged or if respirations appear obstructed; the latter tends to cause a rise in intracranial pressure.

Burr holes may be necessary and a flap turned back to evacuate blood clot if intracranial pressure rises; if the pressure is thought to be due to oedema of brain attempts are sometimes made to draw fluid away from the brain by osmosis, and to that end intravenous dexamethasone, mannitol, frusemide, urea or triple plasma may be used.

A course of antibiotic or chemotherapeutic drugs may be ordered if infection is feared (or is established). In this case the nurse must ensure that the patient received adequate fluid; neglect of this could result in crystallization of the drug in the kidneys. If bladder drainage by catheter has been necessary or if there seems a risk of chest involvement, the appropriate antibiotic will be prescribed after culture and sensitivity tests have been carried out on the urine and sputum.

350 SURGICAL NURSING

A physiotherapist can do a great deal to prevent serious chest infection or stiffness or deformity at joints when unconsciousness is prolonged and, together with an occupational therapist, can speed rehabilitation when the convalescent stage is reached.

Fatal results are due to pressure on the vital centres of the brain. Recovery may occasionally be followed by fits due to pressure on the motor centres. The fits are epileptiform and the condition is known as Jacksonian or traumatic epilepsy. Personality changes may also occur after a head injury.

Fractures of the base of the skull are more serious than fractures of the vault. They may be associated with haemorrhage into the orbit and under the conjunctiva, causing 'black eyes', and bleeding from the nose or ear, according to whether the fracture is in the anterior or middle fossa. This relieves pressure on the brain, but may result in the entrance of infection. When there is bleeding from the ear, the *auricle only* should be cleansed if allowed, painted with antiseptic, and a sterile dressing applied to absorb blood and cerebrospinal fluid. Unless specific instructions are given to the contrary it is better to do nothing to the auditory meatus. The ear must on no account be syringed in case infection is introduced leading to septic meningitis. There may be injury to the cranial nerves, especially to the facial nerve, resulting in facial paralysis.

All these cases of head injury with serious damage to the brain may need to remain in bed for some time and must have careful nursing and a gradual convalescence, particularly avoiding any mental strain.

Fractures of the Lower Jaw

Fracture of the lower jaw is generally compound into the mouth. Symptoms include:

1. Pain on movement of the jaw.
2. Difficulty in speaking and closing the jaw.
3. Dribbling of blood-stained saliva.
4. Irregularity in line of the teeth.
5. Crepitus on movement of the jaw.

Treatment

If the patient has an adequate complement of teeth the oral surgeon will wire his jaws together by attaching horizontal eyelet wires to his top and bottom teeth, then 'lashing' them together with vertical wires. Otherwise splints are made (resembling artificial dentures without teeth) and these are placed in position and are fixed together. Generally immobilization continues for about six weeks.

Nursing care

There are three very important aspects of nursing care to be considered.

Care of the airway. Suction equipment and wire cutters must always be available by the patient in case he should vomit. If this occurs it may be necessary to cut the vertical wires so that the airway may be easily and rapidly cleared, but suction alone is usually adequate. The surgeon will attach new vertical wires as soon as practicable.

Oral toilet. Initially a sterile syringe and tube (a Quill tube is very useful) are used to irrigate the mouth with a suitable lotion, then a small, soft 'baby' toothbrush and toothpaste is introduced. The patient is taught to keep his mouth clean so that he may continue doing this after discharge home.

Nutrition. A liquid diet containing adequate food values and calories is administered and the patient and his relatives will be told by the dietician how an adequate level of nutrition can be maintained when he has been discharged. This diet basically consists of fortified milk, egg, soup, baby foods and normal food that has been passed through a liquidizer. Attempts at talking are not allowed and a pad and pencil must be provided for the patient to make his wants known.

Fractures of the Clavicle

A fracture of the clavicle is extremely common. It is generally due to indirect violence resulting from falls on the shoulder or hand, but may be produced by direct violence from a kick or punch. It generally occurs at the junction of the outer and middle thirds. The shoulder is drawn downwards and forwards by muscle contraction and the weight of the arm. The patient supports his arm and bends his head towards the affected side to lessen the pain by relieving the drag on the fragments.

352 SURGICAL NURSING

The aim of treatment is to restore the alignment of the bone while healing is taking place. This is done by bracing both shoulders back and holding them in this position by means of a figure-of-eight bandage which crosses over in the midline of the patient's back. This bandage must be tightened frequently as it tends to loosen gradually, even though a close-weave bandage is used. If the patient is confined to bed for some other reason the surgeon may decide that this bandage is not necessary if he is being nursed flat on his back. Healing usually takes place in about three weeks.

Fractures of the Ribs

A fracture of the ribs may be due to direct or indirect violence. It may be complicated by injury to the lung, pericardium or heart, and, in the case of the lower ribs, liver, kidneys or spleen. These complications are liable to occur in cases due to direct violence, as in gunshot wounds and car accidents, when the fracture may also be compound.

Simple fracture gives rise to pain, which is increased by deep breathing and coughing. It is due to indirect violence which compresses the chest.

The patient is treated for shock. As soon as shock has subsided, the patient is allowed to get up to lessen the risk of chest complications. Some surgeons inject hydrocortisone locally. The ribs unite very satisfactorily in spite of the fact that there is constant movement. Antibiotic cover is used and the physiotherapist will teach and encourage the patient to perform breathing exercises to reduce the risk of chest complications developing. If excess mucus is present in the patient's respiratory passages then a vibrator will be applied to the chest wall to loosen the mucus so that it can be expectorated more easily.

Complicated and compound fractures are not strapped, as there is risk of increasing the injury by driving in the fragments. If the lung is injured, the patient coughs up blood and dyspnoea and cyanosis may be severe, as the pleural cavity may fill with blood or air. The patient is nursed sitting up; a sputum cup is provided and sputum saved for the doctor's inspection. Oxygen may be ordered.

If the injury permits air to enter the pleural cavity on inspiration, but is valve-like and prevents it from escaping, the pleural cavity on that side will become gradually filled with air under tension: this will ultimately displace the heart and embarrass the breathing, with fatal results. As first aid an airtight petroleum jelly dressing should be

FRACTURES

applied with Elastoplast as quickly as possible. Pneumothorax must be relieved by a hollow needle being introduced into the pleural cavity and tubing attached to an underwater seal in order to allow air to escape and prevent complete disorganization of the action of the heart and lungs.

Complications

Pneumothorax. This must be relieved by inserting a needle into the pleural cavity and allowing the air to escape via tubing and an underwater seal. This may be necessary to prevent complete disorganization of the action of the heart and lungs.

Haemothorax is present when the injury has allowed blood to enter the pleural cavity. This is also removed by means of an underwater seal.

Haemopneumothorax. A combination of both of the two above complications.

Surgical emphysema. Due to the fracture, air may enter the tissues and is recognized by swelling of the area accompanied by a 'cracking' sensation when gentle pressure is exerted on the involved tissue.

Flail chest. This is the most serious complication occurring when the integrity of the majority of ribs on one side of the chest wall is lost. Paradoxical breathing occurs and this is not compatible with life unless it can be stopped. The treatment is by means of positive pressure ventilation until normal respiratory movements are possible and this may be for about six weeks.

Fractures of the Spine

A fracture of the spine may be due to a sudden excessive movement or blow to the spinal column, as when a person falls from a height and the impact is transmitted through the body to the vertebrae. Lesions also occur when a 'whip-lash' injury to the cervical vertebrae occurs in certain types of car accidents and when a person sustains a direct heavy blow on the vertebrae.

The damage may be minor when the only treatment that is required is for the patient to be nursed flat in bed without a pillow, but it may be serious, in which case complex total care is necessary.

The fracture may be complicated and cord damage may be present. This damage ranges from compression to complete destruction of the spinal cord by crushing or severing. The extent and site of the injury determines the type of total care which will be necessary. Damage to the cord may have the following results.

1. *Paralysis* of all muscles supplied from the cord below the site. This will be spastic, except for muscles supplied at the site of fracture, and involves the sphincters.
2. *Anaesthesia* of all tissues below the site of fracture.
3. A *trophic condition* of those tissues which have lost their nerve supply because their nerves are derived from the part of the cord which is injured. This results in trophic bedsores, attacking not only the usual pressure areas, but even the skin over the soft parts, such as the calves. Over the pressure areas the tissues may rapidly slough to the bone, and the bone itself may be involved, unless thorough and frequent preventive treatment is carried out with suitable support.

If the cord is crushed, these symptoms will be permanent; if they are merely due to pressure, stainless steel spinal plates may be used to immobilize the region: they are attached to both sides of the spinous processes.

Treatment

If the fracture has resulted in neurological involvement, surgery may be necessary to relieve the pressure, by means of the spinal plating previously mentioned, but only in the lower thoracic/lumbar regions. If the lesion affects the cervical vertebrae skull traction by means of Blackburn or Crutchfield's skull calipers may be used, the patient being nursed on a hospital type bed which has a firm mattress supported by fracture boards. Very careful, supervised 'turning' has to be carried out by skilled members of the health care team as the spine *must* be kept in correct alignment; sometimes a neurosurgeon will wire the cervical vertebrae to give stability. In this case traction may not be needed.

When a patient has sustained neurological involvement he must be turned two-hourly day and night. Neglect of this will result in the development of trophic ulcers. Turning also helps to prevent the development of chest and renal complications resulting from the stagnation of fluid in the chest and kidneys. On occasions a Stryker frame is used to make the turning easier but it can cause the patient anxiety.

Complications

1. *Hypostatic pneumonia.*
2. *Trophic bedsores.*
3. *Cystitis*, followed by ascending infection, resulting in pyelitis and pyelonephritis resulting in uraemia.
4. *Permanent paralysis* below the site of fracture.

These are the common causes of death in these cases, but the outlook has been greatly improved by sulphonamides and antibiotics. Patients with permanent paraplegia are treated by the physiotherapist and trained to sit up and get about with walking calipers or in wheel chairs, which may be mechanically propelled; they are trained by occupational therapists to make their lives as full as possible and to help support themselves. In selected cases where the patient is extensively paralysed POSSUM (patient-operated selector mechanism) (from the Latin *possum*, 'I can' or 'I am able') equipment will be used to give him a certain degree of independence. Centres are available where specialized rehabilitation can be undertaken.

Fractures of the Pelvis

These fractures are of two types:

1. *Minor.* In this case the fracture does not interfere with the integrity of the pelvic ring.
2. *Major.* The fracture does interfere with the integrity of the pelvic ring and various complications may result:
  a. Rupture of the bladder.
  b. Rupture of the urethra.
  c. Concealed haemorrhage caused by bleeding from the fracture site.

A fracture of the pelvis is due to crushing by direct violence or to indirect violence in 'run-over' accidents, when it is often broken in the front on one side and at the back on the other. It may be complicated by injury to the urethra, bladder, rectum, vagina or sacral nerves.

If the urethra is injured a catheter is passed and tied in till healing occurs, when dilators must be passed to prevent stricture from scar contraction. If the bladder is involved suprapubic cystotomy will probably be necessary and for rectal injuries colotomy is advocated to prevent infection of the sacral nerves, as this is liable to result in severe and lasting neuralgia.

Treatment and nursing

If possible the patient should not pass urine before the surgeon arrives, in case the urethra is injured. This prevents extravasation of urine, which is liable to set up pelvic cellulitis, with serious results. If, however, the patient does pass urine, the whole specimen should be saved and if by any chance he passes urine several times the specimens should be kept separate from each other.

The type of fracture or dislocation determines the form of treatment that will be instituted. If it is only a minor fracture, such as when the superior or inferior pubic ramus has been injured, then the doctor will order bed rest either on an orthopaedic bed, which has metal slats instead of springs, or on an ordinary bed, which has fracture boards beneath the mattress. The patient is soon allowed to start sitting up in bed, then in a chair. This is the type of fracture that is seen in the majority of cases.

However, if a major fracture is present, open reduction with internal fixation of the fractures may be necessary. If separation of the symphysis pubis has occurred, a pelvic sling with crossed cords and pulleys may be ordered to help to hold the anterior pelvis together. In other cases of major pelvic fractures, skeletal traction may be used to reduce the displacement.

Lifting and moving patients with pelvic fractures can be very strenuous and the method used depends upon the site of fracture and the degree of pain the patient is experiencing. Generally the patient can help if a monkey pole has been attached to the head of the bed. As a general rule the patients should be lifted rather than rolled and lifting must be done with the help of an adequate number of people and as gently as is possible.

Pressure areas must be observed and given the appropriate treatment and this can be a very long and difficult task if the patient also has multiple injuries necessitating immobilization and traction.

Exercises must be encouraged to prevent muscle wasting occurring and to reduce the risk of chest complications developing. For this reason the physiotherapist will be involved in this patient's care from the time of admission.

Observations are very important in all cases but especially if injury to other structures is suspected.

Fractures of the Upper Extremity

The humerus

The upper extremity is more liable to dislocation than fracture, but fracture may occur at the anatomical or surgical neck. Fracture at the anatomical neck is due to indirect violence; it occurs in older patients and is often impacted. It should be left alone; if it is disimpacted the upper fragment is liable to die.

Fracture of the surgical neck is common in adults and young adults from direct violence. The upper fragment is abducted and the lower fragment must be brought into line with it. The arm is sometimes put up on an aeroplane splint, with the arm at right angles to the body and the forearm raised at right angles to the arm, to prevent subsequent disability, which might prevent the patient getting the hand to the back of the head and neck. A similar position may be obtained with a plaster cast with a strut from the chest wall to the arm to support the weight. Extension with a Thomas's or Jones's splint may be required. In children, separation of the epiphysis may occur. Fractures of the shaft are also abducted to a right angle, as the deltoid muscle pulls the upper fragment out, except for those at the lower end round the elbow joint. These are put up in full flexion and pronation by figure-of-eight turns round arm and forearm with flannel bandage strengthened by strapping. A special sling is applied. After a few days the elbow is gradually extended a little more each day, using a 'collar and cuff' sling. Care must be taken to prevent interference with the blood and nerve supply.

The radius and ulna

Fractures of the upper extremities of these bones are treated in the same way by full flexion and pronation to ensure a good range of movement afterwards, except for fracture of the olecranon process. This is put up in extension and, as with the patella, open operation is generally required to prevent fibrous union, as periosteum gets between the fragments. Screw, nail, wire or kangaroo tendon may be used to keep the fragments together.

Fractures of the shaft are generally put up in supination, in which position the bones lie side by side in the forearm. Fractures may be set and a plaster splint applied; some surgeons advocate plating to make early movement safe without displacement. The object is to

358 SURGICAL NURSING

prevent adhesions between tendons or muscles and bone so that the hand remains useful.

Colles's fracture at the lower extremity is very common in elderly people. It is due to falling on the outstretched hand. The radius breaks about 2 cm above the wrist and the lower fragment is carried upwards and backwards, forming a characteristic lump at the back of the wrist. The styloid of the ulna is generally torn off. The lower fragment is also rotated and abducted backwards (dinner-fork deformity) and the fracture impacted, so that the radial and ulna styloid processes are on the same level.

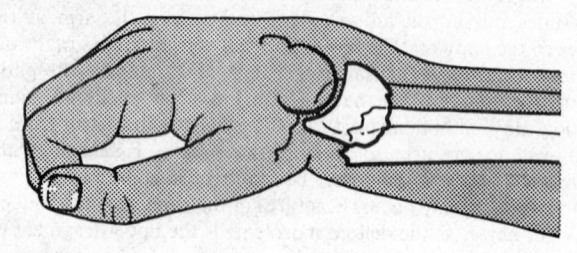

FIG. 50. Colles's fracture, showing the characteristic 'dinner-fork' deformity resulting from displacement of the radius.

TREATMENT AND NURSING CARE

Slight swelling will be present and this will increase following manipulation, so if the patient has a ring on a finger the ring must be removed and put in a safe place. The backward displacement and tilt is then corrected by manipulation under an anaesthetic; the wrist is supported with a plaster of paris back slab held in place with an open wove bandage. After 24 hours, if oedema is not marked, the plaster of paris bandage is completed. This method is used so that the bandage can be easily cut if swelling becomes severe after manipulation.

Supervised finger and shoulder exercises are commenced, particular note being taken of the elderly patient who may be very reluctant to extend the fingers, but this must be done otherwise disabling stiffness may develop.

A check X-ray is performed weekly for three weeks as the fracture sometimes displaces even though it has been immobilized. Union is usually satisfactory in four to six weeks.

Fractures of the Lower Extremity

The femur

Fractures of the neck. At the upper extremity of the femur, fractures of the neck are common. There are two varieties:

1. *Intracapsular fracture* occurs chiefly in old people as a result of indirect violence from slight accidents, such as tripping over the carpet or a step. It occurs because the bone has become brittle from trophic changes due to age. The fracture is frequently impacted. The risk lies in the fact that, because of the state of the bone, there may be non-union; also if the fracture is just distal to the femoral head there may be necrosis of the head since the major part of its blood supply, coming via the neck of the femur, will have been cut off. Intracapsular fracture with abduction occurs in younger patients from direct violence and is comparatively rare.

2. *Extracapsular fracture* occurs in adults and young people, and is due to direct violence from a heavy fall on the greater trochanter. Impaction is common.

In both cases there is shortening and eversion of the limb.

Treatment depends upon the age of the patient. In the elderly patient, confinement to bed for any length of time is liable to prove fatal from hypostatic pneumonia; in the early part of this century that was the usual outcome.

Nowadays treatment of these patients is almost invariably operative, even for patients in their eighties, the dangers of operation being less than those of prolonged immobilization.

It has become relatively common during the last few years to excise the femoral head and replace it with some form of stainless steel or vitallium prosthesis, e.g. the Austin Moore prosthesis. This consists of a femoral head which is used to replace the 'natural' head of the femur. These give excellent results even in very aged patients.

Postoperatively, providing the patient's vital signs are satisfactory, he will be assisted out of bed into a chair on the first day and weight-bearing will commence under the supervision of a physiotherapist on the third day.

Usually a suction drain is in position to prevent haematoma formation. It is removed on the second day, sutures being taken out when the wound is healed, as a rule on the tenth day.

The general nursing care is aimed at the prevention of complications such as chest lesions and pressure sores.

360 SURGICAL NURSING

Fractures of the shaft may be due to direct or indirect violence and are treated by extension in a position of abduction with the hip and knee flexed, as required, to bring the fragments into line. In fractures of the upper third, the upper fragment is drawn up by the iliopsoas and the hip must be flexed, while in the lower third the lower fragment is drawn backwards by the gastrocnemius and the

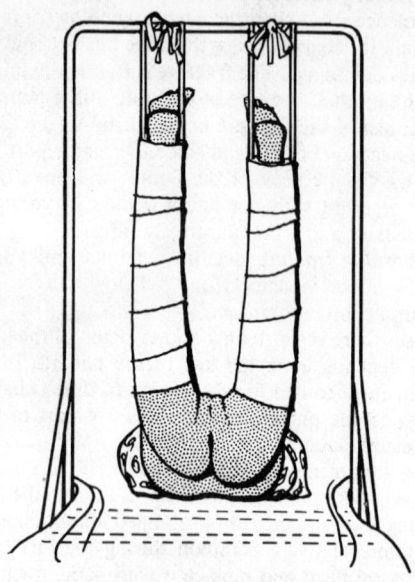

FIG. 51. A gallows extension for applying traction to the legs of infants and young children. Note that the buttocks are raised from the bed so that the weight of the body provides counterextension.

knee must be flexed. Extension may be applied by strapping or by skeletal traction, the latter allowing greater weight to be applied where there is much displacement. On the whole, sliding skeletal traction is used, particularly for relatively young men of good physique who have very powerful muscles exerting a strong pull on the bone fragments. A weight of up to 9 kg may be needed to overcome this and prevent deformity and shortening.

For infants Bryant's method of extension is employed to facilitate changing the napkins and keeping the part clean. A beam is put up over the bed and the limb extended by weight, strapping and pulleys in a vertical position at right angles to the body. Both limbs are put up and sufficient weight attached to keep the infant's buttocks just clear of the bed, so that their weight provides the counterextension. In most instances a folded napkin can be placed under the child's buttocks. It rarely needs to be applied in the conventional way; bulky material between the legs would have an undesirable effect at the fracture site.

The patella

There are two main types of fractures of the patella and the type determines the treatment:

1. *Transverse fracture*, caused by violent contraction of the quadriceps muscle while the knee is flexed.
2. *Comminuted fracture*, caused by a direct blow to the patella such as when the knee strikes the dashboard in a car accident.

The patient's knee is swollen, bruised and painful, and in a transverse fracture a space may be felt between the fragments. The extensor mechanism of the knee will be disrupted.

A transverse fracture is treated by open surgery and fixation of the fragments, then immobilization of the leg in a plaster of paris cylinder or a back splint. If the patient is elderly, a patellectomy will be performed. If a comminuted fracture is present, then because of the risk of osteoarthritis developing the patella is also removed. The knee is then firmly bound in wool with a crêpe bandage and a plaster of paris cylinder or a back splint is applied.

In both types of fracture, if displacement is not present, aspiration of the haemarthrosis will be performed then the joint is immobilized.

The tibia and fibula

Fractures of the tibia and fibula may be due to direct or indirect violence. Fractures of the tibia are prone to be compound, as the bone is so close to the skin. Fractures of the fibula alone cause little displacement. *Pott's fracture* (*external rotation*) is a fracture of the fibula about 7 cm above the ankle, with tearing off of the internal malleolus of the tibia or tearing of the internal ligaments at the ankle-joint. There is also outward and backward displacement of the talus. It is due to violent outward turning of the ankle joint. It is generally put up in plaster with the foot at right angles to the leg.

SURGICAL NURSING

The limb may be used, provided the splinting prevents deformity, and this hastens repair. In this case the plaster must be converted into a 'walking plaster' by the incorporation of, say, a 'rocker' or Böhler iron. It is liable to be followed by osteoarthritis of the foot joints.

DISLOCATIONS, SPRAINS AND STRAINS

Dislocations

A dislocation is a displacement of the articular surfaces at a joint. It is generally due to violence, but may be congenital. Congenital dislocation is liable to affect one or both hips and is due to the acetabulum not being normally developed. It becomes obvious when the child begins to walk, causing limping or a peculiar waddling gait if both hips are affected. The affected limbs are abnormally short and movement very free. It is treated by manipulation followed by putting the limbs in plaster in a position of abduction and fresh plasters are applied at intervals of two to three months until the limb can be brought into correct position. This may result in satisfactory development of the acetabulum; if it fails, plastic operation may be undertaken, followed by rest in plaster.

Dislocation due to violence most commonly affects the shoulder, the jaw and the joint at the base of the thumb, but if the violence is sufficient any joint may be dislocated. Nowadays this applies even to the hip since with the greater speed of road and air transport the force of impact in any accident is much greater.

Signs and symptoms

1. *Pain*, *swelling* and *bruising* at the site.
2. *Deformity*, though this may quite quickly be masked by swelling.
3. *Abnormal position* of the limb.
4. *Loss of movement* at the joint.

Treatment

Reduction is carried out as early as possible; an anaesthetic will be necessary to relax the muscles, as a general rule, unless reduction is carried out at once or the muscles are atonic. The bone is manipulated into correct position, the manipulations varying according to the joint; immobilization is necessary till the capsule is healed. The bone may be fixed by means of strapping, firm bandages, splints or even extension if dislocation tends to recur. Local applications of cold lessen swelling and relieve pain and are useful first-aid measures. Movement may be employed as soon as it can be done without risk of displacement, usually after seven to ten days, to lessen the risk of the formation of adhesions, which will permanently limit the range of movement.

Sprains

A sprain is the tearing or over-stretching of the ligaments of a joint. The ankle is most frequently affected, as a result of a violent outward or inward twist.

Signs and symptoms

1. *Acute pain*, described as 'sickening' in severe cases.
2. *Swelling* at the site.
3. *Bruising*—this may not appear at once.
4. *Deformity*.

Treatment

1. *Rest* to the part in severe cases.
2. *Support* by firm bandages or plaster of paris in severe sprains.
3. *Application of cold* to the site, e.g. evaporating lotion with exposure to the air.
4. *Movement*, passive and active, and possibly massage, which will hasten recovery and promote more rapid absorption of blood clot and lymph. In the case of severe sprains, movement, especially weight bearing, is not allowed until X-ray proof has been obtained that there is no fracture.
5. When the part is first used, *strapping* may be applied for a sprained lateral ligament of the ankle. The strapping should start on the lateral side of the dorsum of the foot and pass inwards and then under the sole and up the outer side of the leg, holding the foot in slight eversion. Two more layers are then applied and a circular turn to hold their upper ends in position. This will prevent the movement of inversion but will not impede any other movement nor

364   SURGICAL NURSING

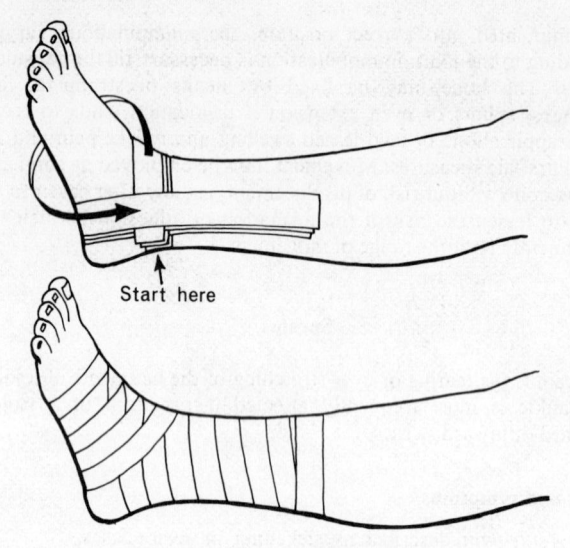

FIG. 52. The method of strapping a sprained ankle.

the circulation in the foot. Use narrow strapping 2–3 cm wide and apply in figure-of-eight pattern, starting low over foot and ankle with the first turn and working upwards. Bandage towards the affected side to evert the foot if the ankle is sprained on the lateral side and to invert it if the sprain is on the median side.

Strains

Strains are usually considered to be comparable to sprains but of less degree, i.e. involving stretching of ligaments and tendons rather than actual tearing; swelling and bruising are usually much less marked.

25

Plastic Surgery

In the repair of extensive wounds and burns, and for the treatment of deformities, the surgeon can often do much to assist healing and to restore the normal shape and structure of the damaged parts. This repair work is known as plastic surgery. The plastic surgeon has been assisted greatly during the last few decades by the tremendous advances that have taken place in the understanding and use of shock therapy, fluid replacement, electrolyte balance and anaesthesia. The nurse must, however, always remember that the patient's physical trauma will be associated with a great deal of psychological trauma and the repair of this forms a very important part of treatment.

SKIN GRAFTS

Much of this repair work necessitates the use of grafts. Sometimes flaps of living tissues from the neighbourhood of the wound can be manipulated by the surgeon to replace the lost tissue; for example, a flap of skin from the forehead may be raised up and brought down to reform part of the cheek or nose. On the other hand, the injury may be so extensive that there is no suitable undamaged tissue in the surrounding area, so that a donor area must be found on some other part of the body: it may even be necessary to obtain skin from another individual, but this is less satisfactory. Skin from another person will almost always be rejected ultimately, but makes a useful temporary covering to exclude infection. Skin or other tissue, such as cartilage or bone, transplanted in this way is called a graft. Grafts may be (*a*) free or (*b*) pedicle.

Free Grafts

A free graft consists of a piece of skin or other tissue completely severed from its original attachment and applied to a carefully prepared surface. If a free graft takes in a satisfactory manner it will have its own blood supply in between seven and ten days. During the first two to three days the graft lives on the tissue fluid, then capillary buds grow into it during the following three to four days. The use of fine suture material also assists this process as it does not damage the tissues. The graft is kept in position with sutures; if it is allowed to slip, or is dragged away from the surface in lifting a covering dressing, the newly formed blood vessels and tissues will be injured and the graft is likely to die. It may also be destroyed by infection, since it has no blood supply temporarily and therefore no power to fight infection. The older antiseptics reduced its vitality and lessened the chances of success, but the newer drugs, particularly penicillin powder in lactose, can be sprinkled on the raw surface to be grafted before the skin is applied without injuring the tissues. As a result the chances of successful grafting are much better than they were, though the greatest care is still necessary to ensure freedom from reinfection, at both the donor and the recipient surfaces.

Free grafts may be either:

1. *Split skin grafts*, thin or thick, where the graft is cut through the papillary layer of the dermis so that it consists of the cuticle or epidermis, with small portions of the true skin.

2. *Full thickness grafts*, in which the whole thickness of the skin is used, extending to the fatty tissue.

The type of graft taken depends upon the needs of the situation. Usually the donor sites (in decreasing order of choice) are the inner aspects of the thighs, the arms and the lower leg. Other sites may be used if the areas of choice are not available, such as when caring for a patient with an extensive burn or scald.

Where the surface to be covered is large, 'pinch' or 'postage stamp' grafts may be used. For the pinch graft many small areas of skin are pinched or lifted up with a hook and cut off with a scalpel: this leaves smaller donor areas to heal, but this method is rarely used. For the postage stamp graft, a large skin graft is cut up into small squares after sticking it to sterile greased paper (the papers from boxes of *tulle gras* are very useful): this makes the skin easy to handle and prevents the edges turning under. The value of numerous small pieces of skin in place of one larger piece lies in the fact that new epithelium grows from every cut edge of the skin; therefore, if one large piece is cut into many smaller pieces and these are distributed over a large raw area, it heals more quickly than if one large graft were placed in the centre. Many surgeons now prefer to use strips of skin about 1 cm wide instead of postage stamp grafts. Also the collection of discharge, which may occur under and dislodge a large graft will be avoided, as the serum, blood or pus can readily escape. These forms of grafting do not give such a good cosmetic effect and are therefore used on parts of the body that are normally covered by clothes, in cases where the skin loss is so great that the area cannot be completely grafted; they are therefore particularly used following severe burns.

Full thickness skin grafts do not 'take' as well but are of better texture and give a better cosmetic result; they are cut to the exact size and shape of the area to be covered and are sutured in position.

Pedicle Grafts

In certain circumstances a free graft is not suitable, for example a free graft will not 'take' if there is not an adequate blood supply in the recipient area. This situation arises if there is tissue loss over bare bone and large areas of fibrous tissue. In these circumstances the surgeon will raise a pedicle graft to cover the involved area.

This pedicle graft consists of a piece of skin raised up as a flap and, if necessary, stitched into a tube, the free end being either attached directly to the surface requiring grafting or transferred there by a third area, if the distance is too great. For example, a flap from the abdomen may be used to repair a burnt elbow, a flap from the thigh to repair a heel or ankle, or one from the chest to repair the chin. To repair the nose and forehead, pedicle flaps may be raised on the abdomen, and the free end attached first to the patient's wrist. After 14–21 days the graft will be getting a sufficient blood supply from the wrist and can be detached from the abdomen, this end now being stitched to the surface requiring repair. After a further interval, when this end has become adherent to the wound and the blood supply to it is established, the other end is severed from the wrist and the tube spread out to cover the wound and stitched in place. By these means, nose, cheeks, lips and eyelids can be reconstructed and extensive deformities be largely overcome.

Pedicle grafts may be:

1. Local flaps from adjacent skin.
2. Direct flaps such as cross leg, cross arm and cross finger.
3. Indirect transferred flaps such as tubal pedicle flaps.

Local flaps. When this method is used the surgeon attempts to match the skin colour and texture with that of the recipient area. It is also a much quicker method, taking about one week to heal.

Direct flaps. This operation is performed in two stages. The first stage takes about three weeks and consists of the period of time when the flap is attached to both its donor and recipient areas. The patient may be nursed in a position that is potentially uncomfortable as the freedom of movement involving the affected areas is greatly impaired. The second stage is when the graft is detached from its donor area and has been attached completely to the recipient area. This takes about two weeks, so the patient's treatment takes about five weeks in all, providing that recovery is uneventful.

Indirect transferred flap. This form of treatment takes a longer period of time as the flap has to be swung to an entirely different part of the body so that the direct flap method cannot be used. It usually takes about eight weeks. The flap remains attached to the donor site and is attached to an intermediate host (area of the patient's own body). This takes about three weeks. The donor site end of the flap is then detached and is attached to the recipient area. This phase lasts about three weeks. Finally the flap is detached from the intermediate host and is attached to the recipient site; this takes about two weeks.

If this method is used plus tubal pedicles then the period of treatment lasts even longer as the tubal pedicle has to be raised and formed while it is still attached to the donor site and this period lasts about three weeks. The tubal pedicle is then attached to the intermediate host in the same way as the indirect transferred flap. In this latter method treatment lasts about eleven weeks in a straightforward case.

Tubal pedicles are now being used increasingly less.

Cartilage grafts, grafts of bone or moulds of dental stent may be used to give shape to the nose or face, according to the extent of the destruction. False noses, ears, and false eyes can be made of the new plastic acrylic resins in some cases, where repair by plastic surgery is impossible. Early results after extensive grafting are often discouraging, as the surgeon must allow for shrinkage of the tissues as they contract.

Technique of Skin Grafting

For good results in grafting the essentials are:

1. The skin chosen must match the surface to which it is to be applied, in texture and colour, as far as possible.

2. The donor area must be carefully prepared, using non-irritating antiseptics such as cetrimide; skin marks made by the surgeon must not be removed; the aniline dyes may be used, in oily solution, for dressing the raw surface.

3. The recipient area must be as clean as possible; cultures may be taken before grafting; the use of saline baths, or irrigations, with penicillin powder in lactose as an insufflation, is a satisfactory treatment for a burnt or raw surface before the graft.

4. Where possible the blood picture should be normal beforehand, as grafts will not take if the patient is anaemic. In emergencies, transfusions may be required. A high-protein diet is also essential.

5. After grafting, dressings must be carried out with strict aseptic technique: it is usual to apply *tulle gras* with a pressure pad or covered with warm saline packs, and to change the packs only, four- or six-hourly, for four to five days; alternatively, dry sterile gauze may be applied.

6. The graft is sometimes stitched in place, but the surgeon relies on a firm dressing and bandage to keep the graft in position and to prevent blood and serum from collecting under it. The bandage must not be tight enough to restrict circulation. Where a tubular pedicle graft or flap is used ingenuity is required to prevent any drag or pressure on the attachment which would interfere with the blood supply or cause movement. The nurse should watch the circulation in the pedicle. Sometimes the surgeon may order the nurse to massage the pedicle gently to increase the blood flow through it. Sometimes the parts are encased in plaster of paris, for example, to hold the foot in position when grafted to a flap raised on the thigh. In other cases strapping or Elastoplast is applied, e.g. to secure an arm to a flap raised on the trunk. Pads will be required to prevent pressure on tubular grafts.

7. As treatment is prolonged and the patient often severely disfigured or crippled, the psychological approach is most important.

SURGICAL NURSING

The patient is liable to acute depression, may resent sympathy of the wrong kind, and is afraid he will not be able to earn his living and support his family if married; if unmarried, he will fear that a normal life is not possible for him. The nurse must treat him naturally like other patients, help him to help himself, encourage him without raising false hopes, and do everything she can to occupy his time in the best possible way. Various types of occupational therapy may be useful, both diversional, or for the specific purpose of finding out what talents the patient has; these may be trained during the long periods of waiting between operations to prepare him for a new trade or business when treatment is completed, if such a change is necessary.

26

X-Ray Examinations

When working in an X-ray department the nurse is responsible for general patient care. She will have to care for patients of all age groups who are to undergo X-ray investigations. Some will be outpatients and others from the wards in the hospital. They may be very ill, or feeling quite fit, but all will be unsure and may even be afraid. Patients in hospital are all under stress and need reassurance, and this is very necessary in this department. In the rooms some of the examinations are done in the dark, and, to the patient, the equipment hanging overhead, the flashing lights and the noises can be very frightening.

It is very important that the patient is given a simple explanation of the procedure and what will be expected of him; this will allow him to cooperate and to appreciate the reason for the events which take place.

Preparation for X-ray examination will vary in different hospitals and, like all such procedures, is subject to change.

General Rules

All patients for X-ray examination other than those of the skull or the extremities should be dressed in a cotton or woollen gown and pyjama trousers free from buttons, pins or metal fastenings. Artificial and real silk show in the X-rays. Dressings containing opaque material such as kaolin, metallic ointments or jaconet should be replaced by a dry gauze dressing in the ward. Zinc oxide strapping should not be used to secure either dressings or bandages; they should be fixed with Micropore tape.

It is important that the patient should be sufficiently warmly clad, especially if waiting is necessary between taking of different films. Jewellery and safety-pins should be removed. If the head is to be X-rayed dentures should be removed and, in the case of women and girls, hair clips or bandeaux.

Splints which are applied to limbs to be X-rayed should be left in position and the department informed if they may be removed for the X-rays to be taken.

Patient's notes and previous X-ray films should be taken with him to the department. In frightening or painful procedures the doctor will prescribe diazepam or pethidine 50 mg to be administered in the ward or in the X-ray department.

The patient should empty the bladder before leaving the ward; a woman who is menstruating should be asked to secure her sanitary towel with tape or a piece of bandage rather than with the usual type of elastic belt.

Whenever a radiopaque contrast medium has to be injected quickly, as in intravenous pyelography, a test dose should be given the day before in the ward by the doctor because most of these preparations contain iodine to which the patient may be allergic.

Preparation for Abdominal X-rays

All radiopaque medicines should be stopped 48 hours before X-ray. These include, amongst others, bismuth, iron, iodine and all tablets. An aperient is given two nights before X-ray, e.g. two tablets of vegetable laxative or two bisacodyl tablets or any aperient that the patient is used to taking. Effervescing salts should be avoided. An enema is given the day before the X-ray if the aperient is not successful; alternatively suppositories may be used. No further aperient is given but a rectal wash-out may be ordered, to finish three hours before the X-ray is taken. The patient, if possible, should remain up and active in order to prevent the accumulation of flatus. The aim of this preparation is to free the intestines of faeces, flatus and radiopaque material. This preparation is suitable for all X-rays of structures within the abdomen, e.g. for cholecystogram, pyelogram, aortogram.

X-RAYS OF THE DIGESTIVE TRACT

All examinations of the digestive tract are done in the dark in the screening room so that the passage of barium in the digestive tract can be watched continuously and X-rays taken when desired. The darkness may cause the patient some difficulty and the operators, who are used to it, may fail to realize the patient's point of view. Elderly people suffering from arteriosclerosis may become confused when their vision, as an aid to orientation, has been taken away from them.

The table may be vertical with a step for the patient to stand on and it may be tipped back into a horizontal position so that the patient is lying on his back. Modern apparatus enables the operators to move the patient very readily from the upright to the flat position. A laxative must be given to the patient following the use of contrast media in the alimentary tract. This will help to relieve the constipation caused by Hypaque, which would otherwise be very distressing.

Barium swallow. No special preparation is essential but the patient should have nothing to eat or drink for two hours.

Barium meal. General preparation for abdominal X-rays is needed and the patient should having nothing to eat or drink for six hours prior to the examination. The patient must be capable of standing for this examination.

Barium meal and follow-through. The preparation is the same but the patient returns to the department at intervals throughout the day, and after 24, 48 and 72 hours. Directions about food and aperients are sent to the ward.

Barium enema. The objective of preparation is to empty the bowel of faecal matter and gas. One method of preparation is for the patient to take one heaped teaspoonful of Isogel granules with fluid three times a day for seven days to soften the faeces, then on the day prior to investigation he has liquids only and an oral aperient. One hour prior to the barium enema a rectal washout of Veripaque 3 g in 1 litre of water is given and this causes a very effective bowel action, so that by the time one hour has elapsed the colon is clear and ready for the barium enema.

Oesophageal dilatation. Before this X-ray the patient is given amethocaine lozenges to suck and is given atropine. Metal dilators of different sizes are used to dilate the oesophagus under X-ray control. Following return to the ward nothing is given by mouth for six hours.

Gastroscopy. The patient is prepared by means of the administration of amethocaine lozenges and intramuscular atropine; diazepam is given to allay the patient's anxiety. Following return to the ward fluids and food must be withheld for six hours. This procedure is mainly carried out when a person is admitted with a haematemesis in order to identify its cause. Screening is carried out if necessary and a biopsy is obtained if required.

X-RAYS OF THE URINARY TRACT

Intravenous pyelogram. The general abdominal preparation is particularly important. Fluid intake should be limited during the twelve hours and forbidden completely in the last six hours before the examination. An intravenous injection of 50 ml of Urografin 325 58% is given, after which a series of X-rays are taken of the kidneys and ureters at carefully recorded intervals of 15 minutes, 30 minutes and 45 minutes. The X-rays are taken with the patient in a supine position. As with other substances containing iodine there is a risk of a reaction when the patient becomes very flushed and has marked skin irritation. If this occurs chlorpheniramine is administered at once.

Retrograde pyelogram. This gives a better outline of the kidney but does not show its functioning. Normally cystoscopy is performed after the patient has been given a general anaesthetic, for which he should be prepared. If a local anaesthetic is used the patient should have nothing to eat for two hours prior to the X-ray although he may be allowed to drink. Cystoscopy is performed in the theatre. Ureteric catheters are passed up to the pelvis of each kidney. The cystoscope is removed and the ureteric catheters are left strapped to the thighs. The patient is then taken to the X-ray department unless there is equipment for taking X-rays in the theatre. The X-ray is best done on a conscious patient. A control X-ray is taken to check the position of the catheters: 7–8 ml of 13% solution of sodium iodide are injected up each catheter and then the X-rays are taken. The patient, especially if he is an out-patient, should be warned that some haematuria may occur.

Micturating cystogram is a very embarrassing procedure for the patient, so great tact is needed. A catheter is introduced into the patient's bladder and all urine is withdrawn, the catheter is then connected to a bottle of Hypaque Sodium 25% and first 500 ml, then a total of 1000 ml, are allowed to run into the bladder; it must be full to the maximum. The radiologist inspects the shape and capacity of the bladder and whether any reflux into the ureters is present.

The table is then tipped so the patient is standing upright and the catheter is removed. The patient then micturates into a container while the radiologist watches the actual flow of urine on his screen. The bladder will be scrutinized for any residue.

Urethrograms are also taken when required in order to detect diverticula of the bladder, dilatation or obstruction of the urethra and similar conditions. Hypaque is again used.

Renal biopsy. The patient is sedated with diazepam and the skin is prepared. The biopsy needle is then introduced so that the specimen may be obtained.

Renal cyst puncture. The technique used is similar to that done for renal biopsy, the aim being to aspirate the contents of the cyst.

X-RAYS OF THE BILIARY TRACT

Cholecystogram. About 4% of gall-stones are radiopaque, so a straight abdominal X-ray is taken first; however, cholesterol is the major constituent of most gall-stones and is not radiopaque. Telepaque tablets may be used or alternatively the patient will be given Biloptin tablets the day prior to X-ray. During the investigation the function of the gall-bladder and biliary tree will be observed before a high-fat 'meal', called Biloptin fatty meal, is given. This will cause the gall-bladder to empty. Calculi will be recognized as the radiopaque medium will show their outline. Before a cholecystogram it is usual for a straight abdominal X-ray to be carried out.

Intravenous cholangiogram or Biligrafin X-ray. This is used when it is important to see the intrahepatic ducts especially clearly.

Following the ordinary abdominal preparation the patient is given a test dose of Biligrafin and possibly a fatty meal; then he is given the full dose of Biligrafin 50 ml in 0·5 litre of 5% dextrose intravenously and then X-rayed at intervals of twenty minutes or more.

Cholangiogram. If possible the full abdominal preparation is given. 40 ml of Urografin 150 30% is injected with a syringe up the T-tube. The abdomen is screened and the passage of the medium up the common bile duct and down the duct into the duodenum is watched and X-rayed.

Biliary stone removal. In the event of stones still being present in the ducts following a cholecystectomy a T-tube cholecystogram is carried out to identify the position of the stones. The T-tube is then removed and a catheter is introduced to the site of obstruction. A basket is passed through the catheter and this is used to 'collect' the stone which is then removed via the catheter. The whole procedure is carried out under X-ray control.

X-RAYS OF THE CARDIOVASCULAR SYSTEM

X-rays of the cardiovascular system involve the injection of radio-paque media into the heart, arteries and veins in order to demonstrate the anatomy and pathology of the circulatory system. They are frequently used before cardiovascular surgery.

The patients experience a very hot, burning sensation as the contrast medium is injected and the nurse must make sure that this discomfort does not cause the patient to move, as the X-rays are taken rapidly.

General Preparation

1. The medium is injected rapidly, therefore a test dose must be given the previous day.
2. A general anaesthetic is given to very nervous patients and children.
3. An appropriate skin area is prepared.
4. A suitable explanation must be given to the patient and a consent form signed.

Types of Examination

Aortogram. A general anaesthetic is given by intratracheal tube and the anaesthetist will inject suxamethonium to arrest respirations at the time of the exposure. If the translumbar route is used the skin is prepared in the region of the twelfth thoracic vertebra. An enema is given to expel faeces and flatus from the bowel. The patient is anaesthetized lying on the back and is then turned into the prone position.

A needle is inserted on the left side of the vertebral column, just below the twelfth rib at an angle, and is introduced into the abdominal aorta. Saline is injected continuously through a polythene tube inserted through the needle. The medium (Urografin 65% or Hypaque 65%) is injected and X-rays are taken rapidly, at a rate of 25 frames in five seconds.

Other X-rays taken in a similar manner include cerebral angiogram, retrograde common carotid arteriogram, cardio-angiogram and peripheral percutaneous arteriograms.

Cerebral angiogram. This may be done under local anaesthetic, the patient being given a sedative, such as diazepam, half an hour before. The patient should have no food for six hours beforehand but may have sips of water. The head must be very carefully positioned and immobilized and the injection of Urografin 65% is made into the internal carotid artery. The patient should be nursed flat, kept quiet and carefully observed for the rest of the day.

Cardiograms. These are most frequently done for infants with congenital cardiac defects and a general anaesthetic is given. In adults they can be done after cardiac catheterization, using a local anaesthetic. An injection of 1 megaunit of penicillin is given one hour before the X-ray and also on the same night. The skin of the antecubital fossa is cleansed and the vein dissected out: a cannula is inserted into the vein and tied in position. Diodine is injected and rapid X-rays of the chest are taken.

Arteriograms. These may be carried out in a planned manner to diagnose certain conditions, e.g. an aneurysm, but in certain circumstances X-rays are carried out on request to detect the actual site of haemorrhage or arterial obstruction, e.g. a mesenteric embolus. A sedative is administered and the patient is placed in the appropriate position on the X-ray table. The Seldinger needle is inserted into the artery and a guide-wire is threaded through the needle and along the vessel until it reaches the site of the lesion. A cannula is then threaded along the guide-wire, the guide-wire is removed and the contrast medium is injected. A series of X-rays are then taken to show the progress of the medium along the artery.

Venograms or phlebograms. These may be done under local anaesthetic because the injection of 50 ml of Urografin 65% into the vein is painful, especially if the patient has a deep venous thrombosis. The patient requires reassurance from the nurse accompanying him.

NEUROLOGICAL EXAMINATIONS

Myelograms. These are taken in order to demonstrate the subarachnoid space around the spinal cord by either the lumbar or the cisternal route.

1. *Lumbar route.* 4 ml of Myodil are introduced following lumbar puncture by the house physician in the ward. The patient is left sitting in bed supported by three or four pillows and taken to the X-ray department in bed. He should be dressed in pyjamas and stockings and may take slippers and dressing-gown.

2. *Cisternal route.* The head is shaved below the occipital protuberance. Myodil is injected by cisternal puncture in the X-ray department. In order to watch the progress of the Myodil, the patient is screened and X-rays are taken in the dark. The patient has to adopt a number of awkward positions; therefore the ward nurse should remain in the X-ray department to reassure him. The procedure may take one to one and a half hours. The care of the patient is the same as after a lumbar puncture, but this reaction tends to be more severe.

Air encephalograms. These are taken to demonstrate the size, shape and position of the ventricles of the brain. The patient may be prepared for a general anaesthetic (or diazepam or pethidine may have been administered in the ward) and is then dressed in pyjamas and socks. If anaesthesia is used an intratracheal tube is inserted. The anaesthetized patient is then lifted on to a stool with a T-support in front and a chin support. The house physician performs a lumbar puncture, sitting behind the patient. Small amounts of cerebrospinal fluid are withdrawn and air is injected. This is repeated, X-rays being taken each time. Approximately 30 ml are injected in all. Air rises in the subarachnoid space and collects in the cerebellar cistern, whence it is aspirated by small foramina into the fourth ventricle. This preliminary procedure takes about one and a half hours. When enough air has been introduced, the patient is lifted back on to the table. The patient's head and shoulders are moved into various positions so that air is introduced in turn into the third ventricle and each of the lateral ventricles. A series of X-ray pictures is taken. This takes a considerable time and the ward nurse is required in order to help lift the patient and support the head. Postoperatively the patient should lie flat quietly throughout the day. Headaches may be relieved by one to three tablets of codeine compound.

Ventriculograms. These serve to give the same information. For them air is injected directly into the ventricles through burr or trephine holes in the skull. It is not done unless the patient is definitely to have an operation later. The whole head is shaved and the patient is prepared for an operation in the theatre under local anaesthetic. A premedication is ordered. Burr holes are made in the posterior portion of the parietal bone. The pressure and quantity of cerebrospinal fluid is noted and some is withdrawn; a biopsy may be taken. 20–40 ml of air are injected into each lateral ventricle. A gauze Mastisol dressing is applied. The patient is lifted into bed with one to three pillows, as directed, and taken to the X-ray department. Here he is lifted on to the table and a series of X-ray pictures is taken as in the case of an air encephalogram. This takes an hour or more and is a long, tedious process for the patient.

Postoperative care is the same as after an air encephalogram. The burr holes are dressed as required.

Encephalography and ventriculography are investigations comparable in the seriousness of their after-effects (raised intracranial pressure) to operations; nurses must not therefore allow themselves to look lightly upon them as 'only examinations'.

EMI Scanner. In this technique radiological information is obtained by scanning the tissue, e.g. the brain. From previous research and knowledge the density of different media is known, e.g. bone and air, so it is possible to produce a detailed picture of the head showing skin, bone, brain tissue and ventricles. This will show tumours and the type can be interpreted, but it does not show the actual blood vessels, e.g. aneurysm.

The patient is starved prior to X-ray and a sedative may be administered as it is an uncomfortable procedure. A general anaesthetic is only used if the patient is liable to be restless.

X-RAY OF THE RESPIRATORY SYSTEM

Bronchograms. A radiopaque substance, usually iodized oil, is instilled into the bronchial tree; this clings to the walls of the respiratory passages. In adults a local anaesthetic is given and atropine will be administered. Amethocaine lozenges are given to suck one hour and then 30 minutes prior to the procedure, but in children full anaesthetic may be required. In the period prior to the examination postural drainage is often necessary to empty the bronchial tree of pus as far as possible. Preliminary testing for sensitivity to iodine is also important.

After the examination the radiopaque substance will eventually be absorbed, but physiotherapy can be employed to assist the patient to expectorate the contrast media. It is important, when a local anaesthetic has been applied to the throat, that the patient is given nothing to eat or even to drink until it is certain that the swallowing reflex has returned; it is also wise to give the first 'drink' of clear water (say 5 ml).

X-RAY OF THE BREAST

Mammography. A low power is used for a longer period of time as conventional X-ray techniques would not show up pathological lesions. If the ducts are to be X-rayed contrast medium is injected into them prior to X-ray.

Thermography. This records heat radiation from the body. Malignant tumours are warmer than surrounding areas and this is detected by the equipment.

Ultrasonography. This method uses sound waves to detect the thickness of breast tissue. The glandular structure reflect sound waves much more than fat so solid structures such as neoplasia and cysts can be demonstrated.

Ultra sound. A lubricant such as liquid paraffin is applied to the skin so that the probe can be moved easily and smoothly over the skin. This probe picks up the ultrasound waves as they bounce from the different body tissues. An image is then formed on a screen and X-rays are taken as required. This procedure is carried out to aid diagnosis of breast lesions. It can also be used in the diagnosis of multiple pregnancies, bladder lesions etc. The patient feels no pain or discomfort.

Further Reading

Aston, J. N. (1969) *A Short Textbook of Orthopaedics and Traumatology*. Philadelphia: Lippincott.

Burke, S. R. (1976) *The Composition and Function of Body Fluids*, 2nd ed. St Louis: C. V. Mosby.

Deeley, T. J. (1970) *A Guide to Radiotherapy Nursing*. Edinburgh and London: Churchill Livingstone.

Deeley, T. J., Gough, M. A. & Fish E. J. (1974) *A Guide to Oncological Nursing*. Edinburgh and London: Churchill Livingstone.

Evans, D. M. D. (1977) *Special Tests and their Meaning*, 10th ed. London: Faber and Faber.

Green, J. H. (1976) *An Introduction to Human Physiology*, 4th ed. Oxford: Oxford University Press.

Hopkins, S. J. (1975) *Drugs and Pharmacology for Nurses*, 6th ed. Edinburgh and London. Churchill Livingstone.

Jameson, R. M., Burrows, K. & Large, B. (1976) *Management of the Urological Patient*. Edinburgh and London: Churchill Livingstone.

Kratz, C. (1979) *The Nursing Process*. London: Baillière Tindall.

Marriner, A. (1975) *The Nursing Process*. St Louis: C. V. Mosby Company.

Mayers, M. G. (1978) *A Systematic Approach to the Nursing Care Plan*, 2nd ed. New York: Appleton-Century-Crofts.

Sutton, D. (1977) *Radiology for Medical Students*, 3rd ed. Edinburgh and London: Churchill Livingstone.

Taylor, S. & Cotton, L. A. (1973) *A Short Textbook of Surgery*. London: English Universities Press.

Thompson, A. D. & Cotton, R. E. (1968) *Lecture Notes on Pathology*, 2nd ed. Oxford: Blackwell Scientific.

Wachstein, J. (1976) *Anaesthesia and Recovery Room Techniques*, 2nd ed. London: Baillière Tindall.

Ward, F. A. (1972) *A Primer in Pathology*, 3rd ed. London: Butterworths.

Index

abdominal surgery, 223
abscess
  acute, 46
  breast, 217
  cold, 53
  incision, 52
  lung, 184
  quinsy, 132
  retropharyngeal, 132
acidosis, 36
acyanotic defects, 200
adenoma of thyroid, 145
adhesions, 256
adrenalectomy, 219
agglutination of red blood cells, 37
alginate preparations, 25
alkalosis, 36
ambulation, 120
amputation
  breast, 219
  leg, 62, 207
anaesthetics, 101
  administration, 105
  complications, 111
  epidural, 102
  general, 104
  hypotension, 109
  inhalation, 105
  intramuscular, 107
  intravenous, 106
  local, 101
  muscle relaxants, 107
  premedication, 108
  rectal, 107
  regional, 102
  spinal, 102
  stages, 104
  topical, 101
anaerobic organisms, 11
anaphylactic shock, 22
aneurysm, 205

angina pectoris, 294
angiocardiography, 187
angiogram, 377
antibiotics, use of, 1, 51
anuria, 69, 70
aortogram (aortography), 376
appendicectomy, 251
appendicitis, 249
arterial disease, 205, 206
arterial disobliteration, 206
arterial grafting, 206
arteriogram, 207, 377
arthritis, 323
arthroplasty, 325
asepsis, hand preparation, 8
atalectasis, 165, 176
atrial septal defect, 202
autoclaving, 6
autonomic nervous system, 291

Bacillus Calmette Guérin, 53
bacteraemia, 49
bacteraemic shock, 19
bacteria, resistant strains, 2
balanitis, 317
Balkan beam, 344
bandaging of amputation stump, 63
barium enema, 373
barium meal, 373
barium swallow, 373
basal metabolic rate, 141
bedsores, 59
biliary colic, 264
biligrafin X-ray, 375
bladder
  affections, 298
  diverticula, 299
  ectopia vesicae, 298
  obstruction of neck, 310
  rupture, 316
  stones, 313

384   INDEX

Blalock and Waterston operation, 198
blood
   agglutination, 37
   autotransfusion, 43
   derivatives, 42
      albumen, 42
      cryoprecipitate, 43
      fibrinogen, 43
      packed cells, 43
      plasma, 42
      platelets, 43
   donors, 39, 40
   grouping, 37
   occult in faeces, 234
   storage, 39
   transfusion, 37
      dangers, 49
boiling (in sterilization), 6
bone lesions, 321
Braun's frame, 343
breast
   abscess, 217
   biopsy, 218
   cracked nipple, 217
   hypertrophy, 222
   male, 222
   mastectomy, 219
   mastitis, 217
   new growths, 218
blood vessels, surgery of, 186
bronchial, *see* lung
bronchiectasis, 182
bronchogram, 379
bronchoscopy, 176
bruise, 11
Bryant's extension, 360
bunion, 333
burns, 66
   classification, 67
   complications, 68
   nursing care, 75
   prevention, 66
   treatment, 70
burr holes, 349
bursitis, 327
burst abdomen, 123

cachexia, 244
calculus, bladder or vesical, 313
callus, 335
carbuncle, 48
carcinogens, 78
carcinoma, 80
   bladder, 314
   breast, 218
   bronchial, 180
   colon, 258
   gastric, 244
   jaw, 138
   kidney, 304
   liver, 269
   oesophagus, 162
   pancreas, 271
   penis, 319
   prostate, 311
   rectum, 288
   scrotum, 319
   stomach, 244
   testes, 319
   tongue, 135
cardiac, *see* heart
cardiogenic shock, 18
cardiogram, 187
cardiospasm, 166, 295
carpopedal spasm, 143
cartilage injury (knee), 331
Celestin tube, 165
cellulitis, 48
Central Sterile Supply Departments (CSSD), 8
cervical rib, 332
Cheatle's forceps, use of, 6
chemotherapy in neoplasia, 86
cholangiogram, 268, 375
cholecystectomy, 266
cholecystenterostomy, 266
cholecystgastrostomy, 266
cholecystitis, 263
cholecystogram, 375
cholecystostomy, 266
choledochotomy, 266
cholelithiasis, 263
circumcision, 317
cleft lip, 133
cleft palate, 133, 134
clips
   Kifa, 121
   Michel, 121
coarctation of aorta, 201
cobalt, radioactive, 85, 86, 157
Code of Practice for Ionizing Radiation, 89

INDEX

colic
  biliary, 264
  intestinal, 255
  renal, 303
colitis, ulcerative, 252
colostomy, 260
complications, postoperative, 121
concussion, 347
congenital abnormalities of urinary tract, 297
  absence of one kidney, 298
  diverticula, 299
  double ureter, 298
  epispadiasis, 299
  extraversion of the bladder, 298
  cystic kidney, 298
  hydronephrosis, 298
  hypospadias, 299
coxa vera, 332
cranial, *see* Head
crepitus, 335
cross-infection, 1
cross-matching of blood, 37
cyanotic defects, 196
cyclopropane, 106
cystectomy, 315
cystoscopy, 297
cystostomy, 314
cytology, gastric, 234

dehydration, 34
Derbyshire neck, 140
Dextran, 43, 71
diabetes mellitus, 48, 57, 96
disc, intervertebral, protrusion of, 327
dislocations, 334, 362
  signs and symptoms, 362
  treatment, 362
double ureter, 298
drainage, 16
  closed chest, 173
ductus arteriosus, patent, 200
dumping syndrome, 244
duodenum
  surgery, 233
  ulceration, 236
duodenoscopy, 235
Dupuytren's contracture, 332

early discharge to care of community, 124

echocardiography, 189
ectopia vesicae, 298
eczema, 215
electrocardiogram, 188
electrolytes, 33, 34
electronic thermometer, 189
embolectomy, 205
embolism, 205
  air, 36
  fat, 336
emphysema, surgical, 353
encephalogram, 378
enterostomy, 261
epididymitis, 318
epispadias, 299
epistaxis, 30
epithelioma, 80
ergot poisoning, 54
exercise tolerance, 188
exophthalmos, 141
extensions, 342

Fallot's tetralogy, 196
fibrillation
  atrial (auricular), 141
  ventricular, 195
fibroscopy, 235
film badge, 90
fissure-in-ano, 283
fistula, 46
  anal, 284
  bronchopleural, 178
  faecal, 229
  tracheo-oesophageal, congenital, 168
flail chest, 353
flatulence, 123
fluid
  balance, 32
  charts, 35
  distribution, 33
foreign body
  bronchial tree, 159
  lung, 185
  oesophagus, 167
  stomach, 248
fractures, 334
  clavicle, 351
  Colles's, 358
  complications, 336
  extensions, 342
  femur, 359

INDEX

fractures (*continued*)
  general care of patients, 345
  healing, 335
  humerus, 357
  jaw, 350
  patella, 361
  pelvis, 355
  plaster of paris, 339, 340
  radius and ulna, 357
  rib, 185, 352
  signs and symptoms, 334
  skull, 346
  spine, 353
  splinting, 339
  tibia and fibula, 361
  treatment, 337
frostbite, 54
furuncle (boil), 46, 47

gall-bladder, 263
  drainage, 266
  surgery, 266
gall-stones, 263, 265
gamma radiation in sterilization, 7
gangrene, 54, 295
  gas, 55
gastrectomy, 240
gastric acid test, 234
gastric cytology, 234
gastric surgery, 233
gastro-enterostomy, 240
gastroscopy, 235
gastrostomy, 166, 248
gastrotomy, 169, 248
Geiger counter, 145
genitourinary system, 296
  congenital abnormalities, 297
  examination, 296
genu
  valgum, 332
  varum, 332
glands of neck, 139
glossectomy, hemi, 135
goitre, 140
grafts
  arterial, 206
  free, 365, 366, 367
  pedicle, 365, 367, 368
  pinch, 366
  postage stamp, 366
  skin, 365
gummata, 322

haematemesis, 31
haematocrit, 68
haematoma, 11
haematuria, 32
haemopneumothorax, 353
haemoptysis, 30
haemorrhage, 22, 238
  arrest, 24
  signs and symptoms, 24
  treatment, 26
  types, 22
haemorrhoids, 285
haemothorax, 353
hallux valgus, 333
hammer toe, 333
head
  injury, 347
  surgery
    after-care, 130
    preparation for, 129
heart
  acute failure, 37
  arrest, 113, 195
  catheterization, 187
  surgery, 186
  rheumatic disease, 191
  transplant, 203, 204
heart–lung machine, 189
Heller's operation, 167
hepatic, *see* liver
hernia, 274
  diaphragmatic, 276
  femoral, 275, 278
  hiatus, 166, 276, 280
  incisional (ventral), 230, 276
  inguinal, 275
  strangulated, 255
  umbilical, 275, 277, 275
herniotomy, 279
hiccough, 123
hour-glass stomach, 239
hydatid cyst, 270
hydrocele, 318
hydronephrosis, 300
hygiene
  personal, 2
  patients, 3
  ward, 3
hypertension, 294
hypospadias, 299
hypothermia, 189
hypovolaemic shock, 18

ileostomy, 262
ileus, paralytic, 165, 229, 232, 255, 257
imperforate anus, 283
infection, 1
  chest, 228
  wound, 229
inflammation, 44
  acute, 49
  chronic, 52
  local, 44
    types, 45, 46, 47, 48
  resolution, 45
  signs and symptoms, 44
  spread, 48
  treatment
    acute, 49
    chronic, 53
infusions, intravenous, 35
  complications, 36
insect bites, 11, 48
intervertebral disc, protrusion of, 327
intestinal obstruction, 253
  acute, 254
  chronic, 258
  mechanical, 253
  paralytic, 254
intubation
  endotracheal, 106
  oesophageal, 165
intussusception, 256
iodine, radioactive, 86, 141
ischaemic heart disease, 191
isotopes, 85

Jacksonian epilepsy, 350
jaundice, 265
Jeffery Communicator, 138
jejunostomy, 262
joint lesions, 321

kidney
  absence, 298
  colic, 303
  congenital cystic, 298
  growths, 304
  horseshoe, 298
  hydronephrosis, 298, 300
  infection, 304
  inflammation, 300

kidney (*continued*)
  pyelonephritis, 300
  rupture, 300
  stones (calculi), 302
  transplant, 305
  tuberculosis, 304
ketamine, 107
Kirschner wire, 343
knee joint injury, 331

laminectomy, 329
laryngeal nerve injury, 144
laryngectomy, 158
larynx
  fissure, 157
  foreign body, 159
leucocytosis, 51
lithopaxy, 314
lithotomy, 314
liver
  affections, 268
  growths, 269
  hydatid cyst, 270
  portal hypertension, 269
  portal pyaemia, 270
  trauma, 269
Logan's bow, 134
lung
  carcinoma, 180
  embolism, 123, 124
  tuberculosis, 170, 179
lymphadenitis, 48
lymphangitis, 48

mastectomy, 219
mastitis, 217, 218
melaena, 31
Ménière's disease, 295
meniscectomy, 331
metastases, 81
micturating cystogram, 374
migraine, 295, 375
mitral incompetence, 192
mitral stenosis, 192
Mousseau-Barbin tube, 165
mouth affections, 132
muscle relaxant drugs, 107
Mycobacterium, 52
myelogram, 329, 378
myxoedema, 144

388 INDEX

National Blood Transfusion Service, 39
neck affections, 139
neoplasms, see Tumours
nephrectomy, 301
nephritis, 70
nephrolithotomy, 303
neurological chart, 348
nitrous oxide, 106
Nursing Process, 92

occupational therapy, 339, 346, 350, 355
oesophagus
 carcinoma, 162
 congenital lesions, 168
 diverticulum, 169
 foreign body, 167
 speech, 159
 stricture, 169
 surgery, 160
oesophagogastrostomy, 163
oesophagoscopy, 161
oophorectomy, 221
operation, see specific operation
orchitis, 318
osteoarthritis, 325
osteomyelitis, 321
osteotomy, 325
oxygen, 71, 106, 108, 114, 124, 352

packed cells, 43
pancreas
 affections, 271
 cysts and tumours, 271
 inflammation, 271
 trauma, 272
 pancreatitis, 265, 271
papilloma, 77, 314
paradoxical respiration, 178
paralytic ileus, 165, 228, 257
paraphimosis, 317
paraplegia, 355
parasympathetic nervous system, 291
parathyroid gland, 145
pedicle graft, 367
penis
 affections of, 316
 phimosis, 317
 trauma, 318
peptic ulcer, 238

pericardectomy, 204
pericarditis, 202
peritonitis, 230
pharyngotomy, lateral, 157
phimosis, 317
physiotherapy
 amputation of leg, 63
 arthritis, 326
 breathing exercises, 119
 bronchiectasis, 183
 fractures, 338
 knee joint injuries, 331
 postoperative chest complications, 119, 121, 122
 protrusion of intervertebral disc, 329
 thoracic surgery, 175, 177
plasma, 21, 32, 42
plastic surgery, 365
pneumonectomy, 180, 181
pneumothorax, 185, 353
portacaval anastomosis, 269
portal hypertension, 269
portal pyaemia, 270
postoperative care, 115
 abdominal, 227
 community care, 124
 complications, 121, 128
 early discharge, 124
 posture, 112, 115, 121, 177
 see also specific operation
post-thrombotic syndrome, 215
Pott's disease, 323
premedication, 108
preoperative preparation, 92
 abdominal, 224
 general, 94
 immediate, 97
 local, 96
 medication, 98
 see also specific operation
pressure sores, 59, 60, 61
prostatectomy, 311
prostheses, 65
protrusion of intervertebral disc, 327
pruritus ani, 290
pulmonary, see lung
pus, 46, 51
pyaemia, 49
pyelonephritis, 300
pyelogram
 ascending (retrograde), 297, 374
 intravenous, 297, 307, 374

INDEX 389

pyelolithotomy, 303
pyloric stenosis, 239
   congenital, 245
pyloroplasty, 241
pylorospasm, 165
pyonephrosis, 302

rabies, 11
radioactive isotopes, 85, 86, 141, 157
radiotherapy, 84
   gamma rays, 84
   isotopes, 85, 86, 141, 157
   nursing care, 87
   precautions, 89, 91
   reactions, 88
   X-rays, 84
radium therapy
   bladder, 314
   breast, 219
   larynx, 157
   malignant growths, 84, 85
   thyroid, 145
radon seeds, 315
Ramstedt's operation, 246
Raynaud's disease, 293
rectum
   bladder, 282, 315
   carcinoma, 288
   examination, 282
   polyps, 288
   prolapse, 285
rehabilitation, 63, 339
renal, *see* Kidney
renogram, 297
reproductive organs, male, 318
   growths, 319
   hydrocele, 318
   inflammation, 318
   torsion of spermatic cord, 320
   undescended testicle, 319
   variocele, 319
resolution of inflammation, 45
respiratory function, 171, 188
respiratory obstruction, 147, 185
rest, in treatment of inflammation, 50
retention of urine, 118, 309
Rhesus factor, 38
rheumatic heart disease, 191
rheumatoid arthritis, 325
rickets, 323
rigor, 41, 48, 49

rodent ulcer, 82
rupture
   bladder, 316
   kidney, 316
   liver, 268, 269
   spleen, 272
   wound, 123

sarcoma, 80, 304
scalds, 66
scalp wounds, 132
Schimmelbusch mask, 105
septicaemia, 48
shock, 17
   clinical assessment, 19
   compensation, 17
   signs and symptoms, 19
   treatment, 20
   types
      anaphylactic, 18
      bacteraemic, 19
      cardiogenic, 18
      hypovolaemic, 18
      uncompensated, 18
skin grafting, 365
   free grafts, 366
   pedicle grafts, 367
speech defects, 133
spermatic cord, torsion, 320
spleen affections, 272
splenectomy, 272
splints, 339
sprains, 12, 334, 363
Staphylococcal Infections in Hospitals, 2, 4
Steinmann's pin, 343
stenosis
   aortic valve, 195
   mitral valve, 192
   pyloric, 239
      congenital hypertrophic, 245
sterilization, 5
   autoclaving, 6
   boiling, 6
   chemicals, 8
   dry heat, 6
   ethylene oxide, 7
   flaming, 7
   formalin, 7
   infra-red rays, 7
   irradiation, 7

390 INDEX

sterilization (*continued*)
    moist heat, 6
    pasteurization, 6
    preliminary cleaning, 5
    ultra-violet rays, 7
Steroid Addis count, 297
strains, 334, 364
strangury, 303
stump bandages, 63, 64
suction
    drain, 16
    tracheal, 146, 154
suppuration, 46
sympathectomy, 207, 293
sympathetic nervous system, 291
syndactylism, 332
syphilis, 322

talipes, 333
tamponade, 195
Teflon, 206
tenosynovitis, 327
teratoma, 87, 304
tetanus, 11, 50
tetany, 143
thermometer, electronic, 189
thiopentone sodium, 106
Thomas's splint, 342, 343, 344, 345
thoracic surgery, 170
thrombo-angeitis obliterans, 294
thrombosis, 229
thyroid gland, 140
    adenoma, 145
    simple goitre, 140
    exophthalmic goitre, 141
    new growths, 145
torticollis, 331
tourniquet, 26, 27
tracheo-oesophageal fistula, 168
tracheostomy, 146
    complications, 156
    preoperative care, 152
    postoperative care, 153
tracheostomy tubes
    Chevalier Jackson, 150
    Durham, 151
    Morant Baker, 151
    Negus, 150
    Parker, 150
    Radcliffe, cuffed, 149

traction
    skeletal, 343
    skin, 343, 344
transfusion
    blood, 37
    blood derivatives, 42
    dangers, 40
transplant
    heart, 204
    renal, 305
transversectomy, 323
trophic ulcers, 57
truss, 277, 278
T-tube for biliary tract operation, 266
tuberculosis, 52, 53, 179
    bones and joints, 322
    glands of neck, 139
    pulmonary, 179
    spine, 323
tumours, 77
    benign, 75
    characteristics, 81
    diagnosis, 83
    effect, 81
    malignant, 79
    treatment, 83

ulcers and ulceration, 57
    corneal, 75
    duodenal, 233, 236
    gastric, 233, 236
    peptic, 233, 236, 237, 238
    rodent, 82
    syphylitic, 59
    varicose, 59, 214, 215
ulcerative colitis, 252
ultra-sound, 235
underwater seal drainage, 173, 353
uraemia, 310
urea concentration test, 297
ureter
    double, 298
    transplantation, 299, 315
ureterocolic anastomosis, 315
ureterolithotomy, 303
urethra
    conditions affecting, 316
    epispadias, 299
    hypospadias, 299
    stricture, 316
    trauma, 318

INDEX

urethrogram, 375
urethrotomy, 316
urinary bladder, 309
    calculi, 313
    enlargement of prostate, 310
    inflammation, 309
    obstruction of neck, 310
    prostatectomy, 311
    retention of urine, 118, 309
    rupture, 316
urinary system, examination, 296
urine, retention, 118, 309

vagotomy, 240
valvular lesions, 191
    aortic, 195
    mitral, 192
varicocele, 319
varicose veins, 212
    injection, 213
    ligation, 213
    stripping, 213
    ulcers, 214
vascular surgery, 205
venogram, 377
ventral hernia, 230
ventricular fibrillations, 195
ventriculogram, 379
vitamins
    B6, 89
    C, 13, 15, 50, 346
    D, 346
    K, 28, 267
Volkmann's ischaemic contracture, 336
volvulus, 256

walking plaster, 341
Wallace's 'Rule of Nine', 67
Whitehead's operation, 287
whitlow, 46
Wilm's tumour, 304

wounds, 10
    after-care, 14
    burns, 11
    burst abdominal, 229
    closed, 11
    contused, 10
    drainage, 16
    haematoma, 11
    healing, 12
    incised, 10
    lacerated, 10
    poisoned, 11
    punctured, 11
    treatment, 13

X-ray examination, 371
    abdominal, straight, 234, 372
    air encephalogram, 378
    aortogram, 376
    arteriogram, 377
    barium enema, 373
    barium meal, 373
    barium swallow, 373
    biliary stone removal, 376
    bronchogram, 379
    cardiogram, 377
    cerebral angiogram, 377
    cholecystogram, 375
    cholangiogram, 375
    EMI scan, 379
    gastroscopy, 374
    intravenous cholangiogram, 375
    intravenous pyelogram, 374
    mammograph, 380
    micturating cystogram, 374
    myelogram, 378
    oesophageal dilatation, 373
    renal biopsy, 375
    renal cyst puncture, 375
    retrograde pyelogram, 374
    thermograph, 380
    ultra-sound, 380
    urethrogram, 375
    venogram, 377
    ventriculogram, 379

Baillière's Nursing Books

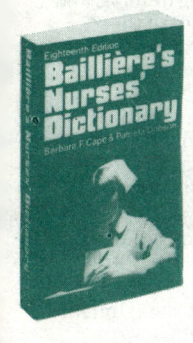

Baillière's Nurses' Dictionary

Cape & Dobson

The 18th edition of this famous dictionary has been completely reset and updated in a new format. It contains hundreds of new definitions, radically revised appendices and new illustrations — an informative, pocket-sized dictionary for student and trained nurse alike.

1974 • 18th edn. • Limp.

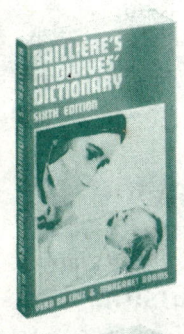

Baillière's Midwives' Dictionary

Da Cruz & Adams

The ideal pocket-sized dictionary for midwives and obstetric nurses. "A little mine of invaluable information...it really does contain the exact definition wanted in a hurry."
Midwives' Chronicle 1976 • 6th edn. • Limp.

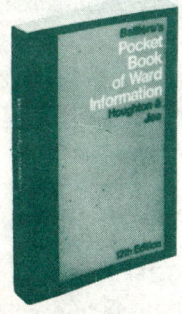

Baillière's Pocket Book of Ward Information

Fully revised and brought up-to-date, this book contains a multitude of useful information likely to be needed by nurses in their day to day work and of particular help to nurses in training.

1971 • 12th edn. • Limp.

The Nurses' Aids Series

nas

The Nurses' Aids Series is planned to meet the needs of the student nurse during training, and later in qualifying for another part of the Register, by providing a set of textbooks covering most of the subjects included in the general part of the Register and certain specialist subjects. The pupil nurse, too, will find many of these books of particular value and help in practical bedside training. The Series conforms to three factors important to the student:

1. All the authors are nurses who know exactly what the student requires.
2. The books are frequently revised to ensure that advances in knowledge reach the student as soon as practicable.
3. The Aids are well printed and easy to read, clearly illustrated, and modestly priced.

Anaesthesia & Recovery Room Techniques/Wachstein
1976 • 2nd edn.

Anatomy & Physiology for Nurses/Jackson
1979 • 9th edn.

Ear, Nose & Throat Nursing/Marshall & Oxlade
1972 • 5th edn.

Geriatric Nursing/Storrs
1976 • 1st edn.

Mathematics in Nursing/Jefferies
1978 • 5th edn.

Medical Nursing/Chapman
1977 • 9th edn.

Microbiology for Nurses/Parker
1978 • 5th edn.

Multiple Choice Questions Book 1
Anatomy & Physiology, Medical, Surgical and
Paediatric Nursing.   1977 · 1st edn.

Mulitple Choice Questions Book 2
Practical Nursing and Personal and Community
Health.   1978 · 1st edn.

Obstetric & Gynaecological Nursing/Bailey
1976 • 2nd edn.

Ophthalmic Nursing/Darling & Thorpe
1975 • 1st edn.

Paediatric Nursing/Duncombe & Weller
1979 · 5th edn.

Personal & Community Health/Jackson & Lane
1975 • 1st edn.

Pharmacology for Nurses/Bailey
1975 • 4th edn.

Practical Nursing/Clarke
1977 • 12th edn.

Practical Procedures for Nurses/Billing
1976 • 2nd edn.

Psychiatric Nursing/Altschul & Simpson
1977 • 5th edn.

Psychology for Nurses/Altschul
1975 • 4th edn.

Sociology for Nurses/Chapman
1978 • 1st edn.

Surgical Nursing/Fish
1974 • 9th edn.

Theatre Technique/Houghton & Hudd.
1967 • 4th edn.

NAS Special Interest Texts
See over

For the Advanced Student

NURSES' AIDS SERIES SPECIAL INTEREST TEXTS

Special Interest Texts will enable the student nurse to study a particular subject in greater detail during training or after basic studies have been completed.

Gastroenterological Nursing/Gribble
1977 • 1st edn.

Neuromedical & Neurosurgical Nursing/Purchese
1977 • 1st edn.

Orthopaedics for Nurses/Stone & Pinney
1978 • 5th edn.

Baillière's Medical Transparencies

* A visual reference library for lecturers and students.

* Of special interest to Nurses and Nurse Tutors are 'BMT 1', on the Anatomy of the Head, Neck and Limbs and 'BMT 2', on the Anatomy of the Thorax and Abdomen. Each set illustrates the major anatomical features of the regions with 21 and 18 slides in full colour.

Other sets of interest to nurses specializing in these topics are **Paediatrics** 'BMT 17' and **Venereal Diseases** 'BMT 9' together with **Other Sexually Transmitted Diseases** 'BMT 19'. 24 slides in each set.

Quizzes and Questions for Nurses

Book A. Medical Nursing and Paediatric Nursing

Book B. Surgical Nursing and Geriatric Nursing

E. J. Hull and B. J. Isaacs

Two new books devised specially to help nurses in training to revise for examination purposes the subjects that they have been studying. The books are similar to the successful 'Do-It-Yourself' Revision series, but are set at a more elementary level. Each chapter is based on an examination question. The 'revision' part of each chapter consists of a quiz, with answers and explanations, covering the material to be revised.

1976 • Book A • 160pp. • 16 Illus. • Limp
Book B • 160pp. • 10 Illus. • Limp

Do-It-Yourself Revision For Nurses
Books 1, 2, 3, 4, 5 & 6

E. J. Hull and B. J. Isaacs

The six books of this series provide a comprehensive framework for revision of the GNC syllabus and developments made since to it. The student reviews a subject of choice, answers questions selected from recent State Final Examinations, and marks her replies against the model answers provided.
'Highly recommended to all student nurses as a planned guide to revision.' *Nursing Times*.

*1970-1972 • **Books 1-6** • 135pp average • illustrated.*

Standard Textbooks

Primary Health Nursing/Lamb
Discribing the work of health visitors, district nur
and all involved in the work of primary health ca
teams.   *1977 · 1st e*

Handbook of Practical Nursing/Crispin
This replaces the well-known textbook by Swire
and is for the pupil and student nurse, written
in a clear, easy-to-read style.   *1976 • 1st e*

Health Visiting/Owen
Combining factual information with discussions
of principles and their application of health visitin
                                        1977 · 1st ec

School Nursing/Slack
Dealing comprehensively with the work of the
school nurse, including medical examinations,
screening, infections and contagious diseases and
health education.   *1978 · 1st ed*

Nursing in the Community/Keywood
Provides a comprehensive account of the various
problems peculiar to nursing outside the
hospital, and describes the organization of a
modern community nursing service.

1977 • 1st edn.

Books for the Psychiatric Nurse

Psychiatric Nursing/Altschul
Indispensable to students training for admission to the Register of Mental Nurses.
1977 • 5th edn. • 400pp. • Limp

Nursing the Psychiatric Patient/Burr & Budge
For students in psychiatric training.
1976 • 3rd edn. • 320pp. • 15 illus. • Limp

Clinical Aspects of Dementia/Pearce & Miller
Focuses on the treatable presenile dementias.
"Extremely useful" — Nursing Mirror
1973 • 160pp. • 12 plates, 15 illus.

Books for the Midwife

Mayes' Midwifery/Bailey
1976 • 9th edn. • 530pp. • 180 illus. • Limp

Obstetric & Gynaecological Nursing/Bailey
(Nurses' Aids Series)
1975 • 2nd edn. • 343pp. • 131 illus. • Limp

For Nurses Working in Intensive Care units

Patient Care: Cardiovascular Disorders/Ashworth & Rose
1973 • 309pp. • 110 illus.

Nurses' Guide to Cardiac Monitoring/Hubner
1975 • 2nd edn. • 66pp. • 37 illus. • Limp.

Cardiology/Julian
1973 • 2nd edn. • 341pp. • 112 illus. • Limp

Nursing Care of the Unconscious Patient/Mountjoy & Wythe
1970 • 104pp. • 11 illus. • Limp

A complete catalogue and current price lists are available on request direct from the publishers.

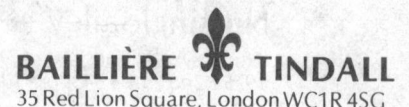

BAILLIÈRE ⚜ TINDALL
35 Red Lion Square, London WC1R 4SG

The details and editions in this list are those current at the time of going to press but are liable to alteration without notice.